Leprosy and Stigma in the South Pacific

Leprosy and Stigma in the South Pacific

A Region-by-Region History with First Person Accounts

DOROTHY MCMENAMIN

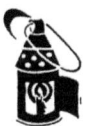

McFarland & Company, Inc., Publishers
Jefferson, North Carolina, and London

LIBRARY OF CONGRESS CATALOGUING-IN-PUBLICATION DATA

McMenamin, Dorothy, 1947–
    Leprosy and stigma in the South Pacific : a region-by-region history with first person accounts / Dorothy McMenamin.
        p.   cm.
    Includes bibliographical references and index.

    ISBN 978-0-7864-6323-7
    softcover : 50# alkaline paper ∞

    1. Leprosy — Oceania — History.   I. Title.
    RC154.9.A1M46 2011
    614.5'460995—dc23   2011031760

BRITISH LIBRARY CATALOGUING DATA ARE AVAILABLE

© 2011 Dorothy McMenamin. All rights reserved

No part of this book may be reproduced or transmitted in any form or by any means, electronic or mechanical, including photocopying or recording, or by any information storage and retrieval system, without permission in writing from the publisher.

On the cover: Rere Abana and his granddaughters outside their home (photograph from author's collection); background © 2011 Map Resources

Manufactured in the United States of America

McFarland & Company, Inc., Publishers
  Box 611, Jefferson, North Carolina 28640
  www.mcfarlandpub.com

Acknowledgments

As the oral historian commissioned to gather archival material for the international history of leprosy project in the South Pacific region, I am privileged to dedicate this book to honor the memory of the courageous people who endured leprosy and willingly shared their life stories by permitting their voices to be recorded for posterity. For researchers interested in knowing more about leprosy in the South Pacific, it is suggested that there is a great deal more to be gained by listening to the oral history recordings than can be conveyed here, especially for speakers of the local languages. Despite the fact that many of the interviews were conducted through interpreters, where the subtleties and nuances of personal expression were often lost to me, the interviewer, the voices of the contributors, between their laughter, tears and even song, provide vivid expressions of the life-long experiences they encountered since the symptoms of leprosy appeared, the traumas that followed diagnosis, separation, isolation and eventually reunion back home. However, after many years of separation, the return home was not always a happy ending because the fears associated with leprosy and its contagion sanctioned the age old legacy of stigma. But fortunately times are changing, and since an effective cure is available, the "face of leprosy" is being erased, and fear and stigma are fading. It is hoped this work provides another step towards hastening a transformation in attitude towards the victims of leprosy.

My heartfelt thanks are due to each of the leprosy sufferers who allowed their stories to be recorded, and to Jane Buckingham and Jo Robertson, who facilitated my commission with the world-wide leprosy project. However, without the assistance and personal contacts provided by Michael Gousmett, Margaret Stacey, and especially the contribution of the late Noeline Harris of the Pacific Leprosy Foundation, the oral history project would not have been possible. My thanks more recently go to the present PLF staff. Together with the leprosy sufferers, who, towards the end of each interview, always asked me to convey their thanks to the PLF board members and especially the donors, I add my appreciation for all the help, encouragement and kindness extended by the PLF staff.

My sincere thanks also go to the individual PLF liaison personnel in the islands, interpreters and everyone who contributed to the unforgettable experience in reaching the interviewees. The introductions by the intrepid Missionary Sisters of the Society of Mary (SMSM) and PLF assistants, with their varied and diverse skills (including driving trucks, irrespective of weather conditions, deep off the beaten tracks of the Pacific Islands, and maintaining internet contact from the urban centers) proved invaluable. All of them went out of their way to accommodate me and make this project possible.

From the time of my first visit to Fiji in 2004 to the most recent to Vanuatu in 2008, there are so many people who deserve my thanks each step of the way. In particular I must thank the staff, residents and friends at Twomey Memorial Hospital in Suva; Sisters Marietta, Josephine and Aquin of the SMSM in New Zealand; the SMSM in Samoa for their wonderful hospitality and party never to be forgotten; Sisters Joan Marie, Goretti, and the SMSM in Tonga who provided me with home comforts when Nuku'alofa city center went up in flames due to civil unrest; Dr. Jacques Michaudel, Sister Noëllie and Dr. Maryse Crouzat in New Caledonia; and Tony Whitley, Carren Bough and Jimmy Andre in Vanuatu. Particular thanks are due to the medical specialists Dr. Desmond Beckett, Marilyn Eales, Dr. Roland Farrugia, Dr. Bruce and his wife Catherine Mackereth, Dr. Brian McMahon, and Sister Betty Pyatt of the Melanesian Mission. To all others not mentioned here but who have assisted me in countless ways, my sincere thanks. Special thanks to my husband Paul for his encouragement and endurance through my ventures, and to our children who put up with my frequent absences, especially Kevin, who transcribed a large portion of the interviews.

Abbreviations and Terms

Ducos/RFC: Leprosarium at Ducos, New Caledonia, named Raoul Follereau Center in 1958.
DDS: Sulphone treatment, available from 1950s.
Lolowai: St. Barnabas leprosarium, Ambae, Vanuatu.
LTB: Leprosy Trust Board (now called PLF).
LMS: London Missionary Service.
Makogai: Leprosarium at Makogai Island, Fiji.
Marsden Fund: Marsden Fund Council, government-funded and administered by the Royal Society of New Zealand.
MDT: Multi-Drug Therapy, available since the 1980s (dapsone, clofazimine and rifampicin).
PLF: Pacific Leprosy Foundation (formerly LTB).
Oxford Project: International Leprosy Association Project, Global Project on the History of Leprosy (funded by Nippon Foundation), Welcome Unit for the History of Medicine, University of Oxford.
RFC/Ducos: Raoul Follereau Center, leprosarium, Ducos.
SMSM: Missionary Sisters of the Society of Mary.
Twomey Hospital: P.J. Twomey Memorial Hospital, Suva, Fiji.
WHO: World Health Organization.

Contents

Acknowledgments	v
Abbreviations and Terms	vii
Preface	1

Introduction	3
The Disease and Its Brief History	5
Historiography	9
Brief History of Leprosy Stigma	12
Missions and Stigma	15
Myth of Stigma and Self-Stigma	16
Growth of Leprosaria and Missionary Involvement	17
Other Leprosaria	19
The Interviews	25

1. Community Through Adversity — New Zealand to Fiji	31
Patrick J. Twomey: Early Encounters with Leprosy	31
Formation of a Charitable Trust in New Zealand	35
LTB/PLF and Leprosy Sufferers in the South Pacific Region	38
Leprosy in Fiji: Historical Background	40
Early Accounts of Leprosy	41
Establishment of the Leprosarium at Beqa	42
Establishment of the Leprosarium at Makogai	43
Conditions at Makogai and the SMSM	45
Sulphone Treatment and Changing Times	50
St. Elizabeth Leprosy Home, Suva	52
P.J. Twomey Memorial Hospital, Tamavua, Suva	53
Testimonies of Interviewees at Twomey Hospital	54
Testimonies of Interviewees Living in Their Own Homes	67

2. Former Penitentiaries as Leprosaria — New Caledonia	73
Historical Background	73
Early Reports and Treatment of Leprosy	74

Involvement of Religious Orders in Care at Belep and Ducos	75
Conditions at Ducos Leprosarium to the Late 1960s	77
The LTB and Other Charitable Involvement at Ducos	81
Leprosy on the Island and at Ducos Since the Late 1960s	83
Continuing SMSM Involvement	91

3. Rise and Demise of Stigma — Samoa   98

Historical Background	98
Early Incidence of Leprosy and Attitudes Toward the Disease	99
Leprosaria at Alia and Nu'utele	101
Removal of Leprosy Sufferers to Makogai, Fiji	103
Samoan Experiences at Makogai and Reintegration Back Home	109
Leprosy Treatment in Samoa Since the Late 1950s	113
PLF Assistance in Samoa	118

4. The Loneliness of Isolation — Tonga   124

Historical Background	124
Early Incidence of Leprosy	127
Fale'ofa Leprosy Clinic at Ngu Hospital, Vava'u	128
Tongan Experiences at Makogai Leprosarium	131
Village of Longomapu, Vava'u	141
Experience of Isolation at Fale'ofa	146
Leprosy Experiences Without Isolation	148

5. The Benefits of Leprosaria — Vanuatu   155

Historical Background	155
Earliest Accounts of Leprosy	157
Melanesian Mission and Establishment of Leprosarium at Lolowai	159
Conditions at St. Barnabas Leprosarium, Lolowai	167
Leaving Lolowai	173
Supporting Accounts of Conditions at Lolowai Leprosarium	174
Incidence of Leprosy and PLF Assistance	176
Testimonies of Leprosy Sufferers	179
Memories of Lolowai	180
Experiences Living at Home with Leprosy	185

Conclusion   191

Minimal Biblical and Missionary Causes of Stigma	192
Leprosaria and Stigma	193
Stigma and Self-Stigma	196

Appendix: The Betty Pyatt Letter	199
Chapter Notes	203
Bibliography	215
Index	221

Preface

How leprosy and its stigma impacted on the lives of those who suffered the disease is explored in five South Pacific nations visited by the author — namely, Fiji, New Caledonia, Samoa, Tonga and Vanuatu. Oral histories were recorded with elderly leprosy sufferers, many of whom suffered decades of isolation at various leprosaria in the Pacific islands. One New Caledonian interviewee had been in residence at a leprosarium for over seventy years. Introductions were facilitated through the Pacific Leprosy Foundation, a charitable organization founded in 1939 in Christchurch, New Zealand. With the assistance of their staff at the leprosy hospital in Suva, Fiji, as well as agents, volunteers and sisters of the SMSM who helped leprosy sufferers in the islands, the author was driven to the homes of the interviewees, often in remote villages, to record the interviews.

The personal testimonies reveal the heart-rending experiences of being diagnosed with the disease, removed from their families, shifted into isolation, their medical treatment, and eventual discharge back home. But the return home was sadly not always to be a happy one. Descriptions of these events implicitly disclose levels of stigma that prevail in the island communities. What becomes evident is that where there is openness and knowledge about the minimal risk of leprosy contagion and the availability of a cure, as has occurred in Fiji and Vanuatu, lower levels of stigma exist. Nevertheless, even in these countries, prior to the availability of an effective cure, fear and horror of the physical effects of leprosy often caused the victims to be cast out or voluntarily leave their homes. This segregation led to groups of leprosy sufferers banding together beyond their villages to help care for each other.

Following the implementation of the policy of isolation in leprosaria by medical officials from the early 1900s despite the initial hardships of separation, it was found that leprosy patients benefited from the better medical facilities available, and particularly enjoyed the opportunities for friendships and camaraderie at leprosaria.

However, if conditions at leprosaria were miserable and the movements of residents restricted by fences visible to the public, as in Samoa and Tonga, leprosy stigma prevailed and was heightened. It was evident that perceptions of stigma varied from region to region and even person to person. In New Caledonia higher levels of stigma were evident because leprosaria had been located at former prison sites and strict isolation enforced. High stigma also prevailed in Tonga because from the earliest days officials linked leprosy with old biblical strictures that asserted leprosy sufferers should be treated as unclean and cast out of their homes and villages. It is important to emphasize that due to the specific focus on the personal experiences of those who suffered leprosy, it is beyond the scope of this research to evaluate stigma in the islands in connection with other diseases and physical deformities.

Following the availability of sulphone treatment in the 1950s, and the improved MDT medication in the 1980s (now freely available worldwide), the disease no longer need be physically disfiguring or disabling when diagnosed and treated early. Thanks in part to the generous donations raised by the PLF to fund medical services at the central leprosy hospital in Fiji and directly assist leprosy sufferers in the Pacific Islands, the huge limitations and corresponding leprosy stigma of the past are fading. As one contributor to the project said, "The time of darkness is ending."

Introduction

A common response by most people when asked about leprosy and its stigma is that leprosy is a disease of the past which caused terrible physical deformities, but because the disease is no longer prevalent, stigma is not an issue. However, if told that they are to meet someone who had leprosy, fear of contagion arises, magnified by fear of the awful physical disabilities associated with it. This fear is unfounded and particularly inapplicable since the mid-twentieth century with the availability of a medical cure that ends contagion by killing the disease-causing bacillus. Early diagnosis, followed by treatment, prevents any possibility of ensuing disabilities.

This fear of contagion and disability lies at the heart of leprosy stigma throughout the ages. It has been perpetuated in the 20th century by images of leprosy sufferers imbedded in the public mind by films such as the epic *Ben-Hur*, which portrayed scenes of a family afflicted by the physical ravages of the disease. More recently the film on the life of Che Guevera, *The Motorcycle Diaries*, vividly dramatized the mutilated appearance of residents at a leprosy colony. These images are horrific, especially in the modern world where physical disabilities are routinely transformed by plastic surgery so that the worst physical deformities are eliminated from public view. In such a world the impact of grotesque physical appearances and any perceived risk of deformity exaggerate and sustain leprosy stigma.

In the past leprosy has often been described as a "fate worse than death," and in today's societies, which thrive on cosmetically contrived beauty, it is hardly an exaggeration to say that gross physical deformities are still viewed as tantamount to a "fate worse than death." Adding to the unfortunate lot of leprosy sufferers, the common use of the word "leper" as an analogy refers to outcasts of society and conjures up notions of ostracism and misery. Greater public awareness about leprosy and its cure (and the realization that global mobility means the disease exists in most countries, but that the risk of contracting it is minimal) is the way to diminish old stigmatic attitudes towards the unfortunate people who have suffered the disease. This research reveals how leprosy affected its victims in five South Pacific nations from the early twentieth century until the present day, and how the discovery of sulphone treatment revolutionized these people's lives. But due to old, ingrained attitudes and ignorance about medical treatments, stigma continues.

This book seeks to extend the battle against stigma by broadening the knowledge and understanding of how the disease and its stigma impacted upon the lives of the victims and their families. In order to locate primary sources and record oral histories with leprosy sufferers, especially the very elderly who experienced isolation prior to the availability of an effective cure, the author visited Fiji in the South Pacific, the Polynesian islands of Samoa and Tonga, and the Melanesian islands of New Caledonia and Vanuatu between 2004 and 2008. The research was initiated and funded, in the main, by the International Leprosy Association Project, Global Project on the History of Leprosy (funded by the Nippon Foundation), Welcome Unit for the History of Medicine, University of Oxford, referred to hereafter as the Oxford Project.[1] Introductions to the individuals who had suffered leprosy were facilitated by the Pacific Leprosy Foundation (PLF), a charitable organization in Christchurch, New Zealand, and its liaison personnel resident in each of the islands. So apart from widening the understanding of the personal experiences of leprosy sufferers, this book forms a useful guide to future researchers utilizing the historical archives deposited at the Macmillan Brown Library, Christchurch, New Zealand.

The oral histories were not recorded with stigma in mind, and it was not the main focus of the questionnaire. However, while recording the interviews, notions of stigma associated with leprosy became evident, and the characteristics that constituted stigma varied from place to place and, sometimes, person to person. It can be argued that stigma, being a reflection of the subjective and possibly even subconscious attitude of the stigmatizer, is more susceptible to psychological than historical enquiry. Nevertheless, various writers have identified historical events and practices as being the causes that have given rise to leprosy stigma, and these events and practices are examined within the South Pacific context. The factors identified as the cause of stigma are:

> (1) Biblical texts and teachings conveyed and perpetuated by Christians and missionaries who aligned leprosy with earlier ideas of sin and uncleanliness, resulting in those with the disease being considered outcasts from society.[2]
>
> (2) Fear of contagion and the mutilating and disfiguring physical characteristics that occur, especially at advanced stages of the disease.[3]
>
> (3) Fear induced by twentieth century medical policies that advocated isolation, which involved the removal of patients from their families and incarceration at leprosaria.[4]

The collection of oral histories has allowed the issue of stigma to be examined more widely — for example, through personal experiences describing the conditions at leprosaria — which has permitted analysis of the impact of these conditions and other associated factors that might have caused stigma. The object has been to set aside preconceptions and, relying only on the oral testimonies of the leprosy sufferers, to examine the degree to which the three above causes contributed towards leprosy stigma in Fiji, New Caledonia, Samoa, Tonga and Vanuatu.

As two of the principal causes of stigma identified above involve isolation of leprosy sufferers at leprosaria, where care was provided by religious orders, leprosaria are an important focus. Accordingly, a section on a few leprosaria worldwide provides a contextual basis for comparison with the central South Pacific leprosarium at Makogai, Fiji. The Makogai leprosarium will in turn be assessed against smaller leprosaria visited in the Pacific islands to ascertain whether these leprosaria caused stigma. To provide an understanding of leprosy sufferers' experiences of the disease, and how it was treated and perceived by the medical fraternity, health care workers and local communities, long extracts of testimonies are quoted to convey the personal dimension of the sufferers' traumas.

The Disease and Its Brief History

Leprosy was more precisely identified and named Hansen's Disease in 1873, after Gerhard Henrik Armauer Hansen of Norway, who identified the disease-causing bacillus, *Mycobacterium leprae*. The *M. leprae* bacillus is related to the bacillus causing tuberculosis, *Mycobacterium tuberculosis*, which attacks the lungs. In leprosy the bacilli attack and damage the nerves under the skin, which can result in paralysis, the loss of sensations, and degeneration of muscles and bone, leading to highly visible progressive disabilities.[5] *M. leprae* attacks the nerves in cooler areas of the body, which are, in the main, the peripheral nerves close to the surface of the skin.[6] This gives rise to visible patches and rashes on the skin, a flattening of facial features, visual problems and loss of facial hair.[7] As a consequence of nerve damage in the limbs, unfelt injuries, especially to the hands and feet, lead to severe physical disabilities aggravated by accidental injuries and repetitive actions in everyday life.[8] Fingers and toes are most easily damaged, and the loss of these digits is a notorious sign of leprosy. The simple repetitious action of walking with anaesthetized leg nerves leads to the later chronic problem of plantar ulcers on the soles, which are extremely difficult to cure and frequently lead to complications that result in amputations.[9] Because the nerves cannot recover, disabilities occur long after the disease has naturally arrested or after medical treatment. For this reason early diagnosis and treatment of leprosy are imperative to prevent nerve damage which later leads to severe physical disabilities.

The long incubation period of leprosy can extend from a few months to twenty or even fifty years, and, together with the varied symptoms associated with different forms of the disease, this has made diagnosis exceedingly difficult historically.[10] The most serious form of leprosy is now clinically identified as multi-bacillary leprosy, also known as lepromatous leprosy, which is a multi-bacillary invasion of the skin, nerves and internal organs.[11] Pauci-bacillary leprosy, also known as tuberculoid leprosy, is the opposite end of the spectrum, where internal organs are not attacked, and the skin and nerves are affected by a solitary or few bacilli.[12] In between these poles lie a varied mix of different presentations of the disease, depending on the degree of specific immunity.[13] Medical classification of these vastly varying forms is defined by the Ridley-Jopling scale.[14] Many cases of leprosy spontaneously cease to be infectious and become inactive, which are commonly referred to as "burnt out cases."

Since Hansen's identification of the leprosy-causing bacilli, it became possible to identify the presence of bacilli in skin samples, confirming a diagnosis of leprosy. Laboratory tests and procedures show the presence of *Mycobacterium leprae* in skin tissues even at the earliest stages of the disease.[15] However, despite extensive research towards the end of the nineteenth century, no successful treatment of leprosy or any form of inoculation had been discovered. At the First International Leprosy Conference in Berlin in 1897 the disease was declared virtually incurable and isolation practices recommended.[16] Various remedies had been tested in an attempt to combat and ease the symptoms of the disease, such as chaulmoogra oil. The oil is extracted from the *Gynocardia odorata* tree and used by early Indian Ayurvedic medical practitioners; it became the treatment most commonly adopted by the British and other medical practitioners for the treatment of leprosy.[17] Chaulmoogra oil was administered orally and later via injections, but its success was very limited.[18] Its taste was most disagreeable, and the injections were administered with thick needles that were so painful as to deter patients. It was not until the revolutionary discovery of antibiotics — in particular, sulphones in 1941 at Carville in the USA — that an effective treatment was eventually found.[19]

By the late 1940s, dapsone, also known as DDS, became the most successful sulphone treatment in the majority of leprosy cases, producing remarkable results and removing the earlier visible marks and skin lesions, although nerve damage remained irreversible. Leprosy was eventually able to be contained, rendering a patient non-infectious, although some patients could not tolerate the prescribed high dosage of sulphones, and relapses did occur. By the 1970s, evidence of serious resistance to dapsone, associated with relapses of leprosy, surfaced worldwide, and the treatment was adapted to counter the problem.[20] The present treatment of Multiple Drug Therapy, MDT, was produced in the 1980s, usually comprising a combination of dapsone, clofazimine and rifampicin. MDT has been proven to effect a more stable and permanent cure, avoiding the earlier problems of drug resistance, and was adopted by the World Health Organization for treatment in their worldwide strategic plan to achieve the elimination of leprosy.[21]

Despite extensive research, the actual mode of transmission of the bacilli is still not definitively identified, although it is medically accepted to be via droplet and/or airborne infection.[22] It has been suggested that a breakthrough in discovering the exact mode of transmission may be helpful in understanding the contagion of AIDS because of the commonalities between leprosy susceptibility and the HIV virus with tuberculosis *Mycobacterium*.[23] Irrespective of the precise mode of transmission of *Mycobacterium leprae*, it is held that leprosy may be a disease of high infectivity but low pathogenicity, thereby suggesting that older ideas of prolonged close skin-to-skin contact necessary for infection might no longer be sustainable.[24]

Dr. Roland Farrugia, retired WHO leprologist and current PLF leprosy consultant, suggests that some societies are more susceptible to leprosy than others, and that ninety-five percent of most societies have differing levels of natural immunity to leprosy; the remaining five (or perhaps ten) percent having some genetic defect that makes them susceptible to leprosy when exposed to the bacillus.[25] This susceptibility, being a genetic weakness, is often passed from parents to their children, and inevitably some children are more prone to contracting leprosy, although leprosy itself is not hereditary. Dr. Bruce Mackereth, in charge of a leprosarium at Lolowai, Vanuatu, in the 1960s, conducted an epidemiological study of leprosy patients. In line with findings from other studies, he noted a strong hereditary factor in that children and siblings of infectious cases were much more likely to be infected and more likely to contract the same form of leprosy than the spouses of leprosy sufferers.[26]

A salient feature of leprosy, with profound impact upon its associated stigma, is that leprosy in itself is not a terminal disease.[27] Even prior to any effective cure being available, leprosy sufferers could live well into old age, but with increasingly serious and outwardly visible debilitating deformities, with death usually attributable to other causes. As explained by the chairman of the PLF Medical Advisory Committee, Dr. Brian McMahon, "People tend to die with it [leprosy] rather than of it."[28] As such, leprosy stigma is due to its epidemiological and etiological characteristics as a mutilating, disfiguring and progressive disease.[29]

Inevitably and historically, the complexity of leprosy led to mystery and public confusion about the disease. As the author Edmond suggests, the western public have remained haunted by past images of the fearful appearance of its physical deformities in advanced cases, frequently portrayed in fictional literature and films.[30] These images are influenced by medieval sumptuary laws which required people with leprosy to signify their presence by various means, such as special clothing and the ringing of a bell. These practices engendered horrific images of leprosy that were perpetuated by images in literature and the media to the public, who in the main were relatively ignorant about the disease. Twentieth century policies of segregation and isolation, intended to prevent contagion, made leprosy a disease out-of-sight-and-out-of-mind, leaving it shrouded in mystery and, in the public mind, often perceived as a disease of the past which no longer existed.[31]

The western medical fraternity, colonial officials and missionaries, right up to the 1950s, were, in fact, fairly ignorant about leprosy also, and their fears of contagion and ideas of segregation influenced the perceptions of South Pacific islanders. The general lack of public knowledge about leprosy, its containment, and its connection with continuing disabilities has contributed to leprosy sufferers remaining objects of dread and, accordingly, objects of stigma in many parts of the world, including the Pacific. Public attitudes towards medicine have been, and still are, molded by medical and scientific knowledge.[32] Once a scientific breakthrough is achieved on the exact mode of transmission, the publicity generated might lead to greater public awareness about leprosy overall and hopefully diminish fears of contagion, which would reduce stigma.

The arrival of leprosy in Polynesia is reported to have been in the mid-nineteenth century and blamed on Chinese immigrants, although these claims are largely unsubstantiated, and there is a lack of evidence to make any definitive claims.[33] It has been suggested that leprosy was prevalent in parts of Melanesia and Micronesia prior to this time, and that the movements of Pacific islanders within the region contributed to the spread of leprosy.[34] It was not until the introduction of western ideas of health and medicine, through missionary activities and colonization, that the incidence of leprosy and its increase was recorded in the Pacific region.

It is not really possible to know how leprosy was viewed by Pacific islanders in the late nineteenth and early twentieth century. The oral history testimonies reveal attitudes towards leprosy sufferers during the mid-twentieth century that likely reflect earlier attitudes. But it is important to note, as pointed out previously, that attitudes of leprosy stigma vary from place to place and even person to person. Another limitation to the overall assessment of stigma in the islands is that the attitudes towards other diseases are not available for comparison. Whether attitudes differed according to the severity of different diseases, and/or are the same as attitudes towards leprosy, lie outside the scope of this research.

There have been very few cases of leprosy diagnosed in New Zealand, and from 1925 until the discovery of sulphones, these cases were transferred to the leprosarium established on the island of Makogai in Fiji.[35] Even prior to the advent of sulphones, with isolation and the level of care available at Makogai, Dr. Austin, the medical superintendent at the leprosarium from 1930 to 1951, reported that the incidence of leprosy in Fiji had fallen, and the increased numbers of patients discharged annually from Makogai by 1948 were "good propaganda" for leprosy.[36] This is in contrast to the Hawaiian situation, where it was reported that the incidence of leprosy continued to rise despite compulsory confinement.[37] The subsequent dramatic improvement in the treatment of leprosy and fall in incidence of cases worldwide since the availability of sulphones in the 1940s and MDT treatment in the 1980s led the World Health Organization (WHO) in 2000 to aim for an elimination level of leprosy at less than one case per 10,000 population in the five year period leading to 2005.[38] As will be shown, this level of elimination has been achieved in most of the South Pacific region, although not yet in many other parts of the world.

Historiography

There has been a recent burgeoning interest in the historiography of leprosy worldwide, which to a large extent has been propelled by the Oxford Project to locate and retrieve archival material. Similar oral history projects and explorations for archival records have resulted in parallel research worldwide, which has contributed to a flourishing of leprosy historiography.[39]

The research initiated by the Oxford Project in the South Pacific region has encompassed hitherto unexplored areas of historiography in Tonga and Vanuatu, and extends the boundaries of earlier works on leprosy in Fiji, New Caledonia and Samoa. An enormous contribution to the historiography of leprosy in Fiji was provided by Sister Mary Stella in *Makogai: Image of Hope* (1978) and Sister Joan Morris' dissertation *They Came to Makogai* (1966), both of which provide a background to leprosy in Fiji. In 1999 a documentary video produced by Bob Madey and Larry Thomas recorded the recollections of leprosy sufferers as they journeyed to re-visit Makogai.[40] Articles by the author and Jane Buckingham have provided accounts of a visit in 2004 to the leprosy hospital in Suva, Fiji. However, this research builds a much wider and more detailed perspective than that available in those initial articles.[41] Although stigma is not specifically addressed in all these works, the lives of the leprosy sufferers and descriptions of differing events implicitly indicate attitudes of stigma.

A collection of the memoirs (in French) of leprosy sufferers in Ducos, New Caledonia, was edited by Maryse Crouzat and Nicole Forrest, *L'Hymne à la vie: des pensionnaires du Centre Raoul Follereau: Une page d'histoire calédonienne*, which was published and launched at the time of the visit to Ducos in August 2006. Access to these memoirs has been limited by lack of a full translation. Nevertheless, reports and documents obtained from Dr. Crouzat, and filed in the Macmillan Brown Library, provide the background to leprosy in New Caledonia, with details of the recent period being supplemented by the oral histories obtained through the Oxford Project. Likewise, the dissertation of Safua Akeli in 2007, *Leprosy in Samoa 1890 to 1922: Race, Colonial Politics and Disempowerment*, has been utilized to summarize the early policies relating to leprosy in Samoa.

Other publications relating to leprosy in the wider Pacific region are John Miles' *Infectious Diseases: Colonising the Pacific* and Anne Perez Hattori's *Colonial Dis-Ease: US Navy Health Policies and the Chamorros of Guam, 1898–1941*, but these do not focus solely on leprosy nor stigma. An autobiography by Dr. John Valentine provides details of his time at the leprosarium at Tinian in the Northern Mariana Islands, and an oral history with him has been archived at the Macmillan Brown Library relating to this work.[42]

Earlier twentieth century historiography of leprosy in the north Pacific region focused on the Hawaiian experiences of leprosy sufferers isolated at Molokai, and the life and death of Father Damien. These seminal events in Molokai shaped the later historiography of leprosy and have been the focus of numerous subsequent publications, but will not form a center of debate in this research.

More recent historiography has looked at western and colonial politics of segregation, and institutions of confinement, such as prisons for criminals and asylums for the mentally insane, as well as leprosaria for the containment of leprosy sufferers. Jane Buckingham, in *Leprosy in Colonial South India: Medicine and Confinement*, argued that the British government was limited in its powers to confine leprosy sufferers, and that the fragmented nature of colonial authority and penal hospitalization was a source of conflict and compromise, where even the weakest could resist. Differences and similarities in the attitudes of traditional Hindu and western cultures towards leprosy were discussed, but no definitive investigation of what comprised the varying notions of stigma itself was explored. Other publications examining the role of colonial powers in terms of public health and internment include David Arnold's *Colonizing the Body: State Medicine and Epidemic Disease in Nineteenth Century India*, Megan Vaughan's *Curing Their Ills: Colonial Power and*

African Illness, Alison Bashford's *Imperial Hygiene: A Critical History of Colonialism*, and, most recently, Rod Edmond's *Leprosy and Empire: A Medical and Cultural History.*

This work does not encompass or examine the limits of colonial powers in the South Pacific region, but provides narrative accounts of the experiences of leprosy sufferers and the care provided for these people by colonial governments and independent governments in the Pacific from the 1930s into the twenty-first century. It considers how the various institutions of confinement of leprosy sufferers established in Fiji, New Caledonia, Samoa, Tonga and Vanuatu, as well as the role of missionaries at these institutions, impacted upon local attitudes so as to contribute towards an understanding of stigma as it manifests in the South Pacific.

The testimonies included here add to the historical understandings revealed through the African voices reported by Eric Silla in *People Are Not the Same: Leprosy and Identity in Twentieth Century Mali*, where a collection of nearly two hundred life histories were used to elaborate the perspectives of leprosy patients.[43]

Silla spent a year in Mali talking to patients and engaging with the political and social dynamics that shaped the lives of the patients; whereas this research only permitted brief visits to the specified Pacific nations, with no time available for in-depth evaluation of the intricacies of national political and social life upon the lives of leprosy sufferers. Nevertheless, the resilience and vibrancy found among the individuals in Mali have much in common with the lives of leprosy sufferers in the South Pacific region, in that the onslaught of the disease in both regions was followed by isolation within home and local communities by health authorities. In these situations the patients formed their own support groups, which led to the establishment of separate communities.

In 1989 Gussow published a socio-historical study, *Leprosy, Racism and Public Health: Social Policy in Chronic Disease Control*, which traced the values and institutional climate in which leprosy was embedded internationally, and the contemporary forces that were replacing established ideology regarding leprosy care. This publication followed on from earlier articles in 1970 and 1971 by Gussow and Tracy, based on their research with leprosy sufferers and workers at the leprosarium at Carville in Louisiana, USA, which concluded that contemporary ideas relating to the stigma of leprosy was a myth that had emerged in the early twentieth century.[44]

These and other propositions by Gussow and Tracy will be discussed further in the following section on stigma; and, in particular, this research will explore to what extent these ideas are applicable to the lives of leprosy sufferers in the South Pacific region.

Brief History of Leprosy Stigma

Stigma is defined as "a mark of disgrace associated with a particular circumstance, quality, or person."[45] The heart of the cruel stigma associated with leprosy and the attitude towards those suffering from the disease is exemplified in the word "leper" which, when used as an analogy in other contexts, makes explicit the sense that a person is shunned or ostracized from society. No other disease has such a derivative cognate as leper, indicating that that person has a specific disease, apart perhaps from the term HIV-carrier in association with AIDS. Like leprosy in the late nineteenth century, AIDS in the mid-twentieth century gave rise to hysterical fears of contagion and created stigma towards the unfortunate victims. In reviewing public health posters on the risks of AIDS contagion, Sander Gilman reproduced the advertising images used, which attempted to prevent the transference of the virus while at the same time avoiding the creation of stigma towards individuals, as in a poster slogan "It won't kill you to spend time with a friend who has AIDS."[46] If the lessons of history are learned in relation to contagious diseases where death is not imminent, such as in AIDS and leprosy, it should be remembered that in the fight against contagion there is a need to avoid ostracizing the victims so as not to increase their suffering.

In support of a worldwide agenda to de-stigmatize leprosy and remove connotations of those having the disease being ostracized from society, the word "leper" is avoided, apart from its use in specific circumstances (as above and in direct quotations). However, it should be kept in mind that some qualities inherent in stigma are present with all medical conditions that put others at risk through infection, such as influenza and the recent publicity regarding possible pandemics of bird and swine flu. Most people, where possible, would avoid putting themselves at undue risk of contagion, and this was the case with leprosy. The fact that the signs of the disease remained visible on leprosy sufferers who had not been diagnosed nor treated at the early stages but survived into old age wrongly raised fears of continuing contagion. Until leprosy was clinically understood, and medical tests confirmed the presence of active or inactive bacilli, neither the leprosy sufferers themselves nor those around them knew whether there was a risk of contagion or not. Findings from the oral histories suggest that the visible signs, and ignorance about the disease and its transmission, lie at the heart of the stigma of leprosy, rather than biblical proscriptions against leprosy.

Nevertheless, connections persist between what is referred to as leprosy in the Christian Bible and the clinical diagnosis of the disease in the twentieth century, and this has been blamed as the source of stigma. Etiological explanations have testified that the word leprosy in the Bible, and modern classifications of leprosy, refer to different conditions.[47] Browne has shown that the Old Testament Hebrew word ṣāra'at and later Greek world *lepra* are complex and untranslatable terms which embraced concepts impossible to interpret into single words in modern languages, but eventually came to be translated simply by the generic term leprosy, which included several skin diseases.[48] The Hebrew word ṣāra'at originally signified a state of ritual uncleanliness or ceremonial defilement characterized by visible surface blemishes, on a par with the ritually unclean who handled corpses or with menstrual uncleanness.[49] Most references to ṣāra'at were in a ritual context, and to the Israelites, ṣāra'at was a condition amenable only to divine intervention, requiring ritual cleansing rather than a medical cure.[50] The Greek word *lepra* referred to the generic concept of scaliness, either scaly skin or sometimes even scaly walls, with no suggestion of the ritualistic defilement incorporated into ṣāra'at; but in the New Testament *lepra* came to be the equivalent of ṣāra'at.[51] Thus the two words coalesced and were translated simply as leprosy into English and other translations of the Bible. Leprosy remained a generic term until the specific disease was precisely delimited clinically in 1847 by Danielssen and Boeck.[52] The serious prejudice associated with the generic term leprosy was reinforced by transfer of the corpus of ṣāra'at beliefs to the innocent victims of newly identified mycobacterial disease, clinically identified by Hansen as leprosy.[53]

Dr. Desmond Beckett, one of the later medical superintendents at the leprosarium at Makogai in 1960s, had earlier been involved in the care of leprosy sufferers at Makondane leprosarium on the island of Pemba, Zanzibar, and at the Jos Plateau in Nigeria. He clearly points out that the biblical references to leprosy and "leper" were not necessarily the same medical condition as that recognized as leprosy today, although it was probably one of the conditions included in the generic use of the term.[54] Nevertheless, Beckett considers that "the morbid interest in leprosy and the instinctive dread of the condition that is almost universal in the non-medical world, stems from this biblical indoctrination."[55] This view supports the opinion of Brody that the "stigma of leprosy is thus the product of a long tradition."[56]

The level of stigma encountered in the South Pacific, predominantly Christian nations, is reported to be less severe than in some other countries — for example, Japan, which is not a predominantly Christian country and where stigma cannot be blamed on the Bible and Christian attitudes. But it was not until 1996 in Japan that a law enacted earlier in 1953 finally abolished forced segregation, putting an end to enforced isolation of leprosy sufferers in sanatoria.[57] Researchers in the Ryukyu Islands have demonstrated that younger Japanese generations are more likely to take a benign view of leprosy because they no longer witness the deformities caused by advanced leprosy. But older groups believed that leprosy patients should be permanently isolated because they had personally observed the deformities of victims and could not accept that the patients were no longer infectious.[58] This Japanese research suggests that early diagnosis and treatment of leprosy, which avoids later physical deformities, should finally result in the diminishment of stigma. The finding is one that will be shown to be supported by this research. The high level of stigma in Japan, particularly among the older generation, has been attributed to the stringent public policies of isolation, so much so that in May 2001, $17 million were awarded to leprosy sufferers as compensation for their ordeals, and the then prime minister, Junichiro Koizumi, publicly apologized for the wrongs of the previous governments.[59] This compensation implicitly recognizes that isolation of leprosy sufferers contributed to the high stigma. A Japanese benefactor, Yohei Sasakawa, through the Nippon Foundation, has made a commitment to provide the medical treatment MDT to leprosy sufferers worldwide free of charge.[60] The benefit of free medication and efforts to ensure early diagnosis and treatment of all leprosy sufferers should result in the gradual elimination of the awful visible symptoms of advanced leprosy cases. If the conclusion of the Japanese research is correct, this, in turn, will lead to a corresponding diminution of the fears that sustain stigma.

The modern use of isolation as a recognized health practice developed in western societies through the public health in the nineteenth century, which focused on sanitation, hygiene and preventative medicine. Practices incorporating quarantine and isolation had been effectively used to combat highly infectious tropical diseases — so much so that at the First International Leprosy Conference in 1897, in view of the lack of any effective treatment or inoculation, and with the backing of Hansen, segregation was advocated for the confinement of leprosy cases.[61] This was in opposition to the earlier findings in India of the Leprosy Commission in 1893 which considered isolation impractical, with compulsion likely to lead victims of the disease to hide from authorities, as had already been evident with compulsory isolation in Hawaii.[62]

The British medical fraternity and National Leprosy Fund, who were aware of isolated cases of leprosy in Europe and especially in Norway, recognized that the disease was not highly contagious and that the public risk was so low that isolation was impractical, unnecessary and even cruel.[63] Nevertheless, the outcry to segregate leprosy sufferers persisted in the public domain, especially in newspapers and even through literature. Elements of the exotic, bizarre and even horror inflamed the imagination.[64] It is a very basic human trait to fear anything that can cause gross physical harm to the body. Leprosy in western society and literature embodies this horror; yet it also inspires fascination and fantasy regarding the limits of societal taboos.[65] This fascination in fantasy and fiction, it is suggested, has compounded western ideas of stigma and leprosy, the latter being a word steeped through antiquity with morbidity.

With isolation practices advocated for leprosy sufferers, in the twentieth century leprosy stigma became associated with the terrors of being removed from one's home and incarcerated far away without any means of self-sufficiency, as has been suggested was the case initially at Molokai, Hawaii. The section below on leprosaria provides a contextual basis for comparison and an assessment of the leprosarium at Makogai, Fiji. The lack of public health resources to support government policies of isolation and segregation, meant that leprosy sufferers became not only wards of the state, but victims dependent upon the goodwill and philanthropic generosity of individuals. The plight of leprosy sufferers spawned the growth of charitable organizations such as the Leprosy Mission, and in New Zealand the Pacific Leprosy Foundation in Christchurch.

Missions and Stigma

From the earliest days of leprosaria in the South Pacific, most people were reluctant to work with leprosy; only the religious orders were willing to do so, as they saw it as part of their duty to help those in need. It has been suggested by various researchers, including Edmond, that the high level of missionary involvement in the provision of care at leprosaria worldwide contributed to a revival of old biblical stigmatic attitudes.[66] Edmond went on to suggest that the missionaries simply "palliate[d] the worst effects of crude and harsh quarantine," and that patients were merely "educated to accept their life-sentence, abandon all other identities and wait for better things in the afterlife."[67] The oral history testimonies of leprosy sufferers in the Pacific Islands do not indicate that the nuns running the leprosarium at Makogai or other leprosaria gave particular emphasis to the connections between leprosy and biblical ideas of sinfulness or divine wrath. Some interviewees were aware of biblical texts and referred to the fact that leprosy was mentioned in the Bible, but displayed no knowledge that their condition might, in fact, have been different from that referred to in the texts. Others acknowledged that segregation was endorsed by the Bible, which prescribed that those with leprosy should be "sent to the end of the village."[68] This idea perhaps fits with biblical prescriptions that the diagnosis of leprosy meant a life sentence away from the community, which in turn sanctioned their own isolation in leprosaria.

Gussow and Tracy have described the ministrations of religious orders at various leprosaria as a "relationship of missionary activity ... bringing to life of a modern parable"[69] — namely, that of the Good Samaritan, which they suggest re-invoked perceptions of older ideas of biblical stigma by the early twentieth century.[70] Because of this biblical stigma, in the USA from 1920 to the 1940s, a process of destigmatization was pursued, which included renaming leprosy as Hansen's Disease; yet stigma is believed to have persisted.[71] Gussow and Tracy explored these ideas in relation to the situation at Carville leprosarium in the USA, and described the link between the biblical stigma and the present-day ideas of leprosy stigma as the creation of a myth.[72] They suggest that this myth was created or re-created during the period when leprosy was encountered in colonies in the late 19th century, particularly after the identification of *Mycobacterium leprae* in 1873 and the hysteria surrounding the death of Father Damien at Molokai, Hawaii, in 1888. The latter event had been sensationally reported in the western press, with fears expressed that although leprosy had virtually disappeared in Europe during the sixteenth century, it could re-emerge and be re-introduced into the west because it had afflicted a European, the Belgian priest Father Damien. These fears were exaggerated because Hansen's recent discovery was seen as confirmation that people with the disease were sources of contagion, whereas methods of transmission of the disease had previously been uncertain and often erroneously considered to be hereditary.[73]

Myth of Stigma and Self-Stigma

The research by Gussow and Tracy at Carville concluded that since the advent of the effective cure by sulphones, fears about the disease and contagion had diminished, replaced with false ideas that leprosy was a disease of the past — so much so that, in fact, prevailing notions of stigma no longer existed in the public mind. It was further noted that the experiences of those suffering leprosy and those involved in the treatment of the disease reflected no consistent pattern of stigma, but that the years of isolation had inflicted a level of internalization of stigma, referred to as "self-stigma," upon the psyche of residents at Carville.[74] Self-stigma is the internalization of the public perception that those with leprosy should be excluded from normal society, so that leprosy sufferers felt they needed to be segregated because they were contagious and needed to protect the public from any contagion.

Although the above categories are essentially western ideas, to varying degrees they are evident in the South Pacific, either through early colonial contacts and/or conveyed by western medical personnel and missionaries. The use of lengthy extracts from the testimonies of leprosy sufferers will provide descriptions of the experiences following diagnosis with leprosy and their internment at different leprosaria. These will also help to show how leprosy sufferers perceived their social acceptance back in their communities, and to what degree, if any, notions of stigma and/or self-stigma existed. A wide range of personal differences were evident, and leprosy sufferers who appear to have internalized stigma tended to isolate themselves and not mix freely in their local communities. Whether this was entirely due to internalized ideas of stigma, or was a reflection of the real attitudes of the local communities, is the vexed and ambivalent issue in the assessment of stigma. The views of leprosy sufferers also demonstrate a responsible and positive attitude in that several interviewees encouraged their family members, especially children, to be checked regularly for early signs of leprosy. This understanding of leprosy, and the simple, effective treatment now available, is changing old negative attitudes towards leprosy in the Pacific islands.

In attempts to deter stigma worldwide, an official day was nominated in 1954 as World Leprosy Day by the French philanthropist Raoul Follereau.[75] Follereau was the benefactor of leprosy sufferers in several French colonies in Africa as well as New Caledonia, and his initiatives led to the formation of the European Federation for Leprosy (ELEP), which later became known as the International Federation Assisting Leprosy (ILEP).[76] World Leprosy Day was nominated as the last Sunday in January, and in Tonga, Samoa and Fiji on this day leprosy awareness programs are aired on national and local radio stations. The effectiveness of this and various other awareness programs is not easily assessed in regards to the extent the information is actually assimilated by the public. In the long run, such programs do help raise understanding about leprosy and the efficacy of the treatments, reducing misunderstood fears about the disease and its associated stigma.

Growth of Leprosaria and Missionary Involvement

During the eighteenth century the practice of isolating particular groups of people grew, and planned asylums were built in the U.S. for specialized purposes (such as homes for unwanted children); while in Europe such asylums were often located in what were originally monasteries.[77] The name "asylum" was derived from the Greek word for refuge, being places inviolable from without. It became implicit that asylums were not considered places for punishment, but places to effect a cure for the ills of society; therefore, being committed did not necessitate any legal process for removal of people to these institutions.[78] The asylum became a benevolent institution that extended to include places of confinement for leprosy sufferers, earlier referred to as lazarette or lazar homes, utilizing the Christian story of Jesus healing Lazarus and indicating that these homes were to assist and treat leprosy sufferers.[79] These leprosaria were also called leprosy stations or leper colonies. The terms colony and station implied self-sufficient places where groups could live and form a functioning community.

This sanction to endorse segregation of leprosy sufferers, particularly in the USA, led to what has been referred to as the "production of a culture of difference"[80] because the institutions created required staff to care for patients and funding to provide necessary services. In Britain the Mission to Lepers was founded in 1874 and became the prototype for church supported agencies for the care and treatment of leprosy patients.[81] In providing specialized facilities for leprosy sufferers, leprosy became institutionalized, with even a specific name for the doctors — leprologist — and further specialized services developed in line with modern health care practices.

With institutionalization in the twentieth century, leprosy became a zealous and altruistic mission for the church and missionaries, who in turn used their influence and widespread affiliations to raise charitable funding.[82] Since lay people were reluctant to care for those suffering from leprosy in institutions, especially in remote areas, religious orders undertook the work. The commitment and selfless devotion of sisters from different Christian denominations, who provided daily care, involved spending the majority of their lives in remote leprosaria, examples being the Daughters of Charity of St. Vincent de Paul in Carville, USA, from 1896 to 2005, and the Sisters of St. Paul of Chartres at Culion leprosy colony in the Philippines from 1906.[83] For the South Pacific region, the founding pioneers of a Catholic order which came to be the Missionary Sisters of the Society of Mary (SMSM), set out from France. One of these pioneers arrived in New Caledonia in 1864, and by 1892 was tending to the needs of leprosy sufferers.[84] Additionally, the Anglican Melanesian Mission began operating in the islands in 1849, which in the twentieth century led to the establishment of leprosaria. The activities relating to leprosy in New Caledonia will describe the involvement of the missions, which subsequently led to the SMSM becoming the providers of nursing staff and helpers at the leprosarium established at Makogai, Fiji, in 1911. The research of Joan Morris describes life at Makogai in the 1950s and concludes that the leprosarium was not simply a "polyglot of sufferers" but a colony which had formed into a "well integrated community."[85] Testimonies of leprosy sufferers who had been isolated at Makogai will be quoted and support Morris' conclusion. These demonstrate that the facilities available at various smaller leprosy colonies and/or wards or wings established at different South Pacific hospitals to isolate leprosy patients contributed to perceptions of increased or diminished associated stigma, dependent upon the conditions at each leprosarium.

The role and activities of the SMSM sisters at the leprosaria in Fiji, and at the Raoul Follereau leprosarium in New Caledonia (as well as the leprosy care offered by sisters in Samoa and Tonga), are examined to assess and refute the claim by Edmond (referred to earlier) that the religious orders simply palliated the needs of leprosy patients and prepared them for the afterlife. Edmond's view fails to recognize the medical and scientific professionalism which has been neglected in descriptions of charitable activities. The role of the Anglican Melanesian Mission staff running the leprosarium at Lolowai, Vanuatu, will be described in this context, and particularly in view of the comparatively low level of stigma evinced in the islands of Vanuatu.

Other Leprosaria

In order to provide a context for comparing the leprosaria in the South Pacific region with leprosaria cited in earlier historiography, a brief description of some of these institutions follows — namely, Molokai leprosarium in Hawaii, Carville in the USA, and the isolation of the Chamorros of Guam at Culion in the Philippines, plus limited comment on leprosaria set up in India and Singapore. Although insufficient details are provided here to make any real overall comparison between these worldwide leprosaria, the descriptions will demonstrate a difference in the approaches to establishing leprosaria in the South Pacific, particularly Makogai in Fiji, and St. Barnabas leprosy hospital at Lolowai in Vanuatu.

Although isolation may have confirmed fears of contagion in the public mind, leprosaria undoubtedly provided a humane alternative for those who could not care for themselves or had nobody else to care for them, as described in the events cited by Edmond.[86] The ambivalence of isolation is evident with a case of leprosy discovered in London in 1898, the same year as the First Leprosy Conference in Berlin, which had advocated isolation for leprosy cases. Although the *British Medical Journal* noted that there was no need for alarm due to contagion, it pointed out the absence of, and therefore the need for, a dedicated institution to care for those leprosy sufferers who were not able to provide for their own care or had no one else to care for them.[87] Debates in the press relating to isolation continued for some years, and an anonymous correspondent signed "A Leper," who had apparently worked in an "asylum for seven years and become infected,"[88] wrote that those infected wished to take every precaution to prevent any spread of the disease, and that "an asylum offered a secure and known world where patients would not be shunned."[89]

In due course, through a charitable donation, a home was established outside London in the village of Woodham Ferrers in Essex. The first few cases of leprosy were transferred during nightfall to avoid attention, and soon two nurses from a religious order and some monks took up residence to provide care.[90] These events clearly demonstrate that isolation of leprosy sufferers fulfilled a need by providing a place where those requiring help could go voluntarily, rather than isolation being simply imposed or enforced by the authorities. The sick deserved to be cared for when, on occasion, they were turned out of their lodgings and should not be left to literally rot on the streets. It will be shown that similar needs gave rise to the establishment of small leprosy colonies in the Pacific islands, which later coalesced into larger leprosaria with better medical facilities.

In Hawaii, as early as 1865, the forced segregation of leprosy sufferers passed into law, and the remote and difficult to access location of Kalaupapa on the island of Molokai became the site to which the unfortunate victims were banished.[91] Much has been written about leprosy at Kalaupapa on Molokai, and on the conditions and manner in which Father Damien devoted his energies to help those suffering from leprosy; these debates will not be entered into here. Nevertheless, it is important to note that from the earliest days when leprosy sufferers were brought to Molokai, they were unable, for various reasons, to become self-sufficient, partly because the land supposedly available for planting was disputed by locals.[92] Living conditions were miserable, as widely reported after the death of Damien, and in the main the patients had to fend for themselves. The horrors reported worldwide regarding the conditions at Molokai and the horrific plight of the unfortunate victims exacerbated fear of being diagnosed with leprosy, which led to patients resisting or hiding from health authorities.[93] This inevitably increased the stigma associated with leprosy. In Fiji, as will be discussed, a large leprosarium was established on the island of Makogai much later, in 1911; in contrast, it was well planned, with good facilities available, prior to the arrival of patients. The whole island of Makogai was dedicated to improving the living conditions of the residents, who from earliest times took part in gardening and fishing to support a self-sufficient and useful lifestyle — because a life sentence was envisaged on the island.

The first institution in the U.S. devoted solely to leprosy was the Louisiana Home for Lepers in 1894; in 1896 the Daughters of Charity of St. Vincent de Paul came to tend the patients.[94] The Louisiana leprosy station on the banks of the Mississippi River, not far from New Orleans, was a remote and poor region, and patients were brought from distant places and segregated far from their families. The poor district and tyranny of distance put fear into the minds of leprosy sufferers and their families. Because of the strong stigma of leprosy, an atmosphere of stealth and secrecy prevailed in the early years at Louisiana, where the first batch of patients were brought up-river under the cover of darkness to avoid discovery of the purpose of the dwelling by locals.[95] The conditions were such that the patients and sisters had to contend with ignorance and prejudice against the disease that "rendered the stigma even harder to bear than the physical suffering."[96]

By contrast, in Fiji and other Pacific islands, small leprosy colonies had initially been set up nearer the homes of leprosy sufferers, often with impoverished conditions, and the patients were gradually transferred to the larger leprosaria, enabling them to benefit from the wider range of facilities available. In these circumstances, removal by force was unnecessary, although stigma was evident in the problems encountered to secure transportation for the patients. Rather than secret transportation, a few boats agreed to carry such patients, but would signal the presence of leprosy patients by flying a special flag; and the boats were disinfected after the patients disembarked.[97] Hoisting a flag on boats carrying sick or quarantined people was a common practice in colonial ports.

The advantage of establishing larger leprosaria is evinced by the purchase of the Louisiana station in 1921 by the U.S. Government, whereupon conditions improved and it became the national hospital for leprosy in America, commonly known as Carville, the leading center for research into leprosy and rehabilitation of leprosy sufferers. It was here in the 1940s that the phenomenal breakthrough was made — the successful treatment of leprosy by sulphone drugs.[98] This discovery and the commencement of an effective treatment for the disease made a revolutionary improvement in the lives of patients, but the stigma was reported to be harder to eliminate.[99] The stigma attached to leprosaria remained, as Dr. Beckett pointed out, partly because the location of Carville remained where it had been deliberately positioned — between the male and female State penitentiaries, as a means to prevent intermingling.[100] Such geographical locations are naturally perceived as locations for outcasts from society. The location of leprosaria in distant, often impoverished areas, or, alternatively, in prisons (as occurred in New Caledonia), impacted on public perceptions of stigma associated with leprosy sufferers and leprosaria. Fortunately, with the more recent effective treatment of MDT, leprosy is gradually being treated as just another disease at ordinary hospitals, and specialist care specifically for leprosy is situated within the walls of general health providers. Thus the association of leprosy with separation and outcasts from society should cease in the public mind which will bring relief to the victims themselves.

Another example of the tyranny of distance and fear contributing to the perceived stigma of leprosy is seen in the treatment of the Chamorros of Guam, who were transferred to the leprosarium at Culion in the Philippines, which was established in 1901 and became the largest leprosarium in the world.[101] Leprosy sufferers were forcibly gathered by the U.S. Navy in Micronesia, including Guam, and taken to the distant island of Culion. In 1902 the Chamorros were initially segregated at the nearby island of Tumon in Guam, the colony being surrounded by high, barbed wire fences. Iron bars were placed on widows and the doors padlocked at night; but many inmates managed to escape, and family members managed to enter the barricades (which, in fact, perhaps, made the segregation tolerable).[102] Hattori notes that a language reflecting the "criminalization of the ill"[103] is evident in government records, not only in the manner of capture but in living arrangements, which would have confirmed ideas of exclusion and unacceptability in the psyche of patients.[104] Finally, in 1911 it was deemed more expedient to transfer the "inmates" at Tumon to the distant Philippine island of Culion, despite the awareness by officials that the Chamorros appeared accustomed to the disease and were opposed to isolation.[105] The fear of banishment was so great that, it is reported, a blind man with leprosy carried a woman who could not walk on his back, and together they escaped transportation by the Navy and evaded detection for over a month.[106] Exile to Culion continued until 1924, at which time the surgeon at Guam decided that the expulsion policy resulted in worse health conditions for the Chamorros; cooperation was needed for health programs to succeed, and the fear of exile had led leprosy sufferers and other patients to avoid American doctors and hospitals.[107] Leprosy suffers were returned from Culion to the Tumon colony where patients continued to be segregated. These events demonstrate that banishment and exile contributed to the fearful reputation of leprosy, which is also evident in South Pacific regions, raising fears and stigma. The use of force to remove patients undoubtedly aggravated perceptions of stigma in Guam, which did not occur further south in the Pacific, apart from some evidence of forcible confinement in New Caledonia.

Some patients in Guam indicated they took pride in accepting banishment because their action avoided the risk of being the source of contagion to their own families.[108] This double-edged sword of leprosy demonstrates that a level of humane segregation was acceptable to patients; but however brave the idea of pride in accepting exclusion and distant exile may have been, exile raised stigma. Significant stigma is evident in the fact that leprosy patients hid rather than seek medical attention because of the consequences of a diagnosis of leprosy. These findings are partially reflected in the experiences of those in Tonga, where patients who returned from isolation at Makogai faced stigma through exclusion in their own homes — either because they continued to be perceived as a risk for leprosy contagion, or due to ingrained attitudes in their village communities.

Another instance of the conditions of incarceration which would have perpetuated ideas of exclusion and stigma is Buckingham's description of the high walls specially placed around a leprosy hospital built by the British government in Madras, India, ostensibly as a place of voluntary residence.[109] Here patients had to wear red caps, as did criminal prisoners; so instead of being seen as a charitable and benevolent institution, which was at least in part the intent of the medical officer working there, the hospital came to be seen as "a place of terror."[110] Nevertheless, Buckingham suggests that it was the hospital which was stigmatized, not the leprosy patients, as their families continued to visit at the hospital. Another leprosy hospital was established at Port Blair on the Andaman Islands, a well known British penal colony[111] — yet again linking leprosy with the outcasts from society. In New Caledonia, the leprosarium at Ducos was previously a prison, and the stigma of leprosy appeared greater in New Caledonia than in neighboring Vanuatu. The perception of leprosy patients being treated the same as those who were outcasts from society appear to have contributed to a higher level of stigma.

Although leprosy confinement was not compulsorily enforced in India, and institutions were altruistically intended to be places of refuge rather than places of detention, the geographic situation of institutions at penal colonies with high fences around them, and particularly the stipulation of wearing caps like those worn by state prisoners in Madras, would have contributed to the perception of an unwanted people, unworthy and barred from ordinary society. During the earlier days of isolation in Samoa and Tonga, high fences were erected at the end of hospital grounds to contain leprosy sufferers in special buildings, segregating from the main hospital; these areas were viewed with some degree of fear and horror by the general public.[112] Buckingham indicates that in India this culture of difference produced feelings of shame in families with leprosy but mainly the poor and homeless were segregated into the leprosy colonies, while those with families who could provide care were frequently hidden from public gaze in their homes to avoid being shunned by their community.[113] Despite segregation of the poor, Buckingham suggests that patients retained the power of resistance and negotiation, and viewed the leprosy hospital in Madras more as an institution for care and treatment than a place of forced confinement.[114] These findings run counter to the view that leprosy sufferers were merely confined for the public good. Additionally, it demonstrates that leprosaria served the interests of advanced leprosy cases both before and after the availability of sulphones in India and the South Pacific.

In 2005, Loh Kah Seng interviewed elderly leprosy sufferers in Singapore, many of whom had been segregated for several decades, and was told by patients who lived at the leprosarium that because they bore visible scars and disabilities, they had been unable to convince family, friends and the public that their leprosy was cured.¹¹⁵ It was further noted that following the discharge of large numbers of patients soon after the first sulphone treatments, many of those discharged demanded to be readmitted because they had been rejected by their families and had nowhere to go.¹¹⁶ This supports the proposition that the physical manifestations of the disease form one of the core constituents of stigma, and that leprosaria fulfilled a need for leprosy sufferers with physical disabilities. Furthermore, these attitudes cannot be ascribed to Christianity because Singapore is not predominantly Christian.

There are commonalities between the British colonial governments in Singapore and the Pacific Islands. In Singapore a Lepers' Ordinance was passed in 1897 — two years earlier than a similar ordinance implemented in Fiji in 1899, both of which restricted the occupations that leprosy sufferers could hold.¹¹⁷ There are various parallels within the history and approaches to containment of leprosy in Singapore and the Pacific Islands, although in the Pacific Islands confinement was not enforced by the authorities like in Singapore. Centralized leprosaria came to represent places fondly remembered as a home for the residents, providing friendships and a sense of community spirit.¹¹⁸ The Singapore interviews indicated that although their "lives are bad" due to leprosy and disabilities that prevented them from returning to ordinary life, their "luck was good" because they had received care and a place that had become home to them, despite societal rejection.¹¹⁹ This sense of cheerful irony is somewhat echoed by interviewees at Twomey hospital in Suva, Fiji, after the closure of the leprosarium at Makogai; residents were concerned because their hospital was being increasingly used for non-leprosy patients, and they felt at risk of losing their home.¹²⁰

These attitudes of leprosy sufferers, however, can be interpreted differently — that is, as a dependence on institutions reflecting a continued expectation of an entitlement to free care and medical support. This care and ongoing support is available to elderly leprosy sufferers who underwent isolation and had lost support of families and their communities, as well as cases with severe physical disabilities who are residents at various leprosaria in the South Pacific. Certainly the PLF continues to offer support to these people. But with MDT treatment, patients can now be rendered non-infectious within forty-eight hours,¹²¹ and such expectations can no longer be taken for granted, as new cases of leprosy fall within the realm of ordinary diseases. This view is reported by Silla in his research in Mali, where the French leprologist Pierre Bobin, who had previously worked in New Caledonia, noted that in both countries "former patients ... had grown accustomed to receiving free medicines, quality care for ailments unrelated to leprosy ... and considered themselves entitled to these benefits."¹²² Silla's research demonstrates how leprosy sufferers in Mali viewed themselves as a separate group, with their identities rooted in the disease.¹²³ He describes how these people formed an association to fight for their rights to obtain charitable grants donated by the Association Raoul Follereau, little of which had been seen by Malians. Also, when the government sought to take over land earlier allocated as a leprosy village by the former colonial government, the residents fought back, revealing their collective participation in civic life, which Silla suggests demonstrated "the capacity of the disease to define identity as forcefully as more common attributes rooted in languages, religion or ethnicity."¹²⁴ Silla reports that Dr. Bobin viewed suggestions of a collective identity of leprosy patients as an anachronism, as opposed to Silla's contention that scientific advancement and medicine had failed to eradicate the disease and its stigma.¹²⁵ However, Silla also observed that leprosy no longer prevented marriages or caused social isolation, but concluded that stigma "still permeates the society in which they live."¹²⁶ Silla does not specifically identify what constitutes stigma, but suggests that stigma derives from the incurable and chronic nature of the disease.¹²⁷ This tends to support the proposition by Bobin that the separate identity of leprosy sufferers, centering on the disease, was indeed an anachronism in the late twentieth century, since leprosy was virtually curable. Alternatively, identity associated with leprosy could be interpreted as reflecting elements of internalization or self-stigma, as observed by Gussow and Tracy, drawing together a community with close common interests and past experiences.

These historical descriptions of life at some worldwide leprosaria demonstrate that although isolationist policies imposed fear and emotional hardships of separation from loved ones on leprosy sufferers, leprosaria offered opportunities for friendships without any fear of being the source contagion. Living at leprosaria developed a spirit of camaraderie and community. A leprosarium was a place where patients felt they belonged, and for many it became home and a place where some friendships resulted in marriage and family. These findings are paralleled by leprosy sufferers in the South Pacific, and these testimonies will be explored to discover whether, apart from the benefits of leprosaria, leprosaria per se and/or the nursing mission sisters contributed to the idea of stigma.

The Interviews

My first visit was made to Fiji in 2004, followed by visits to Samoa, New Caledonia, Vanuatu and Tonga in 2006, and a further visit to Vanuatu in 2008.¹²⁸ The PLF liaison personnel in the islands usually approached individual leprosy sufferers prior to my visit, and personally escorted and introduced me to the interviewees. A general questionnaire was utilized at the interviews, seeking details of the interviewees' childhood, parents, siblings, schooling, lifestyle, their own adult experiences, occupations, marriage and children, with a focus upon their health. Questions were not specifically directed at experiences relating to the stigma of leprosy, but stigma was implicit in the life stories recounted. Interpreters were frequently used because of my lack of Pacific languages.

The experience of interviewing leprosy sufferers is not easily conveyed, especially the warmth of their reception to a foreigner arriving in their homes, not only enquiring into but recording various private aspects of their lives. I am obliged to recognize that the warmth of my reception may have been linked to the presence of the PLF liaison personnel who facilitated the introductions, having driven me to remote village homes to enable the oral histories to be recorded. The interviewees might have felt beholden to the PLF representatives, who provide assistance from the PLF and report back to Christchurch concerning future needs. In the main, the interviewees appeared pleased and excited to have their stories recorded and were happy to pose for photographs. Matters relating to physical disabilities were indirectly raised by enquiring what problems were experienced later in life due to leprosy.

The first interviews were conducted with thirteen leprosy sufferers living at P. J. Twomey Memorial Hospital in Suva, Fiji, in August 2004. Two of the residents had previously been filmed for a documentary about life at the leprosarium at Makogai and the residents appear to have been happy with the result. There was no apparent apprehension about having their personal life stories recorded.[129] My concern was in doing justice to each interviewee given the restraints imposed by limited time — trying to squeeze in all thirteen interviews and visit other leprosy sufferers in their homes within five days.

Three visits were made to leprosy sufferers in their homes and villages in Fiji. Although prior arrangements had been made to record the oral histories, family members were present in the home, often young children who played nearby and interjected at times. The homes, frequently built with the assistance of PLF donations, were simple two or three room houses close to neighbors or plantations. The open style of homes could not prevent the sounds of trucks clattering past, neighbors talking, radios outside nearby, dogs barking and cocks crowing or fighting. The ideal oral history interview environment of a quiet room with no interruptions was never available in the island homes visited. Conducting oral histories with casual interpreters meant there was little control over what was actually asked and how accurately answers were interpreted. Careful phrasing of questions in English, and innuendoes in the replies, were probably lost through the use of casual interpreters.

The second series of interviews took place in Samoa in January 2006. Sister Marietta SMSM, originally from Christchurch, was the liaison contact and facilitated the meetings with the leprosy patients. A PLF truck, shared with the doctor in charge of leprosy patients, was available to Sister Marietta to drive us to their homes around the island of Upolu. The majority of interviews took place in Samoan homes—*fale*—which are literally open walled buildings with pillars and a roof. The roof provided protection from the sun and rain, and the supporting pillars allowed the cool breeze to circulate through the home. Conducting interviews in these surroundings again meant no possibility of excluding unwanted sounds. The interviewees were very forthcoming with their stories, providing vivid accounts of their experiences, particularly in Samoa. Sometimes the manner of speech was difficult to follow for an outsider new to Samoa, but the majority of interviewees spoke good English.

On the visit to New Caledonia in September 2006 it was discovered that the leprosy sufferers at the Raoul Follereau leprosarium at Ducos, near Noumea, had already had their stories recorded for a French publication, launched during my visit. It was not deemed appropriate by the authorities and care givers that further recordings be made. New Caledonia had stopped receiving funding from the PLF, and the French government provided the care for leprosy sufferers, so there was no PLF contact on the island. A visit to the SMSM mission headquarters in Port Vila, Vanuatu, enabled a meeting and interview with a local SMSM sister, Noëllie, who had worked with leprosy patients throughout her life of service. She then arranged a visit and interview with one of the longest term residents at Ducos leprosarium.

Tonga was visited in November 2006, and Sister Joan Marie SMSM ran a nursing clinic and was the PLF liaison contact at Maofanga on the main island. She made time during her busy surgery hours to introduce me to the doctors who worked with leprosy patients, and arranged for her assistant to facilitate the interviews around Nuku'alofa, who also acted as interpreter. The homes of the interviewees were small *fale*-type buildings, with materials provided by PLF, most homes being relatively remote from nearby villages. On a visit to the northern island of Vava'u, four leprosy sufferers, and a matron of the hospital to which the Fale'ofa leprosy station was annexed, were interviewed. Sister Goretti SMSM was the PLF contact in Vava'u and drove me to meet the interviewees, also serving as interpreter. While visiting Tonga, the research had to be curtailed due to civil political action, resulting in the central section of the capital city Nuku'alofa being burnt down, which I witnessed from small aircraft returning from the northern island of Vava'u to Maofanga. Electricity supplies to the island failed, all businesses and government departments closed, access within the city was restricted and airports were closed to flights for several days.

The visit to Vanuatu in October 2006 permitted only interviews in Port

Vila with staff who had worked at the leprosarium at Lolowai and now resided in Port Vila, together with an interview with Dr. Roland Farrugia, the visiting PLF consultant and former WHO leprologist. Names were obtained of staff of the leprosarium who retired back in Auckland, New Zealand, and subsequent interviews were conducted with Sister Betty Pyatt, and Dr. and Mrs. Mackereth. In 2008 a visit was made to a northern island of Vanuatu to record interviews with leprosy sufferers in Espiritu Santo. Tony Whitley, of Rowhani Baha'i School in Santo and a PLF liaison contact, organized a driver and another fellow Baha'i worker, Carren Bough, to act as guide and interpreter to enable interviews with leprosy sufferers both nearby and deep into the island.

The Melanesian homes were very different than the open, *fale*-styled Polynesian homes, as they were often tall, tapered, windowless huts with dark, cool interiors. As it was the "winter" season in the tropics, and overcast outdoors, interviews were conducted inside the huts where very little light penetrated. Small wood fires were lit on the open ground of the interior for warmth and light. These home conditions revealed how easily leprosy sufferers with anesthetized limbs injured their feet and/or hands while warming themselves beside the embers.

Despite the lively tales and vivid details of the memories of the interviewees, dates and western ideas of time were quite vague in many cases in Vanuatu. Birthdays were often unknown; and with older participants, to obtain an idea of dates, such as when leprosy was contracted and visits to leprosaria occurred, it was useful to ask whether these events occurred "before or after the war," and whether they were children or adults at the time. World War Two had made a huge difference to life in the islands, and several personal accounts were recorded. Other means of dating events involved jogging memories about medical staff at the leprosaria. This lack of personal detail is uncommon among westerners, but it would be quite wrong to assume a corresponding lack of understanding or connection with modern-day life by the Melanesians. Although there was no electricity in many of the homes, with meals being cooked on open fires nearby, comprehension was not an issue. This is particularly evident when the nephew of an interviewee, Mary Alma Namtaktak, joined the photograph session. Immediately afterwards he asked for the memory stick from my digital camera and a few moments later produced the photographs downloaded on his computer. Comprehension and ability were no problem, especially when modern technology was available.

An important feature of this book is that the interviewees are identified and often shown photographed with their families. It is felt that using the real names of the interviewees brings an authenticity, integrity and proper appreciation of the adversity that leprosy sufferers had to overcome — plus the realization that leprosy had not prevented most of them from raising normal, healthy families. The openness with which the life stories were told, whether it involved tears recounting painful separations or joy in witnessing the good health of their offspring, is more likely to dispel ignorance about leprosy and, accordingly, its stigma. It is believed that ending the secrecy previously associated with leprosy will result in an understanding and recognition that anyone who contracts the disease in this day and age no longer need fear or re-live the painful experiences of the past.

The descriptions that follow relating to the conditions at each of the Pacific nations commence with a pithy historical introduction to provide some idea of the differences between the island nations. This is followed by an overview of the history of leprosy up until the period encompassed by the oral histories gathered. Long extracts of individual testimonies provide vivid and detailed descriptions of the lives and experiences of leprosy sufferers, implicitly voicing the level of stigma encountered at various points in their lives. Comments by medical workers and lay people are quoted to give a greater understanding and perception of the conditions and stigma encountered in the islands.

1

Community Through Adversity — New Zealand to Fiji

Before looking at leprosy in Fiji, the life and activities of Patrick J. Twomey (1892–1963) in New Zealand will first be described to outline his growing involvement with leprosy; then the origins of the charity he created, now called the Pacific Leprosy Foundation (PLF), will be detailed. It was these channels of support initiated by Twomey in the 1920s and expanded over the ensuing years, which enabled leprosy sufferers in the South Pacific to be contacted and their life stories recorded in the 2000s. These oral histories are the primary sources utilized in this book.

Initially Twomey became involved with volunteers who assisted leprosy sufferers isolated on Quail Island by the port of Lyttelton, adjacent to Christchurch. The gradual evolution of these voluntary efforts into a national organization, even after these patients were transferred to a central leprosarium in Fiji in 1925 will be traced. The enormous increase in donations raised in New Zealand enabled the support of all leprosy sufferers at the leprosarium at Makogai, Fiji, so that by 1939 a charitable trust needed to be created in New Zealand, named the Makogai Lepers' (NZ) Trust Board.[1] With the subsequent expansion of the Trust Board's activities to assist leprosy sufferers in other South Pacific regions, in 1942 the name was changed to the Lepers' Trust Board (LTB), which was later again changed to the Leprosy Trust Board (LTB) to avoid the ostracizing term "leper." The abbreviation LTB will be used when describing the early activities of the Trust Board prior to its name change in 1991 to the Pacific Leprosy Foundation (PLF).

Patrick J. Twomey: Early Encounters with Leprosy

Having left school at the age of thirteen, Twomey worked as a telegraph messenger to help support his family. Later, to improve his prospects, he learned shorthand and typing and became a clerk with the Wellington Railways.² Feeling drawn to the religious life, he went to Mittagong, New South Wales, Australia, and entered the Catholic novitiate of the Marist Brothers in 1912. He took his vows in 1914 and was sent to serve in Suva, Fiji, where he first encountered leprosy and its debilitating effects.³ Within a few years, ill health forced him to leave the Order, and Twomey returned to New Zealand in 1919. Hoping outdoor work would improve his health, Twomey joined the Christchurch Gas Company as a meter reader, where he met Benjamin Pratt, an elderly benefactor of local leprosy sufferers isolated on nearby Quail Island in Lyttelton Harbor.⁴ Having witnessed the plight of leprosy sufferers in Fiji, Twomey vigorously assisted the efforts of Ben Pratt to collect goods and cash to provide comfort for this small group of leprosy sufferers.

Quail Island had been declared a quarantine station in 1875, and in 1906 the first leprosy patient, Will Vallane from Christchurch, was placed in the large, seldom used quarantine hospital on the island. The Department of Health constructed a special hut for him in 1907. Here he dwelt alone, with his meals prepared and cut into small pieces by the island's caretaker, and the plate then placed on a table by a fence surrounding his home.⁵ Monthly visits were made by a Lyttelton doctor, with occasional visits by Vallane's relatives.⁶ A second leprosy patient, Jimmy Kokere, was isolated in a hut built next to Vallane's, who was then aged sixty and blind. Kokere continued to care for Vallane, even after Kokere was discharged in 1909.⁷ A detailed account of the conditions of leprosy patients who came to be isolated on Quail Island is contained in the publication by the Tamahua/Quail Island Restoration Trust, which shows that by 1924, nine leprosy sufferers were isolated on the island.⁸

Goods and items were donated to patients by people in Lyttelton and Christchurch, including a gramophone player, records, radios, newspapers and magazines, undoubtedly through the efforts of Pratt and Twomey.⁹ A social hall was set up, containing a well used library and billiard table, although the latter was never properly functional. Dr. Charles Upham became a friend of the patients and visited twice weekly.¹⁰ Permission was given for Rev. A. J. Petrie of Lyttelton and some of his parishioners to take a launch to Quail Island to hold services for the patients, and the group carried a piano up the hill.¹¹ At all times a distance of some fifteen paces was maintained between the visitors and patients, as regulations stipulated that no visitor should approach patients closer than six feet or enter any of the huts.¹² It was noted that "if by chance the visitors should overstep these regulations, the patients themselves will advise him of this fact,"¹³ demonstrating that patients had taken to heart the regulations relating to their isolation and the risk of their contagion to others. The comment of a visitor to Quail Island who "felt ... we were visiting ... the New Hebrides and half expected to see a cannibal emerge from the shadows"¹⁴ reflects the general ignorance of the public about

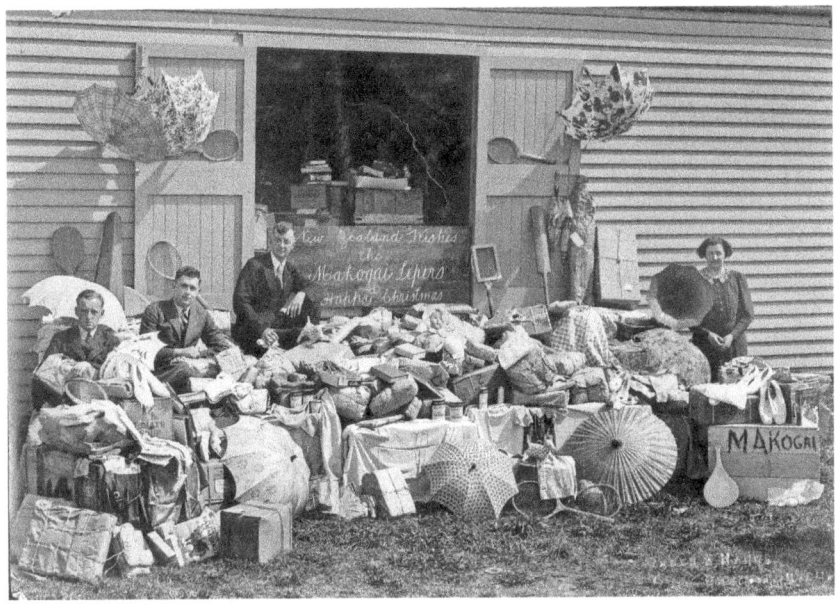

Pat Twomey (center), two helpers and Noeline Harris (right) in Christchurch with charitable goods to be shipped to Makogai.

leprosy, and ideas that leprosy was a disease that was not prevalent in New Zealand or western societies but in distant and remote regions.

Situated in the exposed Lyttelton Harbor, Quail Island conditions were not always ideal for the patients, especially in winter when the sun was lost behind the hills by 2 P.M. By 1925 it was decided that the eight remaining patients on the island should be transferred to the leprosarium at Makogai, Fiji.[15] No evidence was found to support the proposition by Edmond that due to disharmony between patients, staff and locals, the transfer to Makogai was to rid New Zealand of its leprosy problem.[16] The island's exposure to the sea and cold winds, and the problems of providing proper amenities for the patients (compared to the excellent facilities known to be available at Makogai), prompted the move for the benefit of the patients, many of whom were Polynesians who were "very cheerful at the prospect of living in their new island home, and they were hopeful of the future."[17] As the majority of patients were partly Polynesian, the move to a warmer climate would have certainly been welcome, although no doubt the decision was also driven by pragmatic exigencies on the part of the New Zealand authorities.[18] The enormous support of the government, the LTB and New Zealand donors to leprosy sufferers at Makogai increased over the ensuing years.

One of the patients transferred from Quail Island was Ernest Wolfgram, originally from Tonga, who had been sent to be schooled in New Zealand and soon after was found to have leprosy. Following his death in Makogai at age forty in 1948 (prior to the arrival of the new sulphone drugs), Wolfgram was described by Twomey as "a Leper Hero" and "outstanding among men as the oak among the smaller trees."[19] Despite being isolated by the age of sixteen, Wolfgram learned carpentry and other trades through older patients and books, and spent his time at Makogai building furniture, houses and boats, overhauling engines, installing electricity, repairing machinery, teaching music and organizing an orchestra for stage performances by the patients.[20] When asked for details about himself, his written response encapsulates his spirit:

> I dream of building a fast hydroplane — but unfortunately most of my small earnings go to help my old father who is unable to work and my two little sisters. Mother died the year after I got here. I think she and I were the best pals ever.[21]

Individuals such as Ernest Wolfgram have come to epitomize the indomitable strength of leprosy patients isolated at Makogai, and he illustrates the morale engendered by staff and patients themselves at the leprosarium. It is such behavior and spirit at the leprosarium which evoked the long nostalgia and warm memories by the leprosy sufferers who spent many years far from their homes, isolated at Makogai. With the closure of the leprosy colony at Quail Island and the transfer of all New Zealand leprosy patients to Makogai, by 1927 Pratt and Twomey extended their activities to provide for over four hundred residents at the leprosarium.[22]

By 1930, age and ill health forced Pratt's retirement, and Twomey took sole charge of the operation, running the charity from his home with the help of his wife Christine Margaret Farrow, a Masters graduate in botany.[23] Determined to spread the net of the charitable appeal wider, Twomey, during his employment as a gas meter reader, took evening classes for public speaking because he anticipated public appeals for funding would include speeches to clubs and organizations, and promotions via radio. He extended the Christchurch appeal to a national level with a successful nationwide Christmas campaign to raise funds. Each year the annual appeal grew, and the task of writing letters and posting circulars seeking donations likewise expanded. In 1937, through the Catholic Church, the young seventeen-year-old Noeline Harris (née Kieley) was employed as a typist and assistant, working from a small office in the Twomey family home at 172 Bealey Avenue, Christchurch.[24] No canvassers were employed, and appeals were only through radio talks broadcast by Twomey and letters to addressees (selected from the telephone book) soliciting donations, all of which Harris typed. Twomey personally acknowledged all donations.[25] His practice was to dictate letters to Harris, and the typing was then checked by Mrs. Twomey.[26] Harris maintains that without his wife's guidance and assistance, Twomey would possibly not have achieved his phenomenal level of success.[27]

Formation of a Charitable Trust in New Zealand

By 1939, several thousand pounds were being donated annually, and it was deemed necessary to form a charitable trust (registered under the Religious and Charitable Trusts Act of 1908) initially called the Makogai Lepers' (NZ) Trust Board.[28] In 1942 the Trust changed its name to the Lepers' Trust Board (LTB) because the Board decided to extend its activities to help leprosy sufferers in the Solomon Islands and New Caledonia (due to the even larger number of leprosy cases reported in those regions).[29] Twomey received no payment for his services from the early days in the 1920s until, at the request of the LTB committee, in May 1942 he terminated his employment with the Christchurch Gas Company and devoted himself full-time to his position as Secretary of the LTB.[30] At one point a donor had approached the gas company, asking for "the leper man," and from that time the epithet was adopted by Twomey.[31] It was by this title that Twomey became affectionately known in Christchurch, due to the wide publicity he attained by using this moniker in advertisements on Christchurch buses and in his annual letters of appeal to donors. His advertising methods, in fact, mirror current telemarketing practices and advertising on buses today, indicating that Twomey was a publicist ahead of his time. Letters and parcels addressed simply to "The Leper Man, Christchurch" were accepted and delivered by the Post Office to the LTB at one-half the usual postage rate.[32]

Twomey kept donors updated about leprosy with news of his visits to various leprosaria in pamphlets that often included photographs of the recipients with donated goods, or pictures of advanced cases with severe deformities, in order to raise sympathy and solicit funding.[33] Between 1939 and 1944, over 400,000 circulars seeking donations were posted, handwritten on envelopes in distinctive green pen, specifically to the "ladies of the house."[34] In 1943 a record sum of £13,500 was donated to leprosy sufferers, which enabled the LTB to consider funding the rehabilitation of discharged patients.[35] Today rehabilitation is one of the most appreciated forms of assistance to elderly patients, as evidenced by the oral history testimonies. This assistance has enabled a reasonable standard of living for the victims of the disease, who, after discharge, were able to have their own small homes from which they could run various cottage industries, such as growing fruit and vegetables, fishing, sewing or hiring out a donated facility of small copra-drying huts. For those who married, assistance included school fees for their children's education. This ensured that the next generation was not disadvantaged by the long-term effects and disabilities of parents affected by leprosy, which in the past had contributed to a low standard of living for the whole family due to physical disabilities that prevented employment.

In the 1940s there were fifteen committee members on the Lepers' Trust Board, comprising two medical professionals, the Anglican Primate of New Zealand, the Catholic Bishop of Christchurch, solicitors, accountants and a variety of Christchurch businessmen.[36] Twomey had adopted the practice of publishing a full list of donors in New Zealand newspapers, but this had to be discontinued in the 1940s due to lack of newspaper space because of the large number of donors — demonstrating the success of his marketing strategies. The LTB annual balance sheet was published in newspapers for public scrutiny and overall accountability. Twomey's personal integrity and involvement in overseeing the decisions and activities of the Board ensured its success. It has been recorded that the establishment of the LTB was one of the first occasions when the Anglican and Roman Catholic Bishops sat together to discuss affairs of mutual interest, which was an ecumenical pattern that Twomey was keen to foster.[37] In 1942 a decision was made to extend the support from Makogai to include the Solomon Islands and New Caledonia. Allocations of £500 each were granted to the Anglican Melanesian Mission, Presbyterian, Methodist, Seventh Day Adventist and Marist (Catholic) Missions in order to assist leprosy sufferers under their care, and these charitable grants rapidly increased to five figures.[38]

Support for leprosy sufferers was not simply donations of goods or cash to the individuals, but included medical services to care for the patients. Since it was not feasible to set up its own leprosy medical service, the LTB supported general medical teams in the areas, mainly through the churches and government departments to facilitate hospital and nursing care for leprosy patients. Maintaining regular contact with chief health officials and administrators in Fiji ensured that Twomey was kept abreast of reports and surveys of leprosy in the South Pacific region.

A leprosy survey revealed over eight hundred cases of leprosy in the Solomon Islands, as compared to four hundred patients in Makogai. In 1949 Twomey and his assistant, Noeline Harris, traveled via New Caledonia and the New Hebrides (Vanuatu) to establish the channels through which leprosy sufferers could be assisted in the Solomons. Sister Betty Pyatt of the Anglican Melanesian Mission was on the same voyage to take up her appointment as matron of the Godden Memorial hospital at Lolowai, New Hebrides, where Twomey and the LTB subsequently assisted in setting up the St. Barnabas leprosarium (as detailed later in relation to leprosy in Vanuatu).[39]

Twomey and Noeline Harris visited the capital Honiara on Guadalcanal and other islands, including Malaita, where hospital facilities and care of leprosy patients was mainly in the hands of the Melanesian Mission, to which the LTB contributed funds. This practice continues right until the present day because leprosy remains a problem in the Solomons due to remoteness and difficulties with access. Solomon Island self-government was achieved in 1976, and independence from the British two years later. In recent times internal political factions and intermittent civil disorder disrupt the lines of communication and contact with leprosy sufferers. Nevertheless, the Tetere leprosarium and other leprosy clinics operate with the continuing support and nursing assistance of the SMSM and other missions, upon which the PLF rely to maintain support of leprosy sufferers. I had intended to visit the Solomons in October 2006 and, with the assistance of the SMSM sisters stationed in Honiara, record oral histories with elderly patients at various leprosaria who still remember the visits of Patrick Twomey, but civil disorder prompted the New Zealand government to issue warnings against non-essential visits. It also advised that travel was not permitted to outlying areas, which terminated the opportunity to record any interviews. A large proportion of LTB resources had been provided to the Solomon Islands. In addition to the usual financial, medical and material support, three fifty-five-foot diesel-powered launches were presented in 1955, one each to the Anglican, Catholic and Methodist missions to assist communications with the remote regions where leprosy sufferers were known to exist. A hydrotherapy pool was installed at Honiara for physiotherapy to help restore the mobility of patients.[40] The region remains a high priority with the Pacific Leprosy Foundation today because of the high incidence of leprosy.

The visits of Twomey and Harris to New Caledonia and New Hebrides (now Vanuatu) in 1948 are recorded in the respective visits to those islands, and describe the origins of LTB support, together with the subsequent effects upon those receiving assistance. Funding and material goods have regularly been provided to Samoa and Tonga, and the effects on leprosy sufferers are likewise described following my visits to those islands. Twomey also directed leprosy assistance to the Cook Islands, French Polynesia, and Kiribati, although the three island groups are not covered by this research.

What becomes evident from Twomey's earliest ventures into these islands to assist leprosy sufferers is the importance of the personal contacts and lines of communication that he established in order to facilitate assistance to individual leprosy patients. He made it a policy to meet with top government and medical officials in each place to ensure they were aware of the funding available to leprosy sufferers and those working with patients, and to ensure that the best possible help and facilities were offered for their medical care and rehabilitation. Most importantly, it was necessary to nominate someone on the spot who maintained direct regular contact with the patients and reported back to the LTB. Committees for the distribution of funds were set up in each place to ensure even-handed distribution and open scrutiny of the charitable operations.[41] Those most involved in these committees and activities were people associated with church missions and philanthropic organizations, such as the Red Cross and Lions Club; while other altruistic individuals were co-opted as committee members.

In recognition of his service to leprosy sufferers, in 1947 Twomey was made a Member of the Order of the British Empire, and awarded the Medaille d'or des Epidemies by France in 1953 and the rank of *Chevalier of the Legion of Honor*. In 1958 the Pope conferred the Papal decoration *Benemerenti* as a high award for his distinguished service to the sick in the Southwest Pacific. Shortly before his death, Twomey was also awarded the rank of Commander of Merit in the Order of St. Lazarus of Jerusalem.[42]

Twomey's dedication and the travel necessary to establish and maintain the lines of contact between the LTB and leprosy sufferers, including making decisions on how funds could best be applied in the far flung and remote regions on various islands, had serious consequences for Twomey's never-robust health. In 1959 he returned from Melanesia with malaria, necessitating long spells of hospitalization.[43] While in the New Hebrides on tour soon after in 1963, he took ill, was rushed to Suva hospital, and died. It has been said he was happy to end his days in the place where he first encountered leprosy which led him to take up his life's work.[44]

Noeline Harris pointed out that although totally dedicated to his personal mission, Twomey was not always an easy person to work with, earning the reputation of a good fanatic, although she believed that to be a visionary and to follow one's goal with such dedication required an uncompromising spirit.[45] Noeline Harris originally left the LTB and Christchurch in 1954 due to family commitments, as well as difficulties at work. However, after the death of her husband she returned to Christchurch and was appointed a Board member of LTB in 1982, where she continued to serve and work as librarian right until her death in March 2007, age 89. An oral history with Noeline Harris and documents donated by her to the Oxford Project are filed in the Macmillan Brown Library. Twomey's chairmanship of the LTB was taken over in succession by A. S. Geddes, A. H. T. Rose, B. T. McMahon and G. D. Watson. The personal commitment of these individuals ensured the success of the operation in assisting, in a whole variety of ways, leprosy suffers in the South Pacific.

LTB/PLF and Leprosy Sufferers in the South Pacific Region

The mode of LTB support continued the original activities of Pratt and Twomey, providing medicine, bandages, goods, and financial support to individual leprosy sufferers, which later extended to the provision of wheelchairs, homes, grants to set up small businesses and school fees for children. To ensure medical services were available for leprosy patients, grants were also made to governments, hospitals, medical specialists and nursing staff (mainly through church and missionary organizations) in order that the most up-to-date medical remedies were offered. Specialist facilities included surgery for clawed hands, facial deformities, eye operations, amputations, prostheses, purpose-built shoes to protect the feet, x-ray machines, physiotherapy equipment, as well as the fees of specialized staff providing these services. Additionally, scholarships were offered to general practitioners to learn more about diagnosis and treatment of the disease, as well as organizations and researchers attempting to discover a vaccine, WHO leprologists and others researchers in the field of leprosy. Training courses were offered to nurses, laboratory technicians and auxiliary health services to gain and provide the specialized knowledge necessary for identification and treatment of leprosy.

In the Pacific Islands, liaison personnel are essential to maintain contact with patients, and between individual leprosy sufferers and the medical facilities available on their island. To enable this, transport, such as four-wheel-drive vehicles, is provided by the Board to traverse the often unpaved roads and tracks through rough and remote island regions. During the period 1942 to 1977, the LTB distributed over five million dollars to government medical departments, church agencies and leprosy sufferers; in 2005 alone, charitable expenditure totaled over $850,000, the largest expenditures being in the Solomon Islands, with lesser grants to Fiji, Tonga, Vanuatu, Samoa and Vietnam.[46] The incidence of leprosy is very high in Kiribati, but due to major problems in transport and communication, grants had to be temporarily suspended in 2005. Substantial grants were made to the World Health Organisation (WHO) and leprosy consultancies, including the Leprosy Mission and the International Association for Integration, Dignity and Economic Advancement (IDEA), to assist with leprosy rehabilitation outside the South Pacific region.

It has been suggested that the sensational nature of fund-raising appeals by some of the above organizations, often based on "lurid accounts of disfigurements, familial and societal rejection, despair, and poverty"[47] have contributed to false public stereotypes that characterize all leprosy; and that if the relief organizations would stop using these "horror pictures,"[48] the image of leprosy would be more accurately reflected in public perceptions. Although these extreme outcomes only occur with neglected and advanced cases of leprosy, humans innately fear any condition which may have the remotest likelihood of leading to such results, and, of course, such fears undoubtedly produce attitudes inherent in stigma. Yet it was — and is — for these advanced cases that a great deal of funds were specifically raised in order to alleviate their suffering, especially in earlier times prior to the late 1940s and the availability of an effective cure.

A realistic means to raise public funds and at the same time avoid stigma is the use of images of advanced leprosy cases, together with the promotion of knowledge about the cure now freely available to anyone, highlighting that medication prevents all such disabilities with early diagnosis. This message fits PLF attempts to promote public knowledge about the disease and its cure, hastening the end of ignorance which lies at the heart of stigma associated with leprosy.[49] Donors are made aware not only of the material assistance provided to victims but also the provision of specialist medical support required for surgical remedies of the deformities in advanced cases. Photographs of leprosy sufferers, especially with their young, healthy children and family members, are a positive reinforcement of the idea that leprosy can be contained, is not hereditary and poses minimal risk to others. As early as 1930, Dr. Austin, the medical superintendent at Makogai for twenty-three years, observed, "Leprosy is dreaded so much in comparison with other diseases because its manifestations are external and obvious."[50] It is this dread and fear that arouses sympathy and the generous level of donations. There is no doubt that this fear of physical deformity is linked to stigma, but the knowledge that deformities can be averted by early diagnosis and treatment contributes to the demise of stigma. The key to ending stigma is knowledge about leprosy and its treatment.

Leprosy in Fiji: Historical Background

European explorers arrived in the Fijian Islands in the mid-seventeenth to late eighteenth centuries, but fierce cannibalism deterred major European settlements until the nineteenth century, with larger numbers arriving in 1860–1870s. Fiji's first constitution was drawn up in 1865, when seven independent chiefs joined in a confederacy of native kingdoms to form a General Assembly, and the first sitting of the House of Representatives was in 1871. The Council of Chiefs ceded Fiji to Great Britain in 1874, and the first Governor arrived from Australia in 1875. During this year measles killed over 40,000 in the islands, and health became a priority of the earliest colonial government. By 1902 the Trans-Pacific cable linking America with Australia and New Zealand reached Fiji, and the Pacific flying boat service began operating out of Nadi in 1939, making Fiji an important naval and air base during World War Two. These modern communications meant that the Fijian government, including its medical services, was in direct contact with the west and public health policies of the day. Independence was gained in

1970, by which time medical departments had been well established along western lines.

Early Accounts of Leprosy

Leprosy is considered to have been in Fiji prior to European contact, because two Fijian dialects already had indigenous names for leprosy, *sakuku* and *vukavuk*. Additionally, Fijian mythology contained many references to the disease.[51] Until the late nineteenth century, leprosy stones (*vatu ni sakuku*) were owned by keepers of certain clans, who conducted business using the stones, upon request, to create fear and infection.[52] The first recorded mention of leprosy was in 1837 in the journal of a Methodist missionary, who wrote that cases of leprosy were being treated at their Mission.[53] Later, Rev. Moore recorded in 1859 a reputed local cure — that victims be hung head-down in the smoke of a burning poisonous tree.[54] The medical superintendent at Makogai, Dr. Austin, reported that on a stony ridge off the small island of Kia their chief allegedly isolated leprosy sufferers so as to ensure a ready supply of *bokola* — body prepared for the oven — for unexpected guests. This was considered an advance over the common practice of clubbing them to death, both practices undoubtedly signalling strong stigma towards leprosy.[55] Because advanced cases of leprosy were clubbed to death, albeit possibly as mercy killings, the colonial government passed laws prohibiting the practice, which led to complaints in 1891 that the ban had resulted in an increase of leprosy.[56] This treatment of people with leprosy demonstrates a fearful prospect for anyone who felt at risk of contracting the disease and an intolerant stigmatic attitude towards leprosy in the 19th century in Fiji.

By 1907 the medical officer in Fiji, Dr. Bolton Corney, calculated that about 0.8 percent of Fijian deaths were due to leprosy, including a few Indians, although leprosy was reported to be endemic among Indians in Fiji.[57] The Indian indentured laborers brought by the British to work in sugar plantations between 1878 and 1916 were carefully screened for leprosy, and those having or suspected of having leprosy were repatriated.[58] The fears of leprosy led to the Leper Ordinance of 1899, which forbade leprosy sufferers from being employed as bakers, butchers, cooks or any trades having contact with food, drink, drugs, medicines or tobacco, or various other jobs to prevent the victims having contact with society, such as being barbers or domestic servants.[59] Disobedience meant confinement at an isolation station established for non–Fijians at Walu Bay next to the Colonial Hospital in Suva. Otherwise, Fijian patients were to remain in their village homes, or isolated in a house built some distance from their village.[60] This indicates that fear of leprosy was strong among the colonial population. Certainly leprosy sufferers were segregated by both British and Fijian communities in different ways.

Establishment of the Leprosarium at Beqa

Sister Mary Stella, SMSM, has provided an account of events in Fiji from the late nineteenth century, culminating in the establishment of the leprosarium at Makogai. The following is a summary from her book in order to provide a background of leprosy in Fiji and to assess an historical position relating to stigma. The initial segregation of leprosy patients at Walu Bay allowed easy supervision by the resident medical superintendent at the nearby Colonial Hospital, and also access for patients to central Suva. However, local residents began to object to the close proximity of the leprosy hamlet to Suva, although numbers only varied between six to twelve patients.[61] By 1900 it was estimated that there were about one thousand cases of leprosy in the Fijian Islands, and it was advocated that all cases of leprosy be isolated. Walu Bay was too small and unsuitable as a leprosy station if the larger numbers of all Fijian leprosy patients were to be isolated.[62]

Various islands were assessed as possible sites for a larger asylum, and eventually the Soliyaga peninsula, the eastern horn of the island of Beqa, was chosen as most suitable. Beqa was eighteen miles from Suva, close enough for regular medical visits, and with a safe harbor and two natural springs.[63] Despite the objections of residents on Beqa, who did not wish to have a leprosy station on their island, the asylum was eventually permitted by order of the courts.[64] The patients were moved into the new buildings erected at Beqa on Soliyaga on 29 October, 1900, which also housed a warden and cook.[65] The Suva district medical officer visited at least monthly, with more frequent visits by local medical staff on Beqa. Unmarried patients were segregated, and although penal clauses were adopted, the asylum was not intended to be a place of punishment, and patients were expected to perform light duties to be self-sufficient.[66] Although the community was reported to be peaceful, some patients were "clamouring for opium."[67]

By 1907, complaints increased in Fijian districts, usually by European settlers that the patients who had been segregated from their villages were stealing and damaging property (probably attempting to fend for themselves) and generally being "a nuisance."[68] With the pending removal of all leprosy sufferers from districts in all the islands of Fiji, a larger establishment was deemed necessary, as it was not feasible to extend the facilities at Beqa because the neighboring residents opposed the leprosy colony. The attitudes implicit in these events (objecting to the location of leprosy colonies nearby) confirms stigma towards leprosy sufferers.

Since it was not possible to purchase more land on Beqa to accommodate additional patients, and because the conditions of the thirty-six patients isolated on Beqa had deteriorated, a decision was made to seek a larger, more suitable island for the establishment of a leprosarium.[69] The officials responsible for the decision were aware of conditions at leprosaria elsewhere, such as Robben Island in Cape Colony and Molokai in Hawaii. Upon the advice of the Suva medical superintendent, Corney, Makogai was considered to be an ideal site for the new leprosarium, being an uninhabited island with easy access from Suva, with fertile land and a good water supply.[70]

The decision in favor of isolation of leprosy sufferers thus progressed from local segregation to that of isolation in a more distant place. The majority of patients were advanced cases requiring care and assistance; thus the issue of isolation and removal to another island was hardly a matter of any choice for patients but a necessity to provide adequate facilities by the government and medical officers who made the decisions. The resistance by residents in Suva objecting to the close proximity of a leprosy station at Walu Bay, the later objections of Beqa residents, and also the complaints from residents in Fijian districts wanting the removal of leprosy sufferers demonstrates intolerance and fear, pointing to continuing stigma, perhaps with increasing concern about contagion. A reflection of the high degree of stigma by the time a replacement site for Beqa was being sought is the response of citizens of Levuka, who, at the mere possibility of a leprosarium being situated on the island of Wakaya (which was, in fact, ten miles out to sea from Levuka) hurriedly raised a petition opposing any suggestion of a leprosarium.[71]

Establishment of the Leprosarium at Makogai

Once the site of Makogai was agreed upon, the government had to overcome the obstacle of finding nursing staff, because nobody wanted to work with leprosy. It was known that leprosy asylums elsewhere were staffed by Catholic orders, and the Fijian Colonial Secretary requested that the Catholic Bishop seek sisters to serve at Makogai — despite reservations on the part of some officials fearing trouble because the majority of Fijians were Wesleyans.[72] Finally, the services of two European and two Fijian sisters of the Missionary Sisters of the Society of Mary (SMSM) were engaged on the basis of their "qualifications as nurses, irrespective of any religious views they may hold."[73] These sisters, joined by other SMSM nursing and support staff over the years at Makogai, worked with the leprosy patients and administered the leprosarium right through to its closure in 1969. They continued their work at the newly formed P. J. Twomey Memorial Hospital in Suva and remained until the takeover of the hospital by the Fijian government.

The appointment of the SMSM demonstrates that the sisters were requested to work at the leprosarium, rather than the Order itself actively seeking work with leprosy sufferers. This counters the claims that religious orders actively sought positions to emulate the action of Jesus helping victims of leprosy, as in the New Testament, or specifically sought opportunities to re-enact the parable of the good Samaritan, as suggested by various researchers who link the Christian missionary activities with the stigma of leprosy.[74] Connections between Christian activities and leprosy stigma in the Bible may well have been linked, but because of the emphasis given to New Testament teachings by Roman Catholics, the links, if made by the SMSM, were likely to be from the New Testament rather than from ostracizing passages contained in Leviticus in the Old Testament.[75] Rather than as religious teachers, the SMSM sisters appointed to Makogai were chosen because of their training as nurses and their ability to care for the needs of leprosy patients. In short, they had the necessary knowledge to run a specialized leprosarium. This facet of responsibility were also demonstrated later by Betty Pyatt of the Melanesian Mission in Vanuatu. Sister Marietta, SMSM and PLF liaison contact for leprosy sufferers in Samoa, who had begun service as a teacher in Samoa in 1963, maintains that the SMSM simply went to serve "where ever there was a need."[76] And at that time nurses were required at leprosaria.

The transportation of leprosy patients from Beqa to Makogai reveals the high level of fear and stigma in Fiji soon after the turn of the twentieth century, as local Fijians, and other Pacific islanders, refused to carry leprosy sufferers on their boats. Patients were not allowed to travel on the usual boats, even if patients were confined to the deck; so instead, a special cutter was towed, carrying the patients. The cutter was disinfected each time after discharging passengers at Makogai.[77] Stigma is evident in the fact that the medical officer originally appointed to work at Makogai resigned without ever going to the island because he requested special terms which were not met by the government. He had requested a salary almost double the one he received as medical officer on the island of Kadavu, as well as an increased retirement package on the basis that he and his family would face social ostracism because, since it became known he would be working with leprosy, he had been asked "not to call."[78]

Instead, Dr. Hall, an Irish Protestant, was appointed as the first medical officer to work with the Catholic SMSM sisters, taking residence as soon as their new homes at Makogai were completed, the water supply connected, and the main hospital and patients' quarters were ready for occupation. Two Fijian medical practitioners, six warders and twenty indentured Indian laborers responsible for clearing the land, food-planting and road-making were employed. Cattle, sheep, goats and pigs were brought to the island so that the station could be self-sufficient.[79] It took three years from the planning stage to occupation before the first twenty patients from Beqa arrived on Makogai in November 1911, with a remaining twenty patients arriving in December that year.[80] These careful preparations for a self-sufficient lifestyle on the island, together with huts and villages for the male leprosy sufferers, women's quarters, a school and accommodation for children, as well as the hospital, dispensary and staff living quarters, contributed to the success of the quality of life for patients at the leprosarium, as reported by Stella and confirmed by personal testimonies included here.

Conditions at Makogai and the SMSM

After the initial intake of 40 patients from Beqa to Makogai, by the end of 1912 154 leprosy patients were in residence, and by 1919 there were 352.[81] From the 1920s onwards, leprosy patients from other island groups were admitted to the leprosarium, the first being Samoans in 1922. In 1925 the patients from Quail Island arrived in Makogai, followed in 1926 by Cook Islanders, Tongans and a few Solomon Islanders in 1927, and some Gilbertese in 1935.[82] Men and women were segregated, the women being housed in a separate building, while the able bodied males lived in their own villages around the island.[83] Young children lived with the women, while the seriously sick were in special wards at the hospital.

Dr. Austin described Makogai as a beautiful, lush island with a series of rocky ridges, and added that the view from the road above the hospital situated at Dalice Bay was one of the loveliest scenes in Fiji, with

> blues and greens of the lagoon, the white of the surf contrasting with the golden sands, and the red roofs of the buildings, enhancing by contrast the grace and colour of coconut and other tropical trees, provid[ing] a picture to stimulate the most jaded taste.[84]

On clear days, from the higher peaks, the outlines of the main two Fijian islands of Viti Levu and Vanua Levu, as well as some other islands, were visible as a picturesque reef.[85] The terraces of land on Makogai were used as village gardens, coconut plantations and a dairy farm. Even a bakery and soap factory were built, with everything connected by a three-mile road. Two ponies were brought to Makogai to enable the sisters to visit the men's villages dotted around the island each morning to hand out medication and carry out daily health checks. Some years later the LTB supplied motor scooters for this use, which posed a challenge for some of the sisters, as they sometimes rode two or even three on one scooter.[86] On occasion this provided much hilarity for the patients, one of whom said he witnessed a sister "driving up the wall" when she failed to stop her scooter in time![87]

Initially, many of the patients brought to Makogai were advanced cases with terrible ulcerations, so that "the odour could be detected a quarter of a mile away."[88] Caring for the sickest patients was a special task of the sisters, which induced one visitor to comment that "I wouldn't do this for a million dollars," to which the sister replied, "Neither would I," adding that "only Divine love in a human heart" could inspire such service.[89] This indicates the devotion and basic nursing duties involved in the care provided by the SMSM. In 1925 one of the SMSM sisters was found to have contracted leprosy, and she left the sisters' quarters to live at the hospital, where for her remaining thirty years she took over the care of young schoolgirls.[90]

The dedication of the medical staff and SMSM is abundantly evident in the testimonies of leprosy sufferers regarding their isolation at Makogai. Many of the interviewees were taken as children to Makogai, and in the oral histories they referred to the sisters as their "mothers," whose loving care took the place of their much missed mothers back home. The testimonies of SMSM sisters interviewed, and many others spoken to, reflect a corresponding level of warmth for the patients and the lifestyle which they shared, living alongside each other at Makogai. To some extent this is quite extraordinary in view of the strict quarantine rules enforced at Makogai, especially during the years prior to treatment with sulphones, which separated staff who resided in designated "clean" zones, well away from the leprosy sufferers and their living quarters.[91]

Those without leprosy would don special shoes and protective outer clothing when entering what were considered areas of possible contagion, and leprosy sufferers were barred from entering "clean" areas. Noeline Harris, during her visit to Makogai in 1947 (prior to the availability of sulphone drugs), mentioned that she dropped an item while visiting outside the "clean" areas, and that Ernest Wolfgram picked up the item, sterilized it later in special sterilizing equipment that he had personally crafted, and returned it to her in a sterile container.[92] Such rules and procedures indicate a high perception of the contagion of leprosy, demonstrating that fear of contagion by leprosy sufferers was entrenched in the pattern of their lives. These patterns in the daily life of patients, including not sharing crockery, cutlery or personal utensils, would have contributed to the self-perception of their contagion. The testimonies of some interviewees who had been isolated at Makogai indicate that this daily regime developed into habitual behavior.

Discipline at Makogai was strict, and two Fijians were appointed as police to maintain compliance. The doctor's office was used as a court, the main punishments being further isolation — that is, being deprived of mixing with others and/or missing the weekly films — or reduced rations.[93] In the early years a high fence marked the boundary where leprosy sufferers were not allowed to pass. Male and female patients were not allowed to enter each other's living areas, and strict gender separation was enforced (although thirty-seven children were born at the leprosarium).[94] These children were raised by the sisters, with visits permitted by the mothers but no touching allowed. At the age of two, the children were sent to be raised by relatives back home.[95] At specified times men and women could sit together in an open space near the central hospital, and on Saturday afternoons a bazaar was held where weekly trade exchanges occurred between villagers and the women. Highlights in the lives of many patients were the once or twice weekly film nights in the open theater built by Ernest Wolfgram and helpers, funded by the LTB. Despite the relatively harmonious scene depicted by these descriptions, leprosy patients did often suffer depression, and one patient recalled four suicides at Makogai.[96]

Although gender segregation was problematic, two reasons were given to justify segregation. First, pregnancy was known to exacerbate leprosy in women; and second, men outnumbered women at least two to one at Makogai.[97] The interviewees appeared to accept these as valid reasons for their segregation, and also suggested it was needed because otherwise the nuns would be kept too busy tending babies to care for the patients! Additionally segregation meant that young men and women were more likely to have the opportunity to marry after being discharged.

With the long-term isolation of patients, the leprosarium cared for patients well beyond the hospital stage, and the activities at Makogai belie the facile suggestion by Edmond that the sisters merely educated patients to "abandon all other identities and wait for better things in the afterlife."[98] To avoid boredom and depression at the leprosarium, patients were paid small wages to encourage them to participate in work on the island, as well as to accumulate savings either for use after their own discharge or to remit back to their families.[99] The able bodied men living in the villages worked in agriculture and gardening, producing yams, taro, tapioca, sweet potatoes, bananas, pineapples, peanuts and vegetables, as well as rearing ducks and fowls and regularly fishing, providing fresh food for the hospital patients and women. Women washed and mended the men's clothing, and received payment for sewing and embroidering bedspreads, pillow cases and table cloths. All the children attended school, and young men and women were given the opportunity to learn trades and skills which would be of use after their discharge.[100] This in itself provided optimism for their future. For the physical, mental and moral training of boys, a Scouts group was formed, and participation in sporting activities, such as soccer, cricket, tennis and boxing were encouraged. Regular sports days were held for both serious and humorous enjoyment, the training for which was of great value for the physical and general health of the patients.[101] Both a Catholic and Methodist chapel were built for patients, as well as Hindu shrines for the Indians.[102]

Despite the self-sufficient and relatively normal lifestyles fostered at

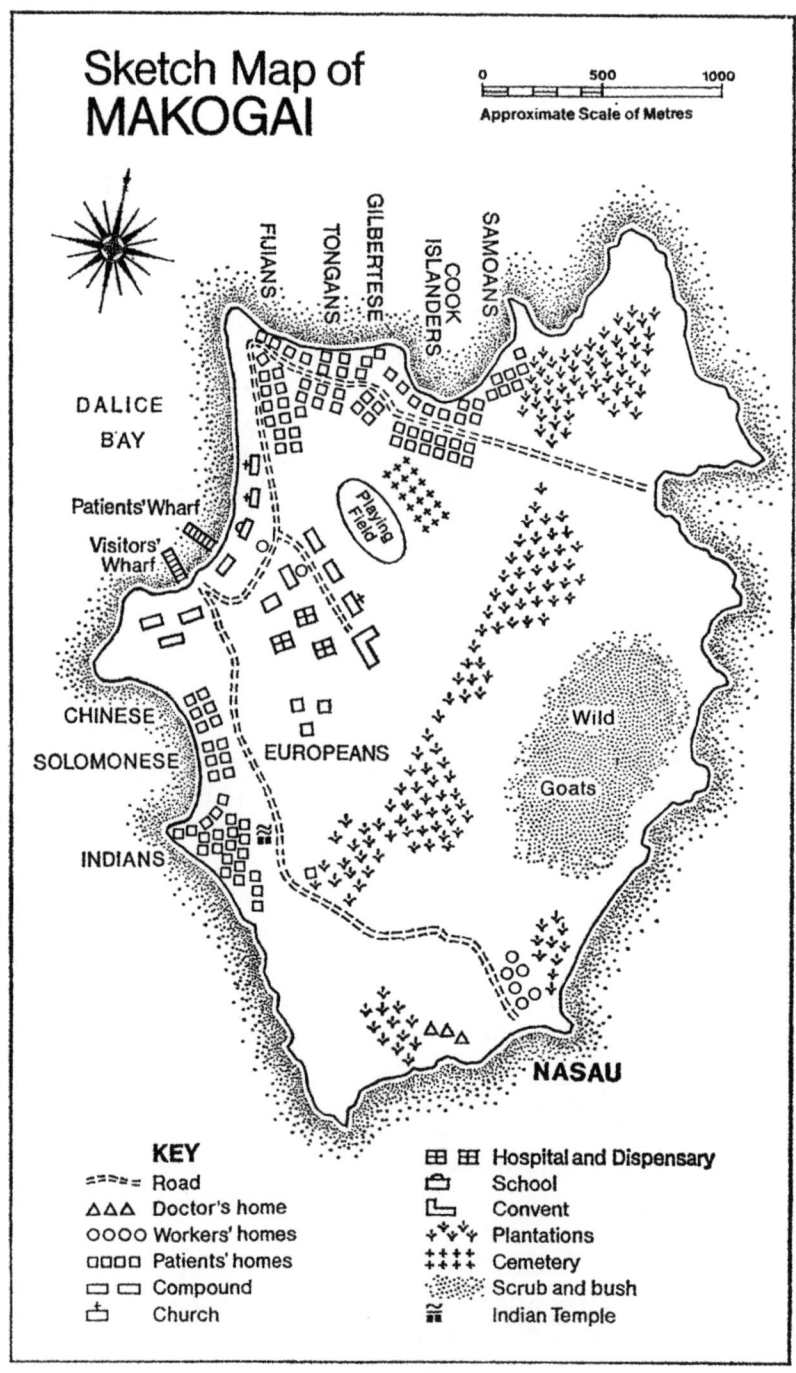

Sketch map of Makogai, reproduced from *Makogai — Image of Hope* with permission of PLF.

Makogai, stigma and fear of contagion continued to be evident among the public. A child with leprosy was selected to present a note to the governor visiting Makogai; and to avoid contact through contagion, the ingenious sisters inserted the note into a bouquet of flowers. But watching journalists noticed this and reported that by means of the note placed in a posy presented by the child, "His Excellency ... was able to obtain possession of the document without it having been handled by an afflicted person."[103]

As this research focuses on the stigma and operation of the institutions of leprosy, it has not encompassed the widespread and dedicated involvement of priests and other male religious orders, as they were not involved in the daily medical care of patients — which was the domain of medical doctors and nurses, the nurses in the main being SMSM. But it is noteworthy to mention that the efforts of Father Damien on Molokai, Hawaii, are paralleled by the dedication of two priests at Makogai. Father Nicouleau was stationed at Makogai in 1913; nine years later he was diagnosed with leprosy and went to live in one of the islander villages, where he died in 1927.[104] Father Le Jeune, a Marist priest from Belgium, arrived in Fiji in 1901; when diagnosed with leprosy in 1935, he was sent to Makogai, where he devoted his energies in service of leprosy patients and died at Makogai in 1951.[105] There is little doubt that those from the religious orders at Makogai, both priests and nuns, would have administered to the spiritual wants of patients and offered advice to those in need with regard to accepting their plight away from family and home and to look to better things in the afterlife, as suggested by Edmond.[106] But the focus in the oral histories remained on leprosy, and apart from asking whether the leprosy sufferers followed any particular religion and whether these beliefs helped them in their lives, detailed questions were not asked about their religious lives and spiritual guidance while at the leprosarium. It was apparent that they were free to follow their own religions at Makogai.

In this regard, the title of the book by Sister Stella, SMSM, is worth noting: *Makogai — Image of Hope*. Even before the availability of the sulphone drugs, Stella conveys a sense of optimism among some of the patients. This optimism is a based on the hope that active leprosy in patients would cease, and they would be discharged. This hope would have been engendered through the efforts of the medical staff and SMSM nurses, and Stella noted that "hopefulness and contentedness are incompatible with despair ... it can safely be presumed that Makogai had become, at least for many of its inmates, an Image of Hope — even if the hope was ... rather dim."[107]

With the advent of the new drugs, an emphasis upon rehabilitation was pursued, and in the 1960s a Jubilee celebration was held, inviting visitors to the island. Also, highly successful exhibition of the handicrafts from Makogai was displayed in Suva, with the *Fiji Times* noting:

> It would have been considered unthinkable that the work of patients at a leprosy hospital should be brought to the outside world for public exhibition. The shadow of the horror of leprosy ... still remained in the community mind. There is now no justification whatever for its darkening influence ... the period of separation is being steadily reduced.... In this atmosphere of hope, there has been at Makogai a quite remarkable flowering of a variety of arts and of craftsmanship.[108]

This report indicates that life on Makogai created an atmosphere of hope by its focus on creating full and useful lives for the patients who looked forward to a future back in their home communities. In sharing the achievements of patients with the public, these activities organized by the staff contributed towards diminishing levels of stigma.

Between 1911 to 1932, admissions to Makogai totaled 1640, of which 253 patients were able to be discharged.[109] This was prior to any effective treatment being available, and was attributed to good hygiene, nursing and personal care, where the disease had been arrested or become inactive.[110] Overall, up to 1969, Makogai statistics show that there were 4185 admissions, over half of this number being Fijians and Indians, with the remainder being from other Pacific islands. A total of 2,343 patients were discharged; and in December 1969 there were only eighty-three patients at Makogai.[111] During the period 1938–1949, prior to the availability of sulphone drugs, about forty patients annually were discharged, being what Dr. Austin described as "good propaganda"[112] for Makogai, which refers to the positive effects upon stigma. The success of the new treatment would have contributed further to such good propaganda.

Sulphone Treatment and Changing Times

Life for patients was transformed in 1948 when it was learned that a new drug for leprosy treatment was available in America. In fact, £800 was collected by the patients at Makogai to purchase the drug through British agencies, as it was not yet available in Fiji.[113] However, the Medical Department soon purchased a limited supply of the new sulphone drugs as a trial, and between the doctor and patients a unanimous decision was made that the most ill should receive the first treatments.[114] As will be shown, this is in direct contrast to the decision regarding administration of the drug in New Caledonia. According to one Makogai patient, the results were "quick and marvellous. All the sores dried up, and the smell which used to be so bad from the wards of the very sick, was gone in a week. Everyone was so excited! We held a big party to celebrate."[115] Even the medical superintendent was "astounded."[116] It was felt that the treatment signalled the end of segregation and would revolutionize attitudes towards leprosy, and that the new name for leprosy, Hansen's Disease, would no longer carry the stigma "attached to leper and leper asylum."[117] The sulphone drug DDS was highly effective in controlling widespread ulceration of the skin, thereby eliminating the need for frequent dressings; but DDS was toxic and could not be tolerated by many patients. Reactions had to be medically supervised, and relapses and reactions monitored. Clinical smears were regularly taken from patients until these showed that the bacilli had degenerated and were eventually eliminated.[118] Morris, who made a study of Makogai conditions in the early 1950s, noted that with any recurrence of the disease by discharged patients, re-admittance was voluntary.[119] This confirms that the facilities at the leprosarium were appreciated by patients, and that confinement was not perceived as being enforced.

At Makogai, once a smear test showed that no bacilli were present, a patient was regularly tested, and if smears remained clear for two years, discharge was granted. Laboratory tests could not determine whether the bacilli were active or inactive, but contagion was deemed at risk whenever bacilli were present. The interviewees often referred to these regular screening tests as simply testing to see if they were "low or high." The time span for testing whether a patient was clear of bacilli was later reduced to one year, and finally six months, as it became clearer that the risk of contagion was minimal. When Dr. Beckett was appointed Medical Superintendent at Makogai in 1957, there were about 730 patients isolated on the island. He recalled that patients could not be discharged until they showed "negative skin scrapings and no recurrence of symptomology for two years," but he soon persuaded the authorities to reduce the period to one year. Beckett also managed to obtain permission for patients to be allowed two weeks leave to visit their family home, which he said was "a bit more of a struggle" due to "conservatism," as some people worried Fiji might be "riddled with leprosy again."[120] This indicates a persisting level of stigma, although undoubtedly much reduced since the early days of isolation, as Beckett recalled:

> I don't know whether it [stigma] had totally disappeared or not but it was certainly much less. I mean I can remember patients coming back from leave and telling me that they'd seen someone they knew coming along the road and they were trying to decide whether to say hello to them again, and suddenly they [the friend] looked at their watch and ... gone along a side road, or something, to get away from them. Other patients said to me, "The worst thing was that I visited some friends and when I left I heard the crash of the cup I had used to have a cup of tea" ... so that nobody else would use it. That sort of thing happened.[121]

Although this indicates a persisting level of stigma, the eventual return of the majority of patients into their homes without an increased incidence of leprosy would have led to a reduction in public perception of contagion, resulting in diminishing stigma. On his appointment as assistant director of medical services in Suva (where he served between 1965 to 1970), Dr. Beckett was the instigator closing the leprosarium at Makogai, not simply because of economic pragmatism (as only 150 patients were at Makogai in the late 1960s), but also because of the trauma that isolation caused to families (since it was no longer necessary to isolate leprosy cases due to the availability of the new sulphone medication).[122]

St. Elizabeth Leprosy Home, Suva

Another important facility operated for the benefit of leprosy patients by the Fijian government and run by the SMSM was St. Elizabeth Home situated at Walu Bay near the Colonial Hospital in Suva, which provided a transit stop and temporary rehabilitation point for leprosy patients. Patients awaiting transport to Makogai were held here, under the care of the SMSM, as well as those discharged from Makogai awaiting transport to their home islands. Most importantly, the home offered a rehabilitation zone between isolation and society, which again contradicts the view that religious orders did little other than prepare those under their care for the afterlife. It is likely that St. Elizabeth Home in many ways helped de-stigmatize both the public views towards leprosy and leprosy patients themselves, as it was situated close to Suva.

St. Elizabeth Home provided an opportunity on the way back from isolation to have contact with the public and society at large without being dependent. Leprosy sufferers lived with others in the same position as themselves, exchanging advice and support in a neutral buffer zone. Patients benefited from their rehabilitative stays at the home, and, in particular, it produced a highly successful outcome for one shy patient returning from Makogai, Semisi Maya. Maya had been diagnosed with leprosy at age twenty-one and spent a total of fourteen years at Makogai, from 1938. Upon discharge, despite being unable to hold paint brushes due to deformities of his fingers, he learned about techniques of painting from one of the SMSM staff.[123] Discovering his natural propensity for art, he was taught to blend colors, and later, using the edges of his hands and hairs on his forearms, he applied shapes such as waves, ocean creatures and plant life, the finer features being drawn by locking a spatula between both hands or in his mouth. His paintings were exhibited in Christchurch, London, Australia and the USA, and are still for sale on fund-raising cards and bookmarks at the PLF.[124] His paintings decorated the walls of the Suva Travelodge as well as at Twomey hospital, which became his home in 1958. Such individual levels of rehabilitation undoubtedly helped leprosy sufferers adapt back into society, reducing stigmatic attitudes of those around them, and also provided a positive self-image after years of segregation. The initiatives of the SMSM are again apparent in helping leprosy sufferers attain useful lives after years of isolation and discharge from Makogai.

Having lost the use of his hands and feet, Semisi Maya later made his home at Twomey hospital until his death. The hospital had come to be a place where those debilitated by the ravages of leprosy, especially with the onset of the frailties of age, could find specialized and necessary medical attention, as well as the companionship of others who shared and understood the complications and hardships imposed by earlier leprosy. To some extent, leprosaria as homes for elderly patients with severe disabilities would have kept alive the elements of fear and stigma associated with leprosy among outsiders. However, ignorance and knowledge are the respective keys for keeping alive or ending stigma; and the elderly residents were able to mix in ordinary society. Visitors came to the hospital, and an exchange of knowledge about leprosy would have been gained, leading to empathy and continuing reduction of stigma.

P. J. Twomey Memorial Hospital, Tamavua, Suva

Twomey Memorial hospital at Tamavua, Suva, had been built at the initiative of the Fijian government, together with LTB sponsorship. Its doors opened following the closure of the Makogai leprosarium in 1969. In 1978 the Fijian Government, the LTB and the World Health Organization formed a tripartite agreement that saw Twomey hospital become used as a Leprosy Training Center for the South Pacific. The hospital continues to operate, combining its role as a training center with its original responsibility for treating all leprosy patients, either as outpatients or residents, temporarily or permanently.

During the 1970–80s the success of sulphone drugs, such as DDS, was found to be limited due to resistance to the drugs, and numerous leprosy relapses were reported worldwide, including in the Pacific region. The importance of Twomey Hospital in treating these relapses, and as a medical training center, became paramount in the South Pacific region. It became a place where leprosy sufferers felt they were entitled to free care and a home, because it had been specifically built for them. By the time interviews were conducted with residents at Twomey hospital, extracts of which appear here, the SMSM had withdrawn their service, and the hospital was taken over by the Fijian government. Due to the diminished incidence of leprosy, the government had begun to use the hospital for tuberculosis patients. This led to a sense of displacement and sometimes an apparent lack of self-worth in the residents at Twomey hospital. The testimonies here cover these aspects and also describe how leprosy patients from Makogai contributed to the establishment of Twomey Hospital, and how it has come to represent home to many patients.

Testimonies of Interviewees at Twomey Hospital

In August 2004, with introductions and assistance from the PLF, interviews were conducted with thirteen residents at Twomey hospital and three leprosy sufferers living in homes in Fiji, varying in age from 51 to 82 years. Eleven interviews were oral history recordings (although the testimony of one resident, Polutele Fatakava, being a Tongan, is included in the details about leprosy in Tonga), and the remaining four interviews comprise handwritten notes. Twelve of the interviewees, three females and nine males, had been isolated at Makogai. Three out of the six women interviewed had never married, and four out of the nine men had not married either. But three of the single women either adopted or had one child, while the men said they chose not to marry or have children because they could not support a family. The male partners of the women were men who had also been at Makogai, while two of the men's wives had also had leprosy. These figures, together with relevant testimonies, indicate that it was not easy re-integrating into their lives after isolation and discharge. To a great extent their exclusion and subsequent friendships, and sense of being part of a special community, particularly at Makogai, predisposed them towards friendships with other leprosy sufferers. The fact that Twomey Hospital opened after the closure of the leprosarium at Makogai led to Twomey Hospital being seen as a home where ex-patients could meet old friends, as well as a place for treatment of relapses of leprosy and the recurrent debilitating health problems that followed leprosy sufferers into old age.

Because of the large number of interviews, only the testimonies which contribute to aspects of the lives of leprosy sufferers not encompassed or duplicated by those obtained in the other Pacific islands are included here. The following extracts are organized in chronological order, providing testimonies by individual patients of their diagnosis, arrival at Makogai, lifestyle at the leprosarium, how isolation impacted on their later lives after discharge, and their experiences dealing with relapses of leprosy. Relapses involved re-admission into Twomey hospital, and details of these problems and events in their lives will be included together with their perceptions of the ongoing support from the PLF.

Two of the interviewees, Polutele Fakatava, originally from Tonga, and Susau Fatiaki Layasewa from Rotuma, a distant island of Fiji, are featured in the documentary *Compassionate Exile*, where they and other ex-patients revisited Makogai.[125] In the documentary, Polutele's description of arrivals to Makogai reflects a high degree of stigma towards leprosy, in that he arrived, aged twenty-three, in 1931 with a group from Tonga on a boat which was flying a yellow flag, signifying that leprosy sufferers were aboard, and that after disembarkation at the special wharf reserved for leprosy sufferers, the boat and clothes were fumigated. He had been told that "people became part of the soil at Makogai."[126] A similar dread of never returning from Makogai is present in several testimonies of those in the South Pacific region who faced exile.

Susau Fatiaki Layasewa (b. 1933) was sent by her father, who was a teacher in Rotuma, to attend school in Suva. Aged about ten, and due to return home for a holiday, she felt unwell, so an aunt sent her to a doctor. Susau's explanation demonstrates that even in 1953 leprosy diagnosis was problematic, and travelling with leprosy difficult:

> My aunty took me to the doctor health office in Suva. He was an European doctor, he check me first before I went to Rotuma ... he said no leprosy. So they let me go for a holiday. My brother ... he told my aunty there that I was very sick. So my aunty ... told them [SMSM at St. Elizabeth's Home] about me and then the boat come from Tarawa bringing patients from Tarawa, so they sent the wireless to the boat to collect me from Rotuma ... it was very hard for patients like myself, just come by boat to Suva.... The boat come to Rotuma and took me Makogai.[127]

Susau's testimony confirms that leprosy patients were unable to travel on ordinary boats, supporting the public stigma also evident in Polutele's comments. She went on to describe her symptoms, reaction to medication, and life on Makogai:

> The itching is in my body, in my skin, it is so itchy that I can't sleep.... I was skin and bone ... my eyebrows are fallen off and my eyelashes, even my eyelashes ... then after that, when I was one year... really I can't take the medicine, too strong for me. The DDS or whatever they call it, the drugs ... I'm so weak, you know my blood is anaemia, and they give me iron tablets ... to make me strong.[128]
>
> We had a long dormitory ward, open like this [as at Twomey hospital] ... but there was a special building for the ones very weak, so I was in that building.... The school had their own building, the women all in the building and a special one for the very sick ones. We are shut, the house close at 6 and

open at 6 in the morning. Six o'clock we have to go inside and lock the doors... our head woman locked the doors ... so sometimes they make fun of us, the men, sitting around, jailbirds are inside. ... The men could go where they liked ... the men have their own village. They have their own house. Women locked in, they stay there, some sewing, sometimes singing, playing cards.[129]

We have our own place, you know what I mean. Like we women, we have our own compound, we do what we want to do. We go fishing, we go picnic.... In the morning we just woke up, we cook our own food. Prepare our breakfast, then you go to take medicine, to the dressing room. After that you came back have your breakfast and things like that, then finish. You do your washing or whatever you want to do. Go to the other island for picnic, fishing, enjoy our world.[130]

On Monday and Thursday we look forward to the film night ... we had shop [at Makogai].... When it is Christmas time we all go and do our Christmas shopping! ... Christmas day we have a Christmas tree. On Christmas day we all have a parcel, imagine 700 parcels under the tree, and the sisters calling out names and entertain us. Dance and things like that.[131]

Susau was discharged from Makogai after eleven years in 1964, and recalls that when Dr. Beckett visited from Suva, it was decided to reduce the waiting period to six months, at which time she returned home to her parents, where she stayed six years. She then returned to Suva to work and married a man she had known prior to and at Makogai, who, she maintains, never had leprosy despite being isolated there for seven years. They lived at her place of employment where she was housekeeper to a long-term European resident of Suva.

In 1989 Susau's husband suddenly died while she was seeking treatment at Twomey hospital. She describes her return to the hospital:

When you have leprosy, when it come back ... cold and shivering and start reacting.... So I came here [Twomey hospital].... I was here in 1989 only for three months.... Nowadays you just take your medicine and then send you home, you take it at home. They don't keep you anymore ... came back in 1992 for about one and a half year and then I went back, and then I came back again in 1993 and in and out like that. And then I came back in 1994, and I am still here. But not taking any more drugs.... I like it here. I mean here you just... do what you want, but home, I haven't got a home of my own, just my sister's and my brother's.... They visit me and I go and see them. And they want me to come but, I think I like it here ... because they have their own families, the children have to be educated, they have own things [i.e. responsibilities].[132]

Susau appeared to be the spokesperson for the patients at Twomey, probably because of her education and literacy in English. Although she chose to live at Twomey because she felt it gave her a measure of independence (not being reliant on relatives), she said Twomey did not compare with the good life at Makogai. Susau did most of the washing for the leprosy patients and helped make breakfast and snacks. She said, "Over here, we just sitting here, going round the veranda and there is nothing to do." She said in earlier days at Twomey, when the SMSM were in charge before the government takeover, patients were paid to perform small chores, including gardening and maintaining the tennis courts. They also enjoyed playing tennis and going on picnics.

However, all this had now changed, with older but fewer patients; the facilities were no longer maintained, and much of the hospital had been given over for use by tuberculosis patients. The leprosy patients felt they were gradually being "pushed out," although they were quite sure the PLF in Christchurch would always support their needs. Susau said:

> Sometimes I told our doctor, who doesn't talk much, he is a very nice but quiet man, the medical officer here, and I told him ... what makes me sad, the way they treated us, as if we are nothing.... We heard that they are going to move us out from here.... They say why are we still here, we are cured, we better to home, why are we waiting, why are we sitting here?[133]

These comments reflect a perceived stance by the Government to save on cost and make space for what were considered to be more needy patients.

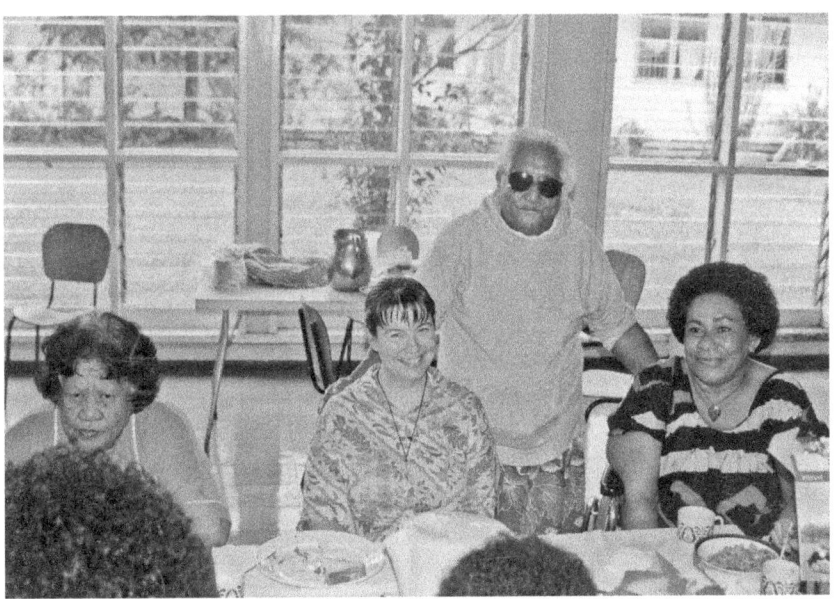

Left to right: Susan Fatiaki Layasewa, Jane Buckingham (researcher), Maria Ita Tetoariki, and Salote Tiko, taken on visit by author to Twomey Hospital in 2004.

It also reflects general health measures to incorporate leprosy as an ordinary part of public health, rather than being served by a separate set of institutions, which it is envisaged will lead to a lessening of fear and stigma associated with leprosy. Twomey Memorial Hospital, however, was a special place created with donations specifically raised to care for leprosy patients and the medical training needed for staff to provide this care. The PLF are committed to assisting these older patients still in residence who suffered early isolation practices and ongoing disabilities due to late diagnosis and/or the later arrival of sulphone drugs.

Nevertheless, Susau's comments, and the comments by other patients, support the argument that older patients who have been institutionalized over long periods find it difficult to fit back into family life. Certainly their physical disabilities cause enormous problems in small family homes, as the subsequent testimonies of Tevita and Salote will reveal. It is extremely fortunate that organizations such as the PLF are in a position to continue offering assistance and, in fact, see it as their duty to do so. It appears that older patients, who, through no fault of their own, had led difficult lives overcoming isolation and ill health deserve these benefits and perceived entitlements in their twilight years. These attitudes of older residents at leprosaria are paralleled by reports of residents at Carville, as well as those in Singapore and Mali, described earlier.

The findings of Japanese research at Ryukyu Islands — that older groups were more resistant to accepting changing views about leprosy — is reflected here to some extent; although it will be evident that it is not simply a matter of being resistant to change, but also that their physical limitations had inhibited the residents from returning to ordinary lives outside the leprosarium, which they had therefore come to see as their home.

Paras Ram (b. 1922), the oldest resident in August 2004, was an Indian Fijian, a widower aged 81. He had been diagnosed with leprosy at twenty-two and was sent to Makogai, he said, on 22 July, 1944. He remained isolated there until 1954. Although he could speak both English and Hindi, he often spoke Fijian to Ward Sister Mana, who kindly interpreted. When Paras arrived at Makogai, the only medication available was chualmoogra oil, which he said was an "injection in the arm.... It hurt very bad ... no good."[134] Later he received "new medicine — DDS, Dapsone ... pills ... every day, one tablet ... much improvement with the tablet."[135] Paras was a reserved man in a wheelchair, having undergone amputations. His memory was clear, and he gave specific details about his treatment and business. He gave a short account of his time at Makogai:

> I go there, and I tell one sister ... [her] face and my mother's face the same. I see her face and think of my mother.... She say, "Oh good, you can just call

me mother.... I look after you." I call sister, mother.... Yeah, good [life] we liked [the life] ... planted peanuts ... sell the peanuts and get paid.... I was very happy with the sisters, they like me.... And I gave them peanuts.... I would go to church, one can go to church, and mandir [Hindu shrine] too ... and family come [to visit].[136]

Having responded positively to Dapsone, Paras returned home, where he subsequently set up his own successful business in 1977 making charcoal by deep, slow burning of wood in wet mud pits, running the business for twenty-five years. During this time he married and had two children, although his first wife left him and his second wife had died. His son was married with children in Fiji, and his daughter lived in New Zealand but visited him whenever possible. However, working long hours stoking fires, then cooling the embers into charcoal, placed him at risk of burns and injury because of anaesthetized nerves in his limbs; these injuries later developed ulcers, which led to amputations and the further problems associated with advancing age.[137] He was almost blind, and he said, "You know what it's like, nobody to look after you at home; after awhile have to come back to hospital, some problems."[138]

Although Paras' story demonstrates a successful return to normal life — running a business and having a family — it is evident that his battle against the effects of leprosy was a solitary and increasingly difficult one. Towards the end of the interview, when asked if he would like to add anything more for the record, Paras whispered and appeared disturbed, with tears in his eyes. But Sister Mana told me not to stop the interview and to wait because Paras wanted to add more. Finally she said, "It is tears of joy ... after all that he went through, until now, that is what he is saying ... he is all right and he is happy."[139] Once the tape was switched off, Paras added that it was so good to be listened to. These quiet emotional statements encapsulate the loneliness and isolation that leprosy can impose on its victims. The generalized aura of stigma contributes to feelings that inhibit speaking freely about their suffering to others, apart from with other leprosy sufferers who understand the shared predicament. No doubt this quiet suffering, associated perhaps with feelings of rejection, is part of all suffering involving rejection; but few other conditions involve such entrenched, albeit nebulous ideas of stigma, making the suffering of leprosy something apart and different from other conditions. Until stigma totally ends, leprosy is not simply another public health concern but represents a social problem. It is for these reasons I feel it is important to attribute this story to Paras Ram personally by name, not under any pseudonym — a story of a proud and reserved man, extremely happy to be in a position to share his experiences.

Maria Ita Tetoariki (b. 1932) was from Banaba, one of the Gilbert Islands. She recalled that as a young girl during the war years when there was no electricity, her grandfather used to ignite a basin full of coconut shells for light. One day she fell in the fire. When she was taken to the doctor for her burns, she was diagnosed with leprosy. However, it was not until some years later that she was taken to Makogai. Although unsure of her dates, Tetoariki thought this was in 1947 when she was about 15. In the interim, waiting transportation to Makogai, she was shifted to live away from the village with other leprosy sufferers. Here the group cooked for themselves and lived as an isolated group for over two years, and she was pleased to get away to Makogai. Her story is explained through translation by Ward Sister Mana:

> Makogai is such a lovely place. She likes the place, she likes the people, she likes the sisters and she is one of the naughtiest girls there! She used to be punished every now and again. The punishment is for them to weed, weed outside or in the garden, or they don't go to the film, no film.... While they were there they feel like home, because of the sisters, how they looked after them, they treat them like their own daughters. While they were still there, the tablet arrived ... and was tested. If it agrees with them to take the medication, they were given the medication. She took the medication for one year but she had [some] reactions.[140]

Tetoariki returned home after the closure of Makogai in 1969 but returned to Fiji in 1982, after which she returned to Rabi, an island in Fiji occupied by the Banabans. The advanced stage of leprosy by the time the new medication was available meant that later problems eventually caused her to return to Twomey hospital. Tetoariki had had no amputations, and the limited deformities to her hands allowed her to enjoy embroidery and knitting, skills which she had learned at Makogai. The anaesthetized nerves around her eyes had been the major problem, for which she had undergone eye surgery, and she was awaiting further surgery at Twomey hospital in 2004:

> She had that [earlier] problem with the eye and they had given her the eye ointment. And she applied the ointment during the night. [Due to lack of sensation in the anaesthetized nerves] ... the container, must have ... pierced her eye, and then the eyeball was removed here [at Twomey hospital]. They put an artificial one in. Now, she had an eye operation last year, and she couldn't see, so we have to take her around. She is losing it again..... Most of these patients, they have eye problems due to the disease.[141]

Ward sister Mana told me she had worked at Makogai with leprosy patients and loved her work, so she continued to work at Twomey hospital. Upon her marriage she left work to have a family, but following her husband's death, she returned to work with the leprosy patients. At the end of the interview with Tetoariki, Mana went on to explain how the leprosy patients felt neglected at Twomey hospital, which was evident in the testimonies of several of the residents.[142]

These views reflect the changes and difficulties faced by older leprosy patients who were part of the earlier age of leprosy when disabilities were caused by untreated, damaged, anaesthetized nerves. Their continued medical needs led to dependence on leprosaria, causing weakened family ties, which instead rekindled old friendships and camaraderie originally found at Makogai, and led to a closely knit community being formed at Twomey hospital.

Tevita Vuni Waqa Soko (b. 1942) was a strong man who had suffered amputations at various points in time to his leg, but who managed to get around quickly and efficiently on crutches. Aged about seven in his village Nukunuku, Tevita felt sick and was taken to a doctor, but it was not until another four or five years that he tested positive for leprosy. At age thirteen in 1955 he was taken by boat, with other people from his island of Lakeba, to Makogai. He remained there eleven years, until 1966, having to wait the minimum two years until he tested clear of the bacillus.[143] He had no recurrence of leprosy and did not need to return to Twomey hospital until 1993, when plantar ulcers led to amputations. He gave a description of Makogai:

> First thing we have to learn there, when you come ... how to look after yourself, wash your clothes, things, brush your teeth and everything. They start from early in the morning ... six o'clock everybody have to wake up. Have a shower ... they have everything there. Then you have to be ready and wait for sister to come and give medicine around at the village.... They dressing [wounds]. If you have any problem you have to run to the hospital, you had a hospital, old men staying there, and they [sisters] can look after....We had physio all the time, every day. Five day or four day we have to go do some exercise there, all of us. One sister specially for physio. *Did you hurt yourself on the island at all?* Yeah, my foot ... only one toe left, my big toe.... I had to go to the hospital and the doctor operate it and take out some bone, getting bad.... We went for the fun job, fishing, other jobs, chicken there to feed and like that. Do the carpenter job ... nobody have to do the work ... after dressing and medicine you free. Free where you want to go, for picnic or three or four people together.[144]
>
> I think about 600 to 700 [patients].... They stay in their own different village, Fijian in one village, these are men, not women.... Indian one, another village Samoan, Tongan, Cook Island. They are from different village. But only the kids and the ladies they stay together.... The school boys, they have their own [place].... [At school] we had six classes, class one to six. About thirty or forty [pupils].... School day was half, eight to twelve [o'clock]. From two to four [pm] we have to go to the plantation with the master and plant some tapioca and anything like that. They call it agriculture, farming.[145]

Once discharged, Tevita returned home to a big welcome with his parents. He worked with his father with cattle and horses, and clearing areas for coconut plantations. In 1985 he came to Suva and worked as a carpenter, utilizing the training he had received on Makogai. Then one of his toes on his other leg turned septic and the bone had to be removed, which led to complications and finally amputation in 1993. However, the amputation was such that a prosthesis could not be fitted, and he needed the aid of crutches to walk.[146] Because of his leprosy, Tevita said he chose not to marry or have children because he did not feel able to properly provide for them. Although a pragmatic view, this may suggest a level of internalized ideas of stigma, as Tevita worked as a carpenter in Suva and did not indicate that he had been excluded from obtaining employment. He had battled leprosy from a young age and had not allowed it to get in the way of an active, vigorous life, but in later years Tevita found himself in the predicament of being dependent on Twomey Hospital. The talk of moving patients out of the hospital caused him to feel demeaned and belittled, and he indicated his awful frustration:

> I not sure, who is making the problem, the government making problem or Ministry of Health ... they keep on to leave hospital.... They draw a permanent list ... all the rest have to go. But most of us say, we not free to stay with our parents, we have no house and thing like that ... how you can move [when you can] hardly move.... I have to bring ... crutch to go inside. But if I have prosthesis leg, I have to take it out, outside, [then] I have to crawl inside.... And I am praying and hoping that it will never come to that, while we are here.... It is like that, it is very ugly to know you are gonna get a life or not. I don't know why they want to keep on moving the leprosy people around, just like a piece of paper, crumpled up, for the rubbish.[147]

Tevita's emotional end to the interview brought him close to angry tears, and was deeply upsetting for me. However, he clearly expressed the difficulties that people with amputations faced, with or without a prosthesis, especially living in simple Fijian homes. There was no space or suitable pathways to the homes for the use of wheelchairs, and once inside it would be embarrassing for both the leprosy sufferer and the family he stayed with, having to deal with the restricted movement in performing ordinary daily routines and ablutions. Good hospitals and leprosaria provided the means essential to a dignified lifestyle, irrespective of the galling handicaps and dependency on an institution.

At 51 years of age, Salote Tiko (b. 1953) was one of the youngest residents at Twomey hospital, a very energetic woman who moved very speedily in her wheelchair. In between her daily physiotherapy exercise regime, she spent her time sewing garments, having more orders than she could keep up with. She was unmarried but had one daughter, who was widowed and had a three-year-old daughter, Salote's grand-daughter. Salote told her story:

> When I was in class eight I start to feel there is a pain on my right foot ... like a boil.... I just used some leaves ... because I was a child I used to use a safety pin ... Usually use it as a medicine because too far from the hospital. You would have to walk to the hospital and during that time, the boil in my right foot it started growing up inside. In 1968 a European doctor came to our island in Lau.... I admitted in the hospital ... and they take my blood and take swab from the wound and they send it over. The result come back and the doctor from Lomolomo told me that you must come to Suva for the next treatment on the next trip of the boat.... I was feel happy because I [want to] be cured and I wanted to join my school.... I came here [Twomey hospital] in 1970 when I was seventeen.[148]

Salote made no mention of difficulty obtaining transport to travel to Suva from her island home, indicating that the level of stigma associated with leprosy had lowered. She went on to describe her predicament:

> But at the time, I had my right side stroke, that was the end of me. *You had a stroke?* Yes, no continue with my school, I can't hold the pen, so my hand weak and I have a dropped leg too, dropped foot.... So it was the first time in 1970 when I saw the [leprosy] patients here, they came from Makogai to here from 1969 to 1970. Oh, I was frightened when I look at them. And even I was frightened to go close to them. And the first time the sisters told me to come and have my breakfast or lunch in the dining room, I feel not like eating when I look at them. I was frightened and then they talk to me.[149]

This, and descriptions by other interviewees at their first sight of elderly leprosy sufferers bearing deformities caused by long untreated leprosy, confirms the fears imposed by the disfigurements.

> First time I came in, I think I stayed five or seven years, and going out to my parents, going out two years and come back to here, I am always in and out like that ... for the treatment. I had to have my review every three months, then after that six months. So, 1982, I finished reviews and in 1983 I was finished with my taking tablets. In 1984 I went back to my island.[150]
>
> But when I went back the wound still in my right foot. When I went back, I enjoy myself staying with my relatives, sometimes do some Fijian medicine to make it, they got it too, it can heal quickly.... I took my sewing to the hotel. I sew something to be used for the tourist and the hotel open and so the manager there, he send me to be the seamstress working in the laundry too. I was working there until 1999 and they found the sugar, I was diabetic. So still the wound on my foot, so when I went to the hospital, they admitted me. They send me back to P. J. Twomey, so I came here and from there I am still in the hospital till now.... In 2002 I had my leg amputated, just because of diabetic.[151]

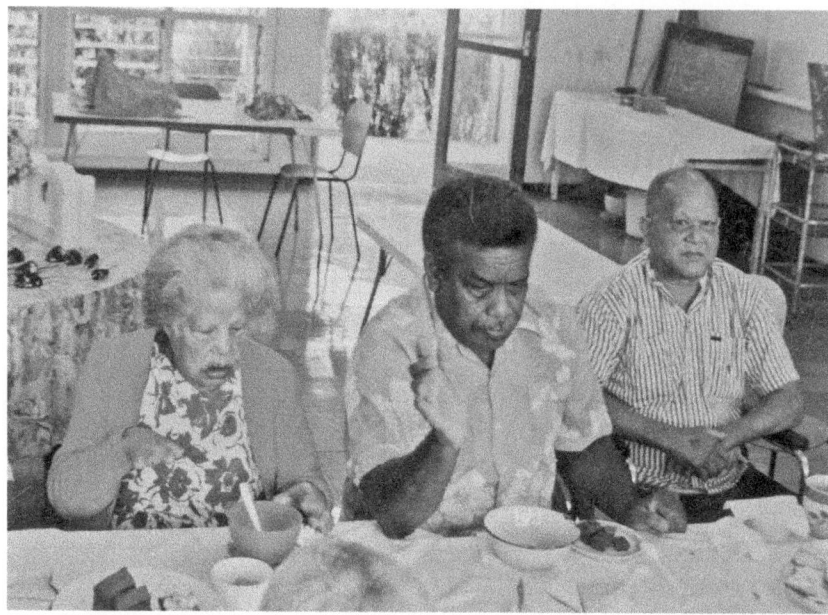

Left to right: Wati Moria, Lenaitasi Musuka and Volau Metuisela having lunch at Twomey Hospital in 2004.

>When I go out I use my artificial leg.... When I am in the hospital I use the wheelchair.... When I am living with my relatives, my aunt's place, sometimes I feel bad when I look at their place and look at me. Because I can't do much housework at home, I have to crawl from here and there. I need a wheelchair and I want to do my clothes business and, so I can't do it because there is no space, because so crowded in the house. The place I sleep, I used to sleep in the ...sitting room, so I have to sleep when they all finish watching TV at night.... My aunty's house ... living with her three sons, their wives and their children ... and my mother and myself.... And my daughter she came over from Viti Lavu and all stay there. Five bedrooms and one kitchen and one living room. Before I went to my aunty's place I always staying in my sister's home.... For me, and that is why I am still in Twomey, the Board [PLF] if they can help me, build a small house for myself and my mother and my granddaughter and daughter to stay in. I think they are the only one that can look after me, and they are the only ones that are close to me.[152]

Although a lot of Salote's problems stemmed from her stroke and later diabetes (a common condition in the Pacific with high carbohydrate diets), her leprosy was the reason she remained at Twomey hospital. As earlier explained by Tevita, the reality of living in family groups meant a loss of independence because their handicaps prevented them from being able to contribute and provide towards the household. Salote was quite desperate to have her own home and continue her own business, but the medical care that she constantly required made that problematic. Twomey hospital provided her space to continue her sewing, the sales of which gave her an important measure of independence. This support and work provided her with a feeling of independence, and the fact that her sewing was in high demand by friends in the outside community signified low stigma towards leprosy.

Lenaitasi Musuka (b. 1950) from Lau, age eighteen, was diagnosed with leprosy and sent to Makogai in 1968 for a few months, and later returned to Twomey hospital for further treatment. In Makogai he lived in the Fijian village. He enjoyed the company, and said the sisters were kind and humorous. He remembered the sister who served in the shop, and recalled, "When we came in, she look down like this, and look at us, 'What you want? You want cigarettes? No!' So when we come, she is very funny."[153] He also suggested I resembled that sister, all this demonstrating a reflection of the good humor with which the sisters interacted with patients.

Subsequently, Musuka married, but his wife died when their second child was young. The children were healthy, but he worried about them, making sure they had regular checks for leprosy.[154] Since 1999 he has had problems with plantar ulcers, and returned to Twomey hospital in 2001 for treatment. He used a wheelchair to move around, to keep his weight off his feet to allow the ulcers time to heal properly. As with all the Twomey patients, Musuka had a beautiful, strong singing voice, and led their hymns at daily prayers.[155]

Volau Metuisela (b. 1937) like Volau was a temporary resident at Twomey hospital because he needed medical attention for a plantar ulcer, which had necessitated a leg amputation. He lived on Lau and worked his family plantation of coconut, kava and sweet potato. Volau was sent to Makogai in 1953, age sixteen, where he stayed ten years, until 1963. His elder brother and sister had been sent to Makokai earlier, and his brother died there.[156] So he was very fearful when he was sent:

> Oh, when I go to Makogai, on that time, I am very worry. I go there, I am dead over there, never come back, I am thinking every time. I am very surprised when I was there, and coming the new medicine, come at that time. And we drink, oh very quick finish the drugs. We take ... small pills.... One year stay there to complete your, what you call, bloods. Still negative ... [no bacilli present]. Negative at one year then you are supposed to go home, leprosy gone. The time we see our name is on the board ... is finish, we look very happy.... Sometime, it goes [up] sometimes six months, one time nearly one year, the last month, and it drop again. You better start again, take the bloods. For the whole year. Oh, we feel very bad on that time. If you drop in the last month, oh.... With me, six months, yeah, two times.[157]

When I was there I was very fit. I am always exercise every time, in the morning. Wake up, exercise, in the evening.... So on the day the doctor tell me yes, Metuisela, you discharged tomorrow, ooh, I never sleep in the night time! I was thinking many years I stay in Makogai, well I go home.... When I go back, soon as I see the island I am very happy, I am crying then, but I am very happy.... Only my mother still alive on that time. My father is died before I go to Makogai. When I go I see my mother very happy, my mother is very happy when I come back ... from the time the doctor tell me I have got diabetes. I drink pills, I never drink sugar and when I eat, I never eat too much, sometimes I eat too much, and my blood still come up.[158]

Volau gave no indication of any stigma on his return home and married three years later, in 1966. He had two healthy children and three grandchildren, despite several cases of leprosy in his wider family. He had looked after his health while working on his plantation, but an accident at home, with a child spilling hot water on his arm, caused a clawed hand.[159] The recent amputation would prevent his outdoor work, but he said he also worked as a minister on his island, an indication of minimal stigma. He had been eight months at Twomey hospital and was ready to return home, although he said he would miss the wheelchair he used at the hospital. He was delaying his return home to Lau, pending the provision of materials granted by the PLF to rebuild his home that had been demolished by a recent hurricane. The provision of materials was being organized by Louisa Nasome, the PLF contact liaison who worked at Twomey hospital.

The description of Volau's stay at Twomey hospital is an example of the service offered to leprosy sufferers in Fiji, which is paralleled by the case of Lome in Samoa, who also spent several months at Twomey hospital for care of ulcers, subsequent amputation, fitting of prosthesis and rehabilitation. Several months, or even longer, are required for such treatments, but the stay is made pleasurable because of the opportunity to meet old friends from Makogai.

The current climate of concern regarding the continued ability to accommodate long-term residents was extremely disturbing to all the residents. They were accustomed to the specialized attention available at Twomey, and were well aware that the facilities had originally been donated for their care. In particular they found that general hospital staff were unfamiliar with the ongoing requirements of leprosy patients, including debriding plantar ulcers. They were uncomfortable with the idea of dealing with staff who, firstly, were unfamiliar with the procedures necessary for their needs, and secondly, made them feel unwelcome. The unwelcome feeling could be attributable to self-consciousness and feeling conspicuous in general wards — these attitudes reflecting ideas related to internalized stigma after so many years of living apart and in institutions. However, despite changes in priority of Fijian health programs, the PLF are committed to ensuring the welfare of all leprosy sufferers in Fiji, and to maintaining the facilities offered through Twomey hospital because it is the leprosy training center for medical staff and supports the prosthetics laboratory, which serves the needs of amputees in the South Pacific region.[160]

Testimonies of Interviewees Living in Their Own Homes

Visits were made and interviews conducted with leprosy sufferers living in their own homes in and around the Suva area. One family consisted of a married couple, the husband Joseph Mai having been on Makogai from 1955 to 1958, and his wife, Venaisi Meto, having been treated for leprosy at Twomey hospital. They lived in the Venaisi's family village, and the PLF had enhanced their livelihood by providing a fishing boat to supplement their own food consumption and sell the surplus.[161] Occasionally the boat was hired to others, and these activities returned a reasonable income for the family and young children. The fact that the family lived close to neighbors who shared their food and the boat indicates that little of the old stigma remained or was directed towards them. Certainly there were no comments indicating stigma.

Another leprosy sufferer, Shah Bahadur (John) Singh, was interviewed in the presence of his son, who indicated he did not understand anything about leprosy. John's wife was away with their daughter who had just borne a second child. The PLF had provided funding for their small home in Suva, and John continued to receive financial assistance because he suffered problems with his eyesight and general health.[162] The family lived close to neighbors, again signifying low stigma associated with John's leprosy.

The third interviewee, Wati Moira, lived with her daughter Josephine and family. Wati, through the translation of Josephine, revealed a very poignant story of her life with leprosy, which will be detailed more fully below, providing another dimension of the difficulties faced by people having suffered leprosy.

Wati Moira (b. 1929) was about twelve when the family learned she had leprosy. Her married daughter Josephine translates her mother's story:

> Spots that were detected on her skin ... even the nurse ... couldn't get herself to tell the parents.... Heard rumour ... daughter is suffering from, they call that in Fijian *matelevu* which means it is a big disease.... They understand that it is leprosy.... People were so frightened of the disease that it contagious ... When they [the parents] prepared her [Wati] to go ... they prepared along

> with her, what we do in traditional culture, was the mat ... for the burial, should they lose her, should she die.[163]

The burial mat especially demonstrates the high level of fear associated with leprosy in the early days, as compared to today.

> Her father was the one who had to take her to Lakeba.... Her father was advised ... go to another [elderly] lady, Salote... who is also suffering from leprosy.... And that is where she went, and they built a little hut where only these two stayed [Wati and Salote], because it was very far away from everybody else.... She didn't like to be reminded that she was sick and she found it very hard to accept that, she was brought down with such a disease because she just wanted to be like everybody else.... [Father] spends the day with her and Salote at their hut, but at night he returns to the main village to go and sleep there. It was prohibited for him to sleep with them at night. But during the day he couldn't tear himself away from the little daughter so he returned. Until he built a little hut beside their home where he could be near them ... [remaining for one] whole year and two months ... due to the ship, unavailability of ships and transportation.... One of the reasons she [Wati] looked forward to go to Makogai was she has had enough of being isolated. She thought of her father leaving behind his responsibility way back in the island, and she has these five brothers to look after, and her mother was alone.... One of the main thing was she wanted to be among people, knowing that, that they were sick people together, but her priority was she wanted to be amongst people instead of being isolated.... But to go Makogai she would be with many people, she had heard people talk about, and hopefully there were children there at her age, and there was no isolation.[164]

The concept that going to Makogai did not represent isolation, as compared to people being separated in their home communities with limited companionship, is interesting. To Wati, living separately nearby was more isolating than living among strangers at a more distant leprosarium. However, being with people sharing a common predicament seemed comforting, and the idea of being part of a community appealed to Wati. This is an aspect of life at Makogai which all leprosy sufferers appreciated, despite the pain of separation from family. Josephine continued Wati's story:

> When they arrived in Makogai the sisters who were looking after them were waiting for them by the wharf. So they received them when they disembarked, and they were taken up to the office, where they were explained things. They were to go to the ladies section ... because of your age you will have to go to the children's section.... They looked up to the sisters as their mothers, and because of that relationship, they felt free to say what they wanted to and all that, just as they could to their mother. But they highly uphold the lives of the sisters for the sacrifice they gave for them.[165]

Memories of Makogai were happy ones, which made it difficult to leave, but also to adjust back to ordinary life, as described:

> [Wati] played netball [and] captained the team.... Makogai was a very rich island, rich in the sea and also rich in the gardens and all that, whereas they don't have to pay for it, and give to the communal life and everybody helped one another. There was no one neglected there. They all assisted and helped one another ... communal life and the richness of the crops, vegetables and fruit and the sea, that's what made them want to stay back there. The unity and the bond that they have had on each other, they know that when they come to Suva, one would be going this way and one there; but there [at Makogai] it was like one big family of them and that's what they said.[166]
>
> It was very hard for them, and especially for those discharged and come to experience the hard life in Suva, financial constraints then, and the families.... That made it very hard.... Some, they were still not sure whether they would be accepted at all or not.... [Wati] says she didn't have problems with the family, with her relatives, but it is with the neighborhood, those who are not family. But directly they didn't... either they stand aside or, you know, make faces like that, or don't stay too long, but she didn't come to problems.[167]

This testimony indicates the actual hardships of adapting to ordinary life after being institutionalized, despite the diminished level of fear and stigma since the availability of sulphone treatment. Wati had remained seventeen years on Makogai, her first visit being from 1941 to 1958. She returned to Suva, and in 1961 had a son, then suffered a relapse and had to return to Makogai for two years, leaving her young son in the care of her family.[168] The testimony recounting the experiences of relapse of leprosy after having a child reveals another dimension of the suffering of isolation for parents and children. Wati's partner and father of her two children had also been a patient at Makogai.

After the first relapse, Wati was released in 1963, and her daughter Josephine was born in 1965. When Josephine was eight months old, Wati had another relapse and again had to return to Makogai for several years, returning to Suva just prior to the opening of Twomey hospital in 1969. This was difficult for her:

> Patients generally were advised, that her blood, or whatever the medical term, is weak for her to bear children, and should she bear children, it would weaken her system.... That is when it will affect her, she will loose her fingers ... deformed and all that. Unlike the first trip when she looked forward [to going to Makogai], but now that she was with the child she didn't want to go, but it was too bad that she had to.... When she had children, the motherly instinct overcame, and she no longer found Makogai the paradise, because her

heart kept returning for her children, so it was a big difference when she started having children. So, she went to Makogai just because she had to be treated, but she wanted to be with her children.[169]

[When Makogai was due to close, Wati] had come ahead of them for a couple of months, because the sisters had asked her to come over here and sew the curtains for the hospital ... and the pillow cases, mosquito nets at Twomey hospital.... It was brand new, it was just newly established.... Twomey was empty then, no one was occupying then. So she was residing at the St. Elizabeth home, down at Walu Bay. She did all the sewing there.... The sisters had asked her if she could stay on and sew shirts, and clothes, and presents, Christmas gifts, for the patients, so she stayed behind and worked three years and did those before she was finally discharged.... She went to live with her brother and her sister-in-law in Suva still. It was a couple of miles away from the main city. She lived with them for awhile, and then I had come over [from grandparents home].... I asked her what was your daughter's reaction. Then she said, "She [Josephine, translating] didn't want to do anything with me [Wati] because all she thought of was her grandparents!" And personally, for me, it was most heartbreaking time ... somebody had come and overthrow my grandparents.... I sort of feared her, I had mixed feelings.[170]

When we first reconciled, was when she was with my uncle, her brother, who was married and was living seven miles away from the main city in Suva. We lived there for a short while.... Life in Suva was so hard, and she was worried how to finance my education.... She learnt from Makogai, sewing, so she sewed and sewed, and the Sisters [through the PLF] assisted her with my education. So being together all those years and seeing the hardship that they go through, and I saw for myself the sacrifice which she had to put up with to make a living for myself, and I came to realize that my grandparents were not going to be able to look after me and my education and all that. I was dependent on her, and that built my love to her, knowing her condition and the effort that she put in, that is really what built the love. That's what makes me want to be with her and return to her all that she has built in me. I was about fifteen when we actually came to live together.[171]

Wati's son, Matui, who had been raised by an aunt, became a missionary with Youth with a Mission and went to Switzerland, where he met and married an American worker.[172] Later he moved and lived in the U.S. When his wife's family learned about Wati's circumstances, they raised a local appeal in the U.S. and financed the purchase in 2000 of the house for Josephine and her family, on the proviso they would also care for Wati and their aunt, which is where they all lived together and where the interview took place.[173] Wati still sewed to earn extra money for the household, selling her embroidery, mats and patchwork bed covers.

Josephine explained the feeling Wati and her family have for friends at Twomey hospital, and went on to convey what Wati wished to express to everyone who had helped her:

> My [Josephine's] children know every name of every patient up there.... They go up and eat out of their hand, and when they eat in the dining room, they think that is their family home. They will go and sit down, they will help themselves to tea and all that, just as if it was home. So Pouli [Pouletele] and the rest of the team, they are not strangers to us. Mum says, "I want to thank them all the way from New Zealand, all the sisters who combined service with them, all the doctors ... also thank Louisa [PLF liaison] who brought you all along today. Because all that is all part of it." She [Wati] is just ever so grateful for them and they are part of her, they are who she is to this very day.[174]
>
> Regarding the project, she says thank you for coming today and for taking her opinion and her story, and she just pray and hope that it will be of great help to you and to colleagues and to whoever will benefit from her story today. She is very grateful and very happy that she is of any assistance in whichever way to this project.[175]

Wati's closing words, through Josephine, poignantly demonstrates her strength and endurance:

> Even though she [Wati] has been diseased with leprosy, the disease does not stop her from having children, and it delights her ... that we are well and that we will continue and that the suffering ends with her. But because we are healthy we do not suffer from that, she is delighted to see her generation go forth, and that the suffering lies with her. And she just hopes that the strength, the determination that she had, it is her prayer, that it will lie with her children in the generation to come.[176]

The richness of life depicted through the above testimonies illustrate the strong friendships and sense of community that arose through common adversity, despite descriptions of the pain of being torn away from loved ones. The care and friendship of fellow companions, the dedication of the SMSM sisters, and the medical services of doctors and staff came together at the leprosarium at Makogai and again at Twomey hospital. The early fear and dread of isolation had faded with the camaraderie at Makogai, and especially later, following the availability of sulphones, leading to the realization that their isolation was temporary. The positive experience at Makogai meant that when the relapses of leprosy occurred due to resistance to sulphones in the 1970s, patients did not hesitate to voluntarily return to leprosaria for assistance.

This voluntary return to leprosaria supports a conclusion that the creation of institutions for leprosy sufferers enriched the lives of patients, provided the opportunities for lifelong friendships, and offered the care necessary for their medical needs at the active stages of the disease and again due to old age in later life. Inevitably these circumstances created a dependency in some leprosy sufferers upon the institutions, rather than upon relatives, because of the free provision of care and the superior amenities available at the institutions (a level of care not feasible in family homes). Nevertheless, stigma and exclusion from society no longer appear to be the reasons for residence at Twomey hospital; instead, the care, friendship and camaraderie that exist there attract the elderly residents. Leprosy sufferers who lived in their home communities gave no evidence of any serious discrimination by the public. They received the support of their families, together with the ongoing and much appreciated assistance of the PLF, which ensured that families with leprosy were not disadvantaged due to the disease.

2

Former Penitentiaries as Leprosaria — New Caledonia

Historical Background

The first European explorer to discover the islands was Captain Cook in 1774, who felt the islands resembled the Scottish highlands and so named them Caledonia. Subsequently, French explorers visited New Caledonia and the Loyalty islands, and by 1840 the sandalwood trade and the abduction of Pacific Islanders (known as blackbirding) operated in the region taking islanders to work on sugar plantations in faraway colonial territories. In 1853 Napoleon III of France annexed New Caledonia, imposed a military regime, and in 1864 founded a penal colony to which convicts were shipped. Conditions on ship over the four-month voyage from the northern hemisphere were miserable. An estimated 40,000 male and female convicts were brought from France, including political prisoners following the 1871 Paris Commune uprising, as well as rebels from France's African colonies. The convicts were isolated on the Ile des Pins, south of the mainland, and at Ile d'Art, one of the Belep islands off the northern tip of the main island. The most dangerous prisoners were incarcerated at a prison built on the main island at Ducos, situated off the peninsula near the main port of Noumea. Following a general amnesty in 1878 and a series of pardons, the majority of convicts were released by 1879.

Subsequently, the penitentiaries at Belep and Ducos, in 1892 and 1918 respectively, became isolation centers for those suffering from leprosy.[1] The policy of segregation and isolating leprosy sufferers was in line with western ideas of hygiene and quarantine, endorsed by the First International Leprosy Conference in Berlin in 1897. The fact that the places of isolation were located at previous prison sites is likely to have introduced and affirmed ideas that leprosy sufferers were unwanted and undesirable people who should be segregated from society, contributing to high stigma. Rather than returning to France, a large proportion of the poor European convicts and other exiles remained in New Caledonia. Known as Caldoches, they took on municipal tasks in abysmal working and living conditions. The correlation between poverty, poor hygiene and diseases is well recognized, particularly with leprosy, and it is the impoverished conditions of the Caldoches which contributed to the unusual phenomenon in New Caledonia — that at the turn of the twentieth century the majority of leprosy patients were non–Melanesian Europeans.[2]

To provide an understanding of how leprosy was dealt with in New Caledonia, the testimonies of a long-term resident at Ducos leprosarium, Honoré Tourte, and that of Sister Nöellie Thiossey, an SMSM nurse who worked with leprosy patients from about 1967 until the present time, will be presented, alongside available sources. The additional testimony of Dr. Roland Farrugia, PLF and WHO leprologist, and former medical superintendent at Ducos in the 1970s, together with the comments of Dr. Jacques Michaudel, an army doctor resident in New Caledonia, will explain how leprosy was handled by the health authorities. Through extracts from these personal accounts and documents provided, that outline government and medical policies relating to leprosy, the government policies to contain leprosy will be described.[3] These sources, together with the SMSM archives, also provide insight into the involvement of missionary orders and the role of the LTB/PLF in providing care for leprosy sufferers. These indicate to what extent government policies and conditions at the leprosaria may have impacted upon stigma, which has remained at a relatively high level in these islands.

Early Reports and Treatment of Leprosy

In 1950 Lonie reported that 71 percent of the leprosy cases in Ducos were Europeans, and 34 percent natives, and that the incidence of lepromatous leprosy was higher among Europeans than Melanesians.[4] This finding is contrary to findings in other Pacific islands where figures for Europeans with leprosy were very low; although with the large numbers of convicts brought to New Caledonia, Europeans represented a large proportion of the population. The high incidence among Europeans is related to the low socio-economic status of the majority of Europeans in New Caledonia, especially Caldoches, as compared to other islands where Europeans represented the elite of the societies, enjoying higher socio-economic living conditions and thereby decreasing their susceptibility to leprosy. Inevitably, in New Caledonia leprosy and its stigma became associated with lower socio-economic groups and those considered undesirables in society.

According to Pierre Bobin, a French leprologist in Noumea, leprosy was brought to New Caledonia by a Chinese seaman some time between 1860 and 1865; the first medically confirmed case was in 1883 with the first European being diagnosed in 1889.[5] As in most other Pacific Islands, the Chinese are blamed for the introduction of leprosy, but as Lonie suggests, the disease could have spread through infected islanders moving around the Pacific region. Within New Caledonia, leprosy initially spread more rapidly among the Caldoches and ex-convicts because of their extreme poverty and terrible living conditions.[6]

Three years after the first European was diagnosed with leprosy, it was decided to establish a leprosarium on one of the northern islands of Belep, to which five hundred patients were transferred and "isolation was total."[7] This French initiative came five years prior to the First International Leprosy Conference in 1897, demonstrating a strict early stance to segregate leprosy sufferers from ordinary society. At Belep patients were left to care for themselves, with occasional visits by a doctor or priest. Shortly afterwards, some care was provided by one of the original pioneers of what later came to be called the Missionary Sisters of the Society of Mary.[8] Six years later, in 1898, the New Caledonian administration decided that the leprosarium should be closer and more accessible to Noumea, rather than at Belep. Due to the increase of leprosy among the indigenous population at that time, the local chiefs were made responsible for isolating leprosy patients, who were housed separately in lazarets close to their own villages.[9]

The European and immigrant leprosy sufferers at Belep, and "one native settlement" (presumably a group of advanced cases), were transported to the Ile aux Chèvres (Isle of Goats), a small island closer to Noumea, north of the peninsula.[10] The majority of the remaining Melanesian patients were sent home to be isolated near their "own tribes of origin." On the Ile aux Chèvres, isolation was again complete, and patients continued to care for themselves and each other, with visits only from priests and the religious.[11] If a serious problem arose, a white flag was raised to alert special quarantine boats on a nearby island, who in turn notified the administration on the mainland to provide medical care from Noumea.[12] These strict isolation practices inevitably contributed to fear of the disease and its contagion, which in turn produced stigma among westerners and locals.

Involvement of Religious Orders in Care at Belep and Ducos

In 1918 the penitentiary buildings at Ducos were acquired for use by the leprosy colony, and the very sick patients from the Ile aux Chèvres were moved to the new central leprosarium established at the old prison.[13] This building now houses a small museum relating to the history of leprosy, with exhibits, photographs and newspaper cuttings set up by the curator, Madam Bobin, probably the wife or relative of Pierre Bobin, the leprologist at Ducos and later in Mali, Africa.[14] Originally the peninsula of Ducos was cut off from the mainland, and access was only by boat across the bay; whereas now the land is connected by a bridge and road to the mainland, making it about a twenty minute journey from Noumea.[15] The area of land around the central leprosarium was fenced off and with large gates. Once again isolation was enforced, and the patients catered to their own needs, with occasional visits only from the religious and a doctor. It was not until 1933 that four nursing sisters arrived at the leprosarium, being from the Cluny and the Missionary Sisters of the Society of Mary (SMSM) orders, who through their devotion reportedly "transformed little by little this ghetto into a hospital."[16]

It is notable, however, that the involvement with leprosy of the original French Order of the SMSM began as early as 1892, with the establishment of the first leprosy colony at Belep. Sister Marie de la Croix from Bordeaux, one of the eleven founding lay sisters of the SMSM (then known as the Pioneers of the Third Order of Mary), arrived in New Caledonia in 1858, and in 1892, after the transfer of leprosy sufferers to Belep, she volunteered to care for the patients.[17] When the government decided to close the leprosarium in Belep in 1898, Sister Marie de la Croix wrote:

> These poor people were crying.... We held these stumps of hand, without fingers. Oh, these unfortunate people whom we loved so greatly, and that we were so happy to console.[18]

To what extent this consolation comprised health or spiritual care, or both, is unclear, but what becomes apparent is that the vocation of nursing gained great appeal within the Order. Another of the founding pioneers, Sister Marie de la Paix, arrived in New Caledonia around 1867, and, together with Marie de la Croix, she worked with the sick on the Ile de Pins, La Conception, Pouebo and the island of Ouvea, although there are no specific mentions of leprosy in the work for which she was later honored.[19] It is likely that this vocational pioneering, especially with leprosy patients at Belep, aroused later SMSM compassion and training of nuns as nurses, culminating in their acceptance of the request to care for leprosy sufferers at Makogai, Fiji, following the establishment of that leprosarium in 1911.

The French Sisters M. Suzanne and Sister Marie Stanislaus were the two founding staff members at Makogai, Sister Stanislaus being the leprosarium's first Superior.[20] Sister Suzanne's interest turned to seeking a cure or vaccine for the disease, and she commenced laboratory experiments on the leprosy bacillus at Makogai, continuing her research from 1938 to 1943 at the Pasteur Institute in Paris and New Caledonia. Her work isolated an acid-resistant germ in an artificial culture, similar to the true leprosy bacillus. It was named *Mycobacterium marianum* in recognition of her work, from which a vaccine was prepared.[21] Sister Suzanne received honors for her pioneering work but died from a brain tumor in 1958 before its completion.[22] Sister Suzanne earlier presented her findings at the Seventh International Congress in Tokyo. Here she met Sister Hilary Ross of the Daughters of Charity from Carville, USA, who assisted in the clinical trials of the *marianum* antigen at the leprosy research laboratory at Carville in 1954. But the trials produced negligible results, as have subsequent trials for a leprosy vaccine.[23] Sister Hilary Ross had trained as a pharmacist and became a research biochemist at Carville, where from 1922 to 1928 she worked on improving the techniques of administering chaulmoogra oil medications. Later, in the 1940s, she assisted in assessing the different sulphone drugs for use in the treatment of leprosy.[24] The parallel research of these two sisters from different religious orders demonstrates a desire to assist in medical research to relieve the physical suffering caused by leprosy, which is far more than being restricted to aiding merely the spiritual life of patients, as suggested by Edmond.[25]

The attraction of serving as a nurse within a religious order is described more recently by Sister Nöellie Thiossey, who stated that for many the service was not simply a calling to receive and provide spiritual guidance, but to provide relief from suffering in everyday lives where there was a need.[26] Sister Nöellie was instrumental in arranging a meeting with one of the longest residents at the Raoul Follereau leprosarium at Ducos, whose testimony follows.

Conditions at Ducos Leprosarium to the Late 1960s

Ten years after the central leprosarium was established at Ducos in 1918, and prior to appointment of inhouse residential nursing staff, the following interviewee aged eight was isolated at the leprosarium in 1928. Honoré Tourte (b. 1920) remained in residence for over seventy years, with a total of only about five years' absence as a teenager, and was interviewed in 2006.[27] Although time prevented a lengthy interview with Honoré, additional accounts of his life and exploits during his time at Ducos are documented in the collection of memoirs of eleven long-term residents and three staff, in a book launched during my visit to Ducos at their annual fair, *kermesse*, at which residents sold crafts, produce and food.[28] Honoré has an excellent memory and was very articulate, despite his eighty-six years and the physical disabilities caused by the ravages of leprosy. The following selections of Honoré's interview serve to illustrate the experience of a leprosy sufferer at Ducos center from its earliest beginnings. He describes the weekly visits by a doctor to administer the chaulmoogra oil injections, and also recounts his experiences receiving the new cure in 1948. These experiences reflect a strong stigma and fear of leprosy, as described through the interpreter, Margaret Dempsey:

> He came here [from Bourail in 1928] when he was eight.... When he was thirteen he went for about [a total of] five years.... In 1940 he came back, and he is here since 1940, until now. About seventy years here. He is one of the last from that time. He knew the beginning of this place.... [There were] eighty people at that time when he arrived.... It wasn't easy, it was difficult, even to come here, because there was no road, and one boat.... No running water, no kitchen, they just had tanks.... The people, they put their own bandages on and they looked after each other.... There was a big fence and people couldn't come here. They rowed boats. There is no efficient treatment at that time. They put them here to protect the population, it was a form of isolation. Because there was no treatment, it was just a matter of protecting the population.[29]

The idea that total isolation was required to "protect the population"[30] is perhaps a rationalization by Honoré that his isolation was necessary to prevent contagion of others by himself, or a repetition of the solution articulated by the health authorities. In the memoirs of other pensioners it is suggested that leprosy sufferers felt the need to go to Ducos to save their families from contagion, as well as the rejection families would face from local communities due to their leprosy.[31] Honoré describes the early years prior to the availability of sulphones:

> There were no nurses, just the people who were less ill looked after the others.... The doctor came twice a week with injections ... chaulmoogra ... very painful.... Twenty years he had that.... He always thought it was going to do something positive, so he didn't try not to have it. Some people did, some people decided not to continue and they stopped. At the beginning it did something, it improved.... And then after, the illness took over. Not like the treatment today where there is a good result.[32]
>
> Always the doctor who did the [chaulmoogra] injections came twice a week.... It was so painful that some people gave up, and they hid. It didn't absorb, in fact ... it was difficult to find a place to do the injection. So that is why some of them hid. They also had to swallow the oil as well. It was pure oil, and he says it tasted awful. There was something else in the injections.... When they gave him injections ... it made him feel ill. It increased the rate of the heart. There was no other treatment.[33]
>
> When he was younger he didn't have a big problem [with leprosy], it was more from 1945 onwards that he had more problems. He said there is always a moment when the illness takes over. For twenty years he controlled the illness, and then ... once the illness takes over the person says there is no point in being treated any more because it is finished.[34]

2. Former Penitentiaries as Leprosaria

Honoré recalls the arrival of the sulphone treatment:

> He was very very ill, it was his last chance in 1948. It was an injection, an intravenous injection. An American treatment ... [administered by] the army doctors.... The doctor only wanted to treat some people, he wanted to experiment, but everybody wanted the medicine, and he said wait, wait, until he took the ones with the least disease. He says that the doctor had selected a few people.... He wanted to test them, because he wasn't sure it was going to be effective. When he saw that it worked well, they gave the treatment to everybody. It worked very well. Especially when they gave an injection.[35]
>
> *Was he in the first batch?* No, afterwards, because he was already too ill. First they took the people who had more chance of surviving. They had to be careful. You shouldn't have problems with your kidneys or anything like that.... Every morning the treatment for four months.... A big reaction. He was very ill and he thought he would never be able to resist, and then finally he resisted, and then it left.... At the beginning ... they had pains everywhere, it was as if the illness exploded because of the treatment. Two and half years his treatment. And till now he has never suffered like that again.[36]

This description of the medical decision to trial the drugs on the least affected patients differs from the unanimous decision between doctors and patients in Makogai to initially trial it on the most advanced cases.[37] It reflects a more authoritarian approach in decision making by the French authorities, as compared to a more open process at Makogai. However, the gender segregation and hygiene rules were less rigorously enforced at Ducos than at Makogai. At Ducos there was no gender segregation, and families lived in self-constructed homes in villages at the leprosarium without strict hygiene surveillance, although the residents were restricted to the fenced area of the leprosarium. Patients were not discharged as at Makogai, so admission to Ducos was a life sentence. These different conditions appear to have imposed different ideas of stigma on the psyche of those isolated at the leprosaria, as well as with the public.[38]

By 1952, two SMSM sisters at Ducos, M. Othilde and M. Irma, contracted leprosy. Sister Irma remained a patient, working among the patients for twenty-five years. In 1956 she was declared free of leprosy, and died, age ninety-five, in 1987.[39] Both Honoré and P. J. Twomey, in his reports relating to Noumea, recall these sisters.[40] In a radio broadcast Twomey spoke about his meeting with Sister M. Othilde, who had been working at Ducos about fifteen years:

> [She] contracted the disease while working there. She has remarkable influence with the 150 native lepers who respect and love her for her great devotion to them. She elected to live with the lepers.... I have seen this sister making her way across the fields to bring in the milk or to feed the pigs ... there is no forty hour week for this worker.[41]

Honoré recalls Sister Othilde being diagnosed with leprosy:

> He [remembers] the sisters ... from 1933.... A sister went swimming, and somebody said she had something on her skin, and somebody said you've got leprosy, and they tested and she had leprosy.... She wasn't a nurse. She did teaching. Sister Othilde, she was the one that had leprosy. After that she came here and she started to look after the people who were ill.... She looks after people with leprosy. She looked after the people who were dying, there were a lot of people who were really at the end, and she looked after them.... They were at the hospital, but some died at home in the houses.... It was not complicated, it was very simple, so when somebody died, they were buried and it was the end. Now it is more complicated. At the cemetery they buried them very quickly, not much formality. *It would have been a sad time for many people sometimes here?* They were used to an environment where there was a lot of suffering, so for them it wasn't really a big problem.[42]

This latter comment is a revealing statement by Honoré because little or no direct comment has been made, in retrospect, on the mental anguish that interviewees routinely must have had to endure while witnessing the terminal suffering of advanced cases of leprosy.

Honoré went on to explain the problems he now has to endure that greatly diminished his quality of life.

> [His favorite pastime was reading] the books at the library. It was a good library, but now there are not a lot of people, before there were more people.... Before there were a lot of activities. Looking after the grounds, building houses, looking after the roads, a lot of work here was done by the people here. There were animals, cattle.... Just in the last fifteen years he has had problems with his eyes; until then there were no problems with them. He said if he had been well treated before he wouldn't have had this problem. [In] 1988, when he started to have problems with his eyes, he saw the optometrist, but the problem is, the damage was already done. With today's treatment it wouldn't have happened. It is the worst handicap, his eyes.[43]

Honoré's comments demonstrate some of the advantages of being placed in leprosaria, especially for young children who benefited from the education facilities available. If children with leprosy had lived in partial isolation in their own villages, they would have been excluded and unable to attend local schools or obtain traditional education in their villages. In addition, comfort and companionship was found in the company of people who suffered from the same condition. Leprosaria in New Caledonia provided an opportunity to create their own community and particularly to support and care for each other; yet at the same time, this undoubtedly caused fear about their own futures as they witnessed the gradual decay of advanced cases and envisaged the same end for themselves prior to the new medication. A salient feature of this testimony is the continued need for facilities at leprosaria because of the continuing disabilities of older patients, especially prior to the availability of sulphones. The leprosaria became home to the residents since they had lost contact with their own families, having had to remain in isolation for many years. Additionally, the strong stigma associated with leprosy often meant that families did not want to maintain contact, and patients had no homes to return to when discharged after the 1970s.[44]

The South Pacific Commission conducted tests in the 1950s to assess the value of the BCG vaccine, *Bacille Calmette-Guerin*, in the Loyalty Islands — namely, Lifou, Maré and Ouvea — which had small stable populations relatively isolated off the east coast of the main island. BCG had proved useful against tuberculosis bacilli *mycobacterium* and was being assessed for protection against *M. Lepra*. Although the results were inconclusive at that point because a longer trial period was deemed necessary, the report provides endemicity figures for each island, being 2.26% for Lifou, 2.99% for Maré and 3.37% for Ouvea.[45] These percentages represent high endemicity levels despite the availability of new treatments. Patients that could benefit from the facilities at the Ducos leprosarium were transferred, and by 1958 all leprosy patients were at Ducos, numbering 300 residents.[46] No details were found relating to patients being discharged from Ducos, and according to Dr. Farrugia, who was in charge in the late 1970s, patients who had been brought to Ducos would spend the rest of their lives at the Center. It is likely that the failure of these trials exacerbated the fear and stigma of leprosy. The gates to Ducos remained firmly closed, and it was not until Dr. Farrugia arrived in 1976 that the gates to Ducos were permanently opened and patients allowed to come and go as they pleased if they were certified as cured.[47]

The LTB and Other Charitable Involvement at Ducos

The published memoirs of the residents at Ducos, *L'hymne à la vie des pensionnaires du Centre Raoul Follereau*, contain examples of the community life, friendships and rivalries at Ducos, including instances of charitable help from outsiders. In particular, the memoirs contain touching reminiscences of the friendships and kindness of American soldiers stationed near Ducos during World War Two.[48] What is perhaps surprising is the reported lack of fear on the part of the American troops, who regularly visited the leprosarium and donated "truck loads of food ... bandages ... water soaked goods ... worthless to the army ... precious to us."[49] One patient indicated there was no fear between the Americans and patients, especially the black soldiers.[50] Medical supplies at the leprosarium were minimal, but during the war years, with the generosity of the U.S. Army handouts, provisions were abundant.[51]

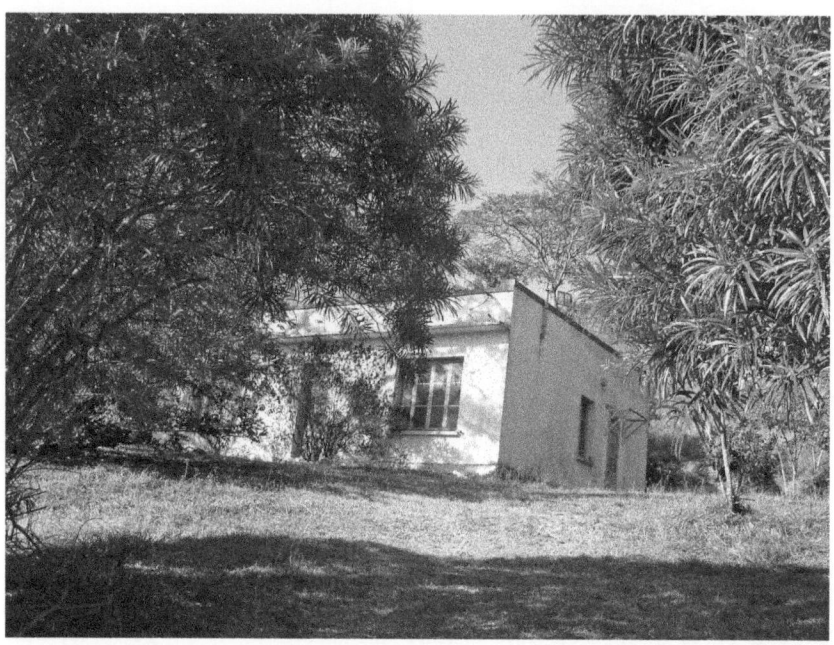

"New Zealand House," a building donated by P. J. Twomey on behalf of the LTB at RFC Ducos.

It was during the war years that a New Zealand soldier stationed in New Caledonia wrote to Patrick Twomey, informing him of the poor conditions of leprosy patients; and in 1944 the LTB sent the first donation of NZ $500 in goods to Ducos.[52] This was a timely intervention, as the American donations ended with the withdrawal of the American troops. Later that year Twomey visited Ducos, as well as a native lazarette at Houailou, and was distressed at the conditions there, which he considered fell far behind the facilities then available at Makogai. It was decided that annual allocations be remitted by the LTB to New Caledonia.[53] It is likely that the poor conditions at Ducos, compared to the facilities available at Makogai, contributed to the higher level of stigma evident in New Caledonia than in Fiji.

Bobin reports in 1952 that the French philanthropist Raoul Follereau visited Ducos, and that same year, with the help of the Red Cross and the Leprosy Trust Board, Ducos became a "proper hospital."[54] Numa Daly of the Red Cross, Henri Bonneaud, Monsieur Potter of the Lions Club and other local Noumean benefactors, together with the administrators of the Ducos Center and Leprosy Trust Board, formed a New Caledonia Support Committee for the leprosarium in 1952.[55] The following year Twomey attended the opening ceremony of an infirmary erected by the LTB, now known as New

Zealand House, and was awarded the Cross of the Legion of Honor for his dedication to the welfare of leprosy sufferers.[56] This is one of the very few honors bestowed on a New Zealander by the French, and a street in Noumea was named *Rue P. J. Twomey, Bienfaiteur,* which still exists today.[57]

Twomey had visited Ducos on a previous occasion, staying at the Center, and in 1949 organized the provision of numerous medical facilities and items for the comfort of patients, including a movie projector, x-ray machine and electrotherapy apparatus, although the latter items caused a few problems since electricity was not available at Ducos until 1950.[58] By Twomey's third visit in 1952, these matters had been resolved, and Dr. Feron was appointed medical resident at Ducos, becoming a friend of the patients. Dr. Feron subsequently chose, along with other benefactors, such as M. Potter, to be buried with the patients at Ducos cemetery.[59] The LTB arranged for two of the nursing sisters and Dr. Feron to travel to Makogai for refresher courses with Dr. Austin, Makogai's medical superintendent, and it is reported that "the cross-fertilisation of the two centres yielded benefits to both."[60]

In 1956 Raoul Follereau visited the Center again, and at his request Ducos participated in 1956 World Leprosy Day, upon which the center opened it gates for the first time officially for one day to Noumeans. Following his generous support of the Center, in 1958 the leprosarium was named the Raoul Follereau Center. By this time Ducos was composed of two villages situated in the valley, N'Bi and N'Du, one for the Melanesians and the other for Europeans.[61] Cattle and pigs were raised at these agricultural villages, and three hundred head and an abattoir were on site. The Melanesians tended the gardens for their own use and for supply to the leprosarium. A school teacher was based at the Center, and there were trade schools for boys, and cooking and dressmaking for the girls to enable the residents to be self-sufficient, these skills not being intended as a useful trade upon discharge as at Makogai. With no gender segregation, the patients married and had children, and there the patients died, with their remains still in a large cemetery at Ducos. Later, the Melanesians and Europeans were regrouped to live together, ending racial segregation, but this apparently caused difficulties and hardship because of the enforced moves into homes built by others and gardens with different produce.[62]

Leprosy on the Island and at Ducos Since the Late 1960s

In the late 1970s, as part of his medical duties while stationed at Koumac in northern New Caledonia, the military doctor Jacques Michaudel visited a remote tribal area every three months, where he tended to the needs of about six leprosy sufferers who lived by themselves.[63] It was a day's trek uphill on horseback to reach the village to administer the medication. Michaudel believed the group had been rejected by their families but chose not to go to the earlier leprosarium at Belep or later at Ducos. Michaudel also visited elderly non-contagious leprosy sufferers who had remained at Belep. He was also flown from Koumac to tend emergencies at Belep — mainly due, he said, to violence stemming from the availability of alcohol, for which Melanesians had little tolerance.[64]

Sister Noëllie (b. 1928) said that as a girl she had been impressed by the local SMSM nursing sisters and chose to become a novitiate and trained as a nurse.[65] Subsequently in 1967/8 she was sent to care for leprosy sufferers at Belep. Sister Noëllie spoke in French, with translations by two English-speaking SMSM, Sisters Danielle and Teresia. Despite the closure of the leprosarium at Belep as early as 1898, Sister Noëllie said she worked with leprosy sufferers in the late 1960s who continued to live on the island caring for one another with no medical facilities on hand, but were visited as required by a doctor from the mainland.

Dr. Jacques Michaudel's description of his duties while stationed at the northern center of Koumac tie in with Sister Noëllie's testimony relating to leprosy sufferers remaining at Belep who were burnt out and/or non-contagious cases. According to Michaudel, regular leprosy treatment was provided by the main hospital in Noumea, and the SMSM sisters ran a clinic on the island.[66] Although no further archival or medical material was available to furnish definitive details, the scenario of small colonies of leprosy sufferers in each of the districts of the main island is likely to have been repeated, operating along similar lines as the descriptions given by Dr. Jacques Michaudel and Sister Noëllie.

Sister Noëllie's mother was a local Melanesian and her father, a Japanese, who was repatriated during the war. She described her understanding of the leprosy station at Belep, which ties in with the introductory background given earlier, as well as her own experiences working with leprosy sufferers at Belep in 1967–69, and at Ducos from 1979 onwards:

> Before, long time ago, people from Belep had been put out from their island and put on the big island, on the main island New Caledonia.... On the island of Belep they put the sick people coming from everywhere else.... So Sister Mary of the Cross [Sister Marie de la Croix] she was there.... Before the Cluny sisters came ... it was a sick patient, a man, who used to care for the other ones. So they looked after themselves and he was looking after the other ones.... The doctor from Koumac used to go to Belep. This was a long time ago, so people used to live in the island like this, no Center, no hospital, and Sister de la Croix went there to look after them. Also one of the patients used

2. Former Penitentiaries as Leprosaria

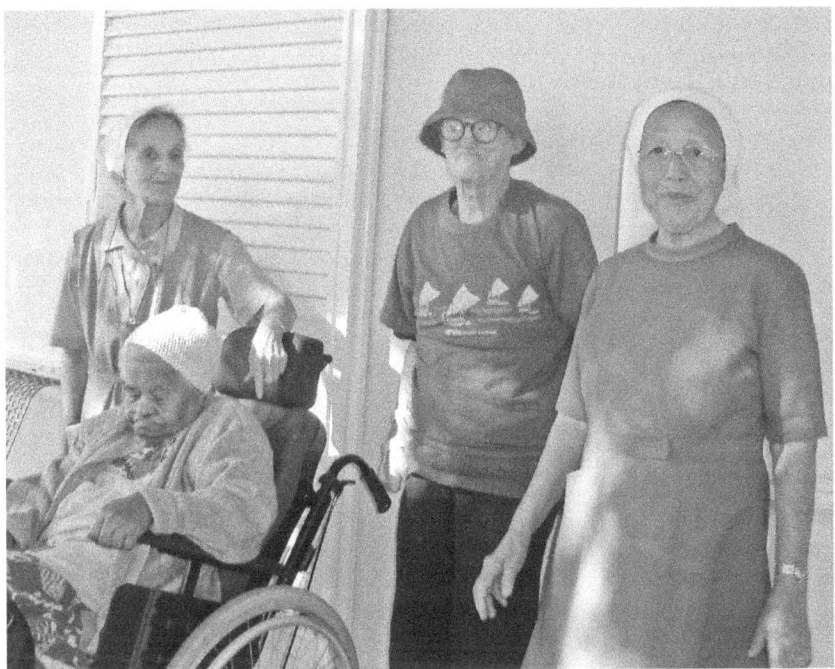

Sister Nöellie Thiossey SMSM (right) and Honoré Tourte (second from right) with others at RFC Ducos.

to assist the other ones ... she was the only one, and another lady, another person helped her. The other one was teaching.... When she needed something, she used to phone to the doctor in Koumac and ask for what she wanted.... [Then] the sick people from Belep they have been sent to small island not far from Raoul Follereau [Ile aux Chèvres]. Because at that time Raoul Follereau was a place for... prisoners.... So when the convicts had been released, the sick people came there, it became a leprosy center. A lot of patients had gone, some of them were still in the village, because they didn't want to come here [Ducos]; they didn't want to leave their village.[67]

At the time we had one sister, Sister Fidelia, an Italian sister ... the military doctor, who depend on them and the doctor asked her to go to Raoul Follereau.... Otherwise someone else could have come and then we would have lost the place. After a time she [Sister Noellie] was in Belep.... And then she went to Pouebo. Pouebo is a hospital in the north and they used to go every two weeks to ... make injections, give medicine to the leprosy in the village.... In Belep it was in 1967–68 and Pouebo 1970.... At Belep, the sick people were in their village.[68]

Dr. Roland Farrugia was the leprologist for the World Health Organization from 1980 until 1999, and since his retirement was appointed as the leprosy consultant for the PLF. He recalled his first encounter with leprosy as a newly qualified doctor at the Raoul Follereau Center in 1976, and described his involvement at Ducos as follows:

> I was posted to New Caledonia as the director of the leprosarium.... I was not particularly happy because I had no desire of doing anything with leprosy.... Because of the length of the flight from Paris to Noumea I had ample time to go back to my [student] notes and start learning again what I had already forgotten.... My interest was in dermatology, but quickly I found out that I was getting more and more involved.... Within a year, I was fully interested in leprosy, and it became something that I really wanted to do.[69]
>
> When I arrived, the Center was a beautiful thing to behold. You could arrive from the top of two valleys, and in the beginning they had given one valley for the natives and the other for the whites — that shows you how many white people had had leprosy. The Center was in the two valleys, and the whole compound formed a peninsula. And at the top end of the peninsula you had a jetty, and people would be brought from Noumea by boat to the jetty with leprosy patients, white or natives. They would [dis]embark from the boat. There was a little cabin with a sentry servant making sure that nobody would escape from the Center. They would be welcomed one way or the other, registered, give them their names and so on, enter the Center and that was it for the rest of their lives.... When I arrived you must remember we had already had three decades of Dapsone, so things were already looking better. We knew ... the disease, the processes.[70]

Dr. Farrugia's testimony confirms the strict enforcement of isolation for leprosy sufferers, who appear to have had no possibility of discharge, irrespective of whether the leprosy might have ceased to be infectious. His testimony goes on to demonstrate the level of expertise of the sisters in tending leprosy patients, and a certain level of protectiveness:

> I met the staff ... composed of Sisters Missionary of the Society of Mary.... I think I did the right thing by telling them straight away that I knew nothing and I was counting on them to show me the ropes, even from the most basic things.... I suppose they said alright we'll do it, so they started showing me really, practically on the skin or on the examination of the face, arms or legs.... We had four sisters ... one sister on duty sleeping at the Center every night.... They would take a week in turns ... come to the Center all day. Oh they were marvellous persons really.... Sister Yves [Cluny order] was the elder one ... she was more or less in charge ... a dominant person, because of her knowledge. To me she was a wonderful teacher.... First of all, I was absolutely puzzled why we had all those people there doing nothing. And the sisters were quite happy to keep everybody under their wings, especially Sister Yves. You know she had her own patients and she would just nurse them like babies. And I remember one ... I suspect had pretended for years to be unable to wash himself and so on, because sister Yves would do it for him every day, so why not? She would wash him, she would put talcum powder everywhere and so on,

and fresh clothes, and ... who was totally inert, would suddenly become alive and go to play cards with the elders. Sister Yves was so attentive.... At the Center we had something like 150 patients resident.[71]

Inevitably, the long isolation led to close relationships between the nursing sisters and patients. This description indicates the care for the physical (and not merely spiritual) needs of the patients by the mission sisters. The sisters' protectiveness did not appear to be totally overwhelming in Ducos, as the changes introduced by Dr. Farrugia, allowing freedom to residents and opening the doors to the public, were not opposed:

> But a few things happened; first of all, the Center had been closed, locked up from real life for decades, the patients were not allowed to get out.... The MDT had not arrived yet. When I got there we still had only Dapsone, so I must point this out. That was really the time when we started finding out that we had more and more resistant cases of the patients to Dapsone, and it became a global problem. That's why ... at the end of the '70s early '80s, they had to devise a new treatment, and it was more than urgent because probably 80% of all cases were already resistant to Dapsone and we had absolutely nothing else. It was the mode of therapy everywhere.... Dapsone still has some value up to now, we still use Dapsone but never as a mono-therapy. Something that you might know with Dapsone was in the history of medicine for leprosy, the first drug against leprosy. Before Dapsone ... chaulmoogra oil and like that, very sticky, itchy and did nothing, absolutely nothing. [Dapsone] resistance started three decades later.[72]
>
> When I arrived I found the situation was absolutely unusual. I must say that in New Caledonia the subject of leprosy is taboo because there is probably not one of all the family of white settlers that didn't have cases of leprosy in their families. *They didn't like to talk about it?* No, because nearly all the families had had leprosy. Apparently it [leprosy] started in Loyalty Islands ... Maré, Lifou and Ouvea.... Nobody knew what it was ... because they had never known it before. But it wasn't just the local Melanesians who were getting leprosy, there were actually a lot of white people as well. Totally unusual ... it's not because white people are not susceptible to leprosy, it's because usually everywhere in the world we have white settlers, the level of living conditions is so much better for whites than the natives. So they escape a lot of infections because they live better. They [people] are more open to infections by [living] crowded in houses, poor nutrition.... In New Caledonia the people were very poor, I mean poor level socially speaking of people, and they more or less adopted the living conditions of the natives, which was very poor hygiene.[73]
>
> I would say [accuracy of] diagnosis was nearly 100% because the treatment had been so bad before the Dapsone, so that everybody had damage in their hands, face, feet, some people were really living wrecks with no teeth, blind.... That lady I'm talking about, when I saw her, she had no fingers, she was blind, she had a problem with her nose and front teeth. She couldn't walk, she had an amputee on one foot and she was living by herself. She had been mar-

ried, her husband was in the Center too, but her husband had died and she was living in a bungalow by herself. We had to give her a servant to look after her because she was totally unable to do anything for herself.[74]

At the Center the people were isolated and the stigma against leprosy was enormous.... There was a lot of little bungalows and people were living there sometimes in couples, married or not married. Some of them had children, we had children with leprosy.... People were in the Center, they wouldn't go out. Even at the hospital the staff especially, the local staff, nurses and so on, wouldn't have anything to do with them, would refuse to do anything or touch them. It was that serious. *What about the families of these people, did they come to visit, was there any contact?* No. *Do you think they were rejected by their families?* Oh, in a lot of cases yes, they were rejected, people were quite happy to have leprosy secluded somewhere and taken away.... *So there was no opposition to this isolation from the families?* No, it was compulsory. It was compulsory anywhere, they would be forcibly taken, and taken to the Center.... If you were diagnosed by a specialist as having leprosy, that was it. The same day you were taken to the Center.... I remember an old lady from one of the white families, she had arrived at the Center when she was a teenager, and she would tell us that one day she was in school when suddenly there was an examination for one reason or the other and the doctor said, "Oh, I must examine that more seriously." And the diagnosis was she had leprosy. And she was taken away from family, school to the Center just like that.[75]

This testimony indicates the high level of stigma prevalent in the public mind in New Caledonia, which was not alleviated but reinforced by the strict isolation imposed by health authorities right into the 1980s.

Both Dr. Beckett, arriving at Makogai in the late 1950s, and Dr. Farrugia, at Ducos in the 1970s, questioned why medically fit and non-contagious people should be kept long-term in isolation facilities, and both implemented changes in policies relating to the internment of such people. In Makogai the changes involved the length of time patients needed to be tested clear of contagion, from a two to one year period, before discharge. Dr. Farrugia indicates that patients had not been eligible for discharge prior to his arrival, and the following extract demonstrates the changes he put in place. The gates were opened, allowing inmates to come and go as they pleased, but the opposition to his changes again indicates the high level of stigma present:

After a little while, when I started to think for myself about leprosy, there was no reason why the patients had to be secluded like that, and I decided to open the Center. First reaction came from the officials from the government, and one day I got a phone call telling me, can you give us the explanation about this and that, why did you allow this one, this one and this one, to get out of the Center? They were seen on the streets in Noumea. And I said yes, I know that because the doors are now open. But they said, "But you must be mad, what are you doing?" I said well look, we have to reason a little bit, they are cured or they are not. If they are cured, what are they doing here? Except that we just support them physically, that's all. So if they're cured, how can I prevent them from going wherever they want, in the streets, talking, touching people and so on, selling their goods, which was totally forbidden at that point in time, and going to the hospital. I said no, if I decided they are cured then they can leave the Center anytime. So it took some time to convince people, even at the hospital. I'm not talking about the doctors, the doctors were medical doctors at that time, all the medical services were assured by medical doctors like myself and they had no prejudice or stigma against leprosy, but the staff in all services, mainly the local nurses and so on, were very difficult to convince. Very hard to change their mind regarding leprosy, but we did.... It was very difficult to change the policy — you had leprosy, you had to go to the Center. I changed that but it took me years.[76]

Here medical knowledge is shown to have taken a long time to impinge on public ideas, as real fear of the disease itself persists:

I guess ... it was a fear, not a fear based on technical knowledge or medical knowledge, it is just a fear of a disease. So they would tell them don't talk about them, don't talk to them. They would do anything, they would burn their houses and everything and so on, and they would certainly not touch anything prepared as food by leprosy patients. But that [stigma] wouldn't apply to doctors for some reason because by the same token it was based on nothing except a feeling for fear of the disease. By the same token there was no fear for a doctor who was in contact with them. *Were they [the public] hesitant about the first fair [annual fair/kermesse instigated by Dr. Farrugia] perhaps?* Oh yes, absolutely. But in other countries it could go much further than that. I saw countries where leprosy patients were being banned from villages.... They were forbidden to bathe or drink the water from the river because that water would come down to other villages.[77]

It appears that the total enforced isolation imposed on leprosy sufferers had contributed to perceptions of dread and fear of leprosy, maintaining a corresponding high level of stigma. Farrugia's testimony supports a conclusion that fear of the disease itself was the main cause of stigma. Policies of isolation, which kept patients out of sight, aggravated fears of contagion that sustained stigma, and not until the general public learned for themselves by exposure to leprosy sufferers that the risk of contagion from these people was very low, and that the disease could be virtually cured, did fear and stigma began to diminish, as explained further by Dr. Farrugia:

Then I went further and I invited people to visit the Center, and I thought that the best way was to have an annual fair. So I did it, and it was a little bit against general opinion and so on. *What was it like the first one?* A success. But I must say not with the locals. It was mainly people from France, who didn't know much about leprosy and had no stigma so they did come.[78]

This suggestion that the French knew little about leprosy and therefore did not associate the stigma with the disease supports the idea proposed earlier that people generally thought leprosy was a disease of the past and they were unlikely to be affected by it. The fact that medical doctors had invited them to the fair at Ducos reassured them that there was no risk of contagion. Further measures were taken in attempting to integrate leprosy sufferers back into the community:

> Now, with help of various key people, we had started the handicrafts at the Center ... ways of supporting themselves because we would sell them. We came quickly to the idea that if they produced enough that could go into the annual fair ... we had that one [a patient volunteer] and he was really a phenomenon of natural skills, of any handicraft possible, he could do anything. We had courses given in the Center from the people who had handicraft shops and that kind of thing in the city. They would come and show people what to do in the handicrafts ... and this one proved himself as a natural phenomenon, and quickly he became so skilled that he did absolutely beautiful, beautiful things. And eventually ... he was set free from the Center ... to have his life and earn a very good life ... eventually became a partner in a shop. The rule that obliged him to stay was actually beneficial to the Center itself, as he was the tool, as it were, to trigger off the development of the skills, so it was really a very positive thing.[79]
>
> The annual fair became something that, more and more, locals eventually accepted.... We decided for the first time to give more and more emphasis to our fair, having more and more things to sell, more and more entertainment. We had groups of dancers coming, singing, dancing, local dancers. And we started having food stalls selling food, drinks and so on, and in a few years it became something.... [Food] was a big step for people ... because food is a very personal and intimate thing.... And when you start to buy food off people who have had leprosy, that is a big step. *How did the sisters and staff at the Center respond to all this, did they like the change?* Yes they did, they could see that there was no real need to keep the old rules and so on. There was no need. They would not participate that much in entertainment but that was alright, but they were perfectly alright.[80]

Dr. Farrugia's testimony indicates that the religious sisters were happy to have the patients under their care allowed to leave the leprosarium and return to normal lives when possible. Sister Yves in charge of Ducos, and Sister Nöellie, whose testimony follows shortly, were both working at Ducos at this time, and despite a lifetime working with leprosy sufferers, neither opposed the changes.

The strict enforcement of isolation of leprosy sufferers in what were previously areas of internment for prisoners might have added to the perceived danger of the disease and its unfortunate victims posing a threat to the community at large. Despite contacts with leprologists in Fiji and the Pacific region, and trials of BCG vaccine in the Loyalty Islands, the New Caledonian health officials appear to have been tardy in ending isolation of leprosy patients, which would have in turn signaled a turning point for the associated problem of stigma. Perhaps the inconclusive results of the BCG tests clouded the issue of contagion, and officials were reluctant to totally do away with isolation. This supports the suggestion that medical mysteries associated with leprosy played a part in sustaining stigma in New Caledonia.

It is not known what attitudes prevailed toward leprosy sufferers within indigenous village communities. But, as in the case of Honoré, patients did not feel able to return home, nor would many have felt it possible to pick up the threads of an ordinary lifestyle or find employment. Therefore, they had little option but to remain at the Center.[81] Ducos continued to serve as a home to these people, especially as they required further treatment associated with the difficulties of aging and paralysis, and the leprosarium provided free daily care and specialist services, such as plastic and orthopaedic surgery and physiotherapy.

Continuing SMSM Involvement

Sister Noëllie provided additional details regarding the lifestyle of the leprosy sufferers at Ducos, and recounted, through the interpreter, her continued efforts to help those still remaining at the Center:

> In 1979, when Sister Noëllie arrived, there were two villages at the Raoul Follereau Center. One for the Melanesians and one for the European sick people ... because they were not mixed. Sister worked in the Melanesian village. In 1986 they put everyone together. Before there were a lot of children, now there are no children.... There was a small house for those who were married.... When she arrived in 1979 there were ten children. They had a school.... When she arrived the sick didn't do the cooking, someone [was employed] there for the cooking. He was helped by sick older people who are not contagious any more. The kitchen was on the Melanesian side, and they used to bring the food to the other side. And for the single people. Those who were very sick, they were at the infirmary, nursing center.[82]
>
> The children, most of them, were Melanesian. The girls were in the house of the Melanesian women. The boys were with the men, Melanesian. At the beginning, the patients who were not contagious used to help for the dressings and also for the cleaning. There was no nursing aid, health care workers. Those who worked in the kitchen, the hospital used to give them a little bit of money. Some Vietnamese, Chinese, even Melanesian, they have a small garden and they sell the produce, vegetables, to the cooking kitchen. So now there is a small store also there, and the one who works in the store, they have small money also.... The oldest one [sister] was Sister Yves.... Every morning you have the care ... seven o'clock started.... Breakfast first, then the care, like now.

> Now it is not so bad, before they had the very bad conditions, ulcers, so you had to make bath, feet first. Doctor used to come three times a week.... The doctor used to come from eight to ten [o'clock] to one village, and from ten to twelve to the other village.[83]

During her working life with leprosy sufferers, Sister Nöellie described two sad cases which made an impression on her, reflecting the strong stigma attached to leprosy. There is no indication of traditional biblical ideas of stigma, but notions of shame and fear of contagion which underlie stigma in New Caledonia:

> The story of two small boys: They arrived by themselves, the father had died, and they were sick, the two of them. This is in 1979–80. So nine years old and seven years old, two brothers, they came to the Center, and the family did not come and see them. Meanwhile, the mother became very sick, here in the hospital. There was a message, this man he wants to bring them to the mother, so he brought these two children to see the mother in the hospital. When they arrived close to the bed of the mother, the mother seems not to see them and not to know them. The doctor was sorry for these two children and asked them if they want to go somewhere. So he took them and went to Tio with another sister of ours, for eight days with the two boys. When they came back, someone asked them if they were happy. "We have been very happy, you want to replace our mother?"[84]
>
> A Chinese, when he came to the Center, his wife get married with someone else. And Sister Fidelia went one day to New Zealand, and she found the family of this man in New Zealand. And the small grandson wants to come here and see his grandfather. And here the grandfather prepare everything to welcome the small boy. At the last moment the grandmother didn't want him to come here.... After this the man let himself go, to die, and maybe this is the cause of him not to fight.... His family didn't say to the rest of the family that he was sick and he was there.... One of his nieces came to Raoul Follereau and she saw the name of this man, her uncle, and she said I want to see my uncle. But the uncle said no. Then someone said, yes you have to see your niece, so he said okay. She looks after him until he died.[85]
>
> They would like to close this Center, but because these people who do not want to go back to their village or their family do not want to have them, they cannot close the Center. One of them has been there over sixty years. They can stay or go back to their family, but maybe they don't want to go, maybe because they have been so long here.[86]

This testimony indicates the tragedies involved in the separation of families, but at the same time it highlights the importance of the leprosarium in their lives. The leprosarium, after so many years of being their home, is the only home they know. Sister Noëllie went on to describe the present situation at Ducos, where the leprosy sufferers expect to end their days, and the arrangements she organized for their funerals:

It is their house, their family house.... Those who are there, because they do not want to go back to their village, and when they die some are buried in the Center, or not far from the Center, and some are sent back to their village. But everything is ready before, and she [Sister Noëllie] is the one who gets everything ready for their funeral, everything. Even for the small money that they have, she look after this so the money will be used at least for the funeral first. [Interpreter: Noëllie is doing a very good job for that, for them.] When one dies, the one in charge contact the family first.... And if the family can do all the arrangements, they do. Otherwise she [Noëllie] is the one who makes the arrangements. Most of the time the arrangements are done before. Everything is okay for all of them now. So the sick people here they are doing small things, and selling, and they get some money from this. And they have realized that the family took all this money and nothing left for the funeral. Now they have arranged everything with this money, and what is left over is given to the family. Now you have a Catholic mass and also the Protestant. So every Sunday you have these two religions present.[87]

Sister Noëllie, having worked with the residents at Raoul Follereau Center for over forty years, helped the last remaining residents tidy up their earthly affairs by ensuring a will was made outlining their wishes, and making provision for their funerals, which in a sense did provide that the leprosy sufferers were suitably prepared for the life everlasting, as proposed by Edmond. During their earlier lives suffering with leprosy, the patients had received physical treatment and daily care from the sisters; but in their autumn years, dealing with the matter of death was a pragmatic means by which assistance was offered to residents by Sister Noëllie to ensure a dignified and orderly departure from this world. It is most likely spiritual matters were also discussed between the religious and the leprosy sufferers, but no reference was made to these affairs in the oral histories. If this aspect was a greater priority of the sisters interviewed, it is most likely that the spiritual benefits would have been mentioned by Sister Noëllie. Instead, what is apparent is a concern for the patients' physical wellbeing and benefits that could be gained to lead a useful life in this world, and for a dignified exit, rather than merely preparation for the afterlife.

The strict regulations pertaining to leprosy and isolation in New Caledonia appear to have contributed to public views and fears towards leprosy, particularly because, as Roland Farrugia indicated, leprosy had affected most families in New Caledonia, giving leprosy a strong and perhaps more terrifying profile, particularly among westerners. The Melanesian leprosy sufferers appear to have had more freedom of movement to return to their villages if they wished, while the Caldoches had less, even no, choice. The poorer Caldoches had little opportunity to find employment in Noumea, where stigma still appears to remain a problem, as is evident in Sister Noëllie's comment that even after her close association with leprosy sufferers at Ducos, whenever she meets old patients from the Center, leprosy is never mentioned:

> When they come to the Center, these old patients, she [Sister Noëllie] welcome them, but she doesn't give them the impression that they have been here.... They don't talk about that.... If the family talk about this, okay, but they will never bring it up.[88]

The strong stigma no doubt stems from the strict policy of enforced segregation, and the closed door policy of the Raoul Follereau Center, despite the philanthropic activities of individuals and groups to provide for leprosy sufferers. Fear of leprosy remained, even as late as 1980, when Dr. Farrugia reported that leprosy stigma was still a serious problem. This tightly closed isolation is late in comparison with what occurred in Fiji and Vanuatu. The difference in Fiji was the closing of Makogai and the establishment of P.J. Twomey Memorial Hospital in Suva in 1969. With the hospital near the center of Suva, and patients free to come and go as they liked, Fijians became more aware of leprosy while at the same time coming to realize that the cured leprosy patients no longer posed a risk of contagion. This realization, confirmed by any lack of resurgence of leprosy in Fiji, would have removed a level of fear of contagion, which undoubtedly lies at the heart of stigma towards leprosy suffers. Although the incidence of leprosy in New Caledonia has fluctuated and gradually fallen over a long period, overall the incidence has remained higher.[89] Conditions on the outskirts of Noumea were poor and overcrowded, and as Dr. Farrugia pointed out:

> When you live in a poor city, overcrowded, in very bad living conditions, bad nutrition and hard work at all times, of course if you are put in presence of somebody who is active and disseminates leprosy bacilli, the chances of catching the leprosy disease is much, much higher.[90]

Dr. Farrugia related a disturbing case, despite the new effective treatments, which perhaps indicates why attitudes towards leprosy were still a problem in New Caledonia, and why advanced cases did not always seek out, or even avoided, treatment:

> We had a case, which was a very difficult case, of somebody who presented a lepromatous form of leprosy, very infectious, and he was a schoolteacher, of all jobs. The fact that he was from an old white family, and he came to me in a state which was really very advanced, married with children.... But it was a problem in all of the country, you know, they wanted to isolate all the children in the school.... They would go to any expense from fear.... He was in the Center and he was a bad case because I suspect he was not regular [at taking his medication] ... not responsible enough, in spite of having that position.... A medical scandal of having a school teacher discovered with leprosy, an advanced form of leprosy ... I believe that he was not regular at all. *So what*

happened in the end? You don't perhaps know? I can't say, I had to bring him back twice to the center, and I left, so I don't know what happened.[91]

This story confirms that old attitudes towards leprosy took a long time to die in New Caledonia. Perhaps, despite re-education and the freedom of leprosy sufferers to go wherever they wanted, it was difficult to change from an environment where, as described by Dr. Farrugia earlier, isolation was compulsory and people were forcibly taken to a leprosarium, usually the same day as the diagnosis. Additionally, the high prevalence of leprosy in most families made the majority of the public feel they were at risk from the disease and its unfortunate victims. In these circumstances, despite the hardships imposed by isolation and separation from family, for leprosy sufferers the leprosarium at Ducos provided a place of long friendships and support in a caring atmosphere under the control of the sisters.

In 1990 the Territorial Hospital in Noumea took over the control of Raoul Follereau Center, and government nurses and staff ran the leprosarium. Some of the earlier religious sisters remained to assist patients for some time, but they had retired by 2006. A report by Dr. Crouzat, in charge of leprosy patients within the dermatology section, indicates that in 1998 there were only seventeen active cases of leprosy in New Caledonia, indicating a decrease in the incidence of leprosy. In 1983 there had been twenty-three new cases, whereas only five new cases appeared in 1998,[92] the overall incidence per 100,000 population being 15.6 and 2.54 respectively. By 2001 the incidence level rose to 3.29 per 100,000 population, with seven new cases that year.[93] These figures are higher than the elimination goal set for leprosy by the WHO of less than 1 per 100,000, and the incidence of leprosy in New Caledonia remains higher than in other South Pacific regions visited. Dr. Crouzat reports that a number of the new cases detected were at the late stage of the disease.[94] This would have contributed to the higher incidence of leprosy in the country, and the detection of leprosy at the late stages would have increased perceptions of fear in the public about the contagion, raising stigma towards the unfortunate victims with visible deformities.

Following the withdrawal of the SMSM and Cluny sisters, replaced by government nurses and staff in 1990, the easy familiarity and closeness between staff and patients is said to have diminished.[95] Although the patients said they now had more in terms of material goods than the earlier days, they preferred the Center being run by the sisters because they had enjoyed helping with the work and maintaining the Center. The government had demolished some of the older buildings, which upset many patients because they had originally helped build these. It was felt that the lack of religion and loss of the close relationship between staff and the patients had erased goodwill.[96] Instead of performing useful tasks, maintaining the grounds and having the independence to grow their own produce and meat, patients were provided with small government pensions. However, with the onslaught of old age and its attendant disabilities, let alone the ravages of leprosy itself, the government policies no doubt are a blessing, as there are no longer the younger, fitter leprosy sufferers to carry on the type of work done in the past. New cases were not isolated or admitted at Ducos but treated at the Territorial Hospital in Ducos.

It appears that the strong pervading stigma remaining attached to leprosy induced some people who had leprosy to hide in order to avoid being ostracized, thus allowing the active bacillus to be dispersed for extended periods. This, Dr. Farrugia suggests, is a contributory reason for the higher incidence of new cases of leprosy in New Caledonia — over four in any one year — as compared to the other Pacific islands visited for this project, and particular nearby in Vanuatu, where for the last three years only one case a year has been reported.[97] Even Dr. Farrugia considered the New Caledonian figures surprising, "considering the level of resources [were] totally different"[98] due to the wealth of the French Government in New Caledonia as compared to the rest of the Pacific countries. Nevertheless, the living conditions in New Caledonia are frequently more crowded and unhygienic for much of the poorer population because of the work undertaken in the prosperous but dirty conditions of the nickel mines operating on the main island very close to Ducos.[99]

The New Caledonian government severed connections with the PLF, and donations from the PLF ceased around the time of strained relations between New Zealand and France during the nuclear tests conducted by the French in 1985 in the Pacific region, which led to the incident involving the *Rainbow Warrior*, the boat containing protesters which was sunk. The New Caledonian government now provides for all the needs of leprosy patients, including the new MDT treatment. Patients are treated in the Territorial Hospital in Noumea, and the Raoul Follereau Center is likely to close when the last remaining residents have passed on. Because the PLF are no longer required to assist with meeting the needs of leprosy sufferers in New Caledonia, no intermediary personnel were available to facilitate introductions to people with leprosy living in their own homes or villages.

The staff at Raoul Follereau were protective of the residents, and as I am unable to speak French, it was not possible to converse freely on my visits to the Center. A visit to the SMSM sisters provided the opportunity to meet Sister Noëllie, who arranged the subsequent meeting with Honoré. Both Dr. Farrugia and Sister Noëllie's comments that families did not wish to speak about leprosy, even though most older families had experienced some leprosy first-hand, confirms a high stigma still associated with the disease. For too long the disease had been kept "out of sight and out of mind," which did nothing to help eradicate stigma, despite the availability of the cure for decades. It is therefore taking longer for the new attitudes towards leprosy to take root and erase the old fears that keep stigma alive. As new cases receive MDT treatment while living in their homes, without isolation and with no significant increase in the incidence of leprosy, gradually the old attitudes should diminish. However, the higher incidence of new cases of leprosy in New Caledonia as compared to the other Pacific islands visited indicates that vigilance is important for public health authorities, and leprosy retains a relatively fearful aspect in the country.

Dr. Crouzat was extremely helpful in providing copies of recent French reports relating to leprosy, but obviously was not in a position to provide introductions to other leprosy sufferers. The conclusion here relating to stigma is therefore restricted to the testimony of the longest staying resident at Ducos, one of the retired SMSM staff members, Dr. Farrugia, who had not returned to New Caledonia since his time at Ducos in 1980, and the reports of Dr. Crouzat. There is a friendliness evident between the dermatological services providing care for leprosy patients at Ducos, which is evidenced by the recording and publication of the memoirs of the last eleven residents at Raoul Follereau Center, as well as the museum set up about the leprosarium and leprosy in the old penitentiary situated at Ducos.[100] No doubt stigma is abating in New Caledonia, as the links with the fearful face of leprosy fade.

It appears that the poor settlers were more affected by the isolation measures than the indigenous villagers. The latter were able to return and live near their villages, or in groups nearby, supporting each other, with regular visits by medical staff. No contacts or information were available regarding stigma associated with these indigenous lifestyles, but the fact that small groups of leprosy sufferers congregated to support each other indicates that segregation took place in village societies, probably associated with stigmatizing attitudes. The formation of small groups of leprosy sufferers tends to be a natural occurrence, as these victims gravitate towards the company of fellow companions who understand the predicament and ongoing effects of leprosy. It is difficult to gauge any stigma associated with leprosy by the public in these more remote regions, but recent medical reports indicate that advanced cases of leprosy were still being detected in the 2000s, suggesting that the stigma associated with leprosy remains high and people were hiding from health professionals until medical attention became urgent. High stigma is also suggested by the comments of Dr. Farrugia and Sister Noëllie that nobody wished to speak about leprosy. However, the good relationship evident between staff at the Territorial Hospital and older patients at Raoul Follereau Center, augers well for the diminishment of stigma, with the free treatment and support for all leprosy patients that continues to be provided by the French government.

3

Rise and Demise of Stigma — Samoa

Historical Background

The islands of western and eastern Samoa, now known as Samoa and American Samoa respectively, were central to a flourishing Polynesian trading community c200 B.C., which included Tonga and Fiji. In 1300 A.D. the Samoans colonized the nearby Tokelau Islands. It was not until the mid-1770s that the islands were spotted by Europeans traversing the South Pacific seeking to expand their lucrative trade. In general, the Samoans were not hostile to foreign visitors, and by the 1840s they had accepted Christianity through the LMS, Methodist and Catholic missionaries.

In 1857 the Germans established a trading depot at Apia, and subsequently the Tripartite Treaty Agreement of 1899 divided the administrative rights over the islands among Germany, the United States of America and Britain. Britain later withdrew from governance, and Germany colonized the islands comprising Western Samoan from 1900 until the outbreak of World War I in 1914, at which time New Zealand troops entered and took over control. The Americans continued to administer the eastern islands, which are still known as American Samoa. In 1947 the Samoan legislative body was granted substantial power by the New Zealand government, and by 1962 Western Samoa became the first Polynesian state to gain independence. In 1997 its name was changed to Samoa.

In 2006 oral histories were successfully conducted recording the experiences of leprosy sufferers from the 1940s onwards, but the search for archival records was in vain. At that time the inspection of historical documents had been suspended pending microfilming of the files due to their fragile condition and fragmentation upon handling, which is a reflection of the difficulties of preserving paper documents in the humid conditions of the tropics. A building dedicated as the Samoan National Archives was yet to be established, and in

2006 the files were housed in three separate buildings, two of which were not even open to access. Once plans to centralize the archives and microfilming are completed, the lacunae in this period of leprosy history may be filled because, in contrast to other South Pacific nations, the colonial government files appear to have been preserved. Some records are held in the archives in Wellington, New Zealand, and these sources were accessed by Safua Akeli in her research into leprosy in Samoa from 1890 to 1922, from which the following early history of leprosy is derived.[1]

Early Incidence of Leprosy and Attitudes Toward the Disease

The growing influence of European colonizers in Samoa in the late nineteenth century occurred at the same time as western health authorities were taking initiatives to control the spread of leprosy in their various colonies following the isolation of the leprosy bacillus, *M. leprae,* in 1873 by Hansen, and especially since the international outcry at the death of Father Damien in 1889 at Molokai, Hawaii. As early as 1890–91 the colonial powers in Samoa extradited Hawaiians living in Samoa because Hawaiians, together with the Chinese, were considered to be the source of leprosy.[2]

The first medically confirmed case of leprosy in Samoa was a Filipino male, recorded in 1893, followed by another five cases confirmed in 1896, one being Chinese and four others classified as European subjects.[3] At this stage none of those diagnosed were Samoans because Samoans lay outside the jurisdiction of the Municipal Council in Apia, who were only responsible for Europeans in the town. Therefore, the health of Samoans in Apia or in the villages were not monitored.[4] As early as 1884, George Turner of the London Missionary Society reported cases of leprosy among the indigenous islanders, and further cases were reported by other missionaries towards the late nineteenth century.[5] It is unknown exactly when Samoans first contracted leprosy, or the extent of the contagion, although early reports indicate that leprosy sufferers lived with their families and retained close contact with them, which is the usual practice of Samoans and their sick.[6] There is no substantial evidence during this early period to definitively know the local attitude towards leprosy, as no written Samoan records exist. The earliest accounts are gained through missionary and colonial records, through which leprosy is traced.

In 1896 legislation was passed in Samoa calling for isolation of people with leprosy, preferably at leprosaria either in Hawaii or Tonga, since a suitable site had not been found in Western Samoa. But this plan did not eventuate, as neither the Hawaiian nor Tongan governments wanted more leprosy sufferers.[7] The German rulers established a general hospital in Apia in 1903 and leprosy patients were isolated in the grounds of this hospital; but once local Samoans were being diagnosed with leprosy, by 1910 negotiations were initiated to build a leprosarium.[8]

This move towards isolation of leprosy sufferers was at odds with customary Samoan practices of maintaining close contact with the ill, including visiting the sick, known as *Asia*.[9] Traditionally, illness was believed to be punishment by supernatural beings, *Aitu*, and leprosy gradually came to be doubly feared because of its severe effects and due to the separation of the sick from their families.[10] It is likely that the combination of these beliefs and practices contributed to heightened fear of leprosy and increased stigma. It is difficult to discern early Samoan attitudes towards leprosy and to what extent it was feared on the scanty evidence available prior to European intervention. Akeli suggests that leprosy "seems to have been a family responsibility without the signs of stigma,"[11] although no evidence is available to support or dispute this claim regarding stigma. The familial closeness postulated by Akeli could have caused the early spread of leprosy within Samoan communities, which, although at one level may have normalized the disease, may also have increased a dread of the awful physical putrescence encountered in advanced cases. The cultural differences between the traditional treatment of the sick and the radical colonial practice of isolation in leprosaria would have undoubtedly raised fears of contracting the disease.

Certainly by the early twentieth century stigma was attached to leprosy, whether through Christian missionary teachings and/or European influences, or the practice of isolation in leprosaria. Early missionary reports observe the presence of leprosy but do not indicate that Christian teachings incorporated ideas that the unfortunate victims should be treated as outcasts due to sin and uncleanliness. The LMS and Methodist missions could have connected ideas of disease being the punishment of *Aitu* with Old Testament ideas of leprosy connected with sin and defilement, conveyed in Leviticus, as occurred in Tonga. Although none of the interviewees connected biblical teachings and leprosy stigma, in his 1984 workshop notes on the topic of leprophobia and stigma in Apia, Dr. Daulako, the leprologist at Twomey hospital in Suva, suggested that "religious preachers through their quoting of the Bible are partly responsible for the present stigma attached to leprosy, and these leaders should be asked to undo the harm they had done."[12] These biblical ideas may have been through European missionaries and/or Samoan pastors and catechists trained in the islands. Daulako's comment indicates that biblical ideas of stigma had arisen at some earlier stage and persisted until as recently as the 1980s.

By 1910, in line with the recommendations of the First and Second International Leprosy Conferences in Berlin in 1897 and Norway in 1909, which called for strict isolation of leprosy patients, the German Samoan government sought to purchase land upon which to build a leprosarium.[13] Proposed land purchases met strong local opposition, but it is unclear whether the opposition was due to the land being sold to the government or for its use as a leprosarium.[14] If the latter, this could indicate fear of leprosy by some who did not wish to have a leprosarium on their land. Alternatively, the leprosarium may have aroused family objection to the alien practice of segregation and isolation. Eventually land was purchased to build a leprosy station at Alia, near Falefa on the main island Upolu, in 1912, where advanced cases were admitted.[15]

Leprosaria at Alia and Nu'utele

The Roman Catholic Mission, established in Samoa since 1845, was involved in the negotiations to set up the leprosy station, and Bishop Broyer, a French national, agreed to provide supervisory staff and building plans.[16] Broyer would have been aware of the service of the French SMSM (originally named The Third Order of Mary) and that one of the pioneers of the Order, Sister Marie de la Croix, had worked with leprosy in New Caledonia.[17] Accordingly, two sisters of this Order, Marie Henry and Marie Christine, were appointed to supervise the establishment of the leprosy station at Alia, with terms and conditions set in place to ensure the economic sustainability of the station, as well as the safety of the sisters from contagion.[18] Sister Marie Henry was appointed senior nurse at Alia because of her nursing experience.[19] This indicates that the focus of the SMSM sisters was to care for the physical needs of patients, in contrast to the proposition that religious orders simply sought to palliate the needs of the sick and prepare them for the afterlife.[20]

After much trouble and negotiation, the leprosarium was completed in early 1914, and twelve leprosy sufferers were moved to Alia, half of these being Samoans and the remainder of mixed or foreign origin.[21] The leprosarium was situated on a very steep hill behind Falefa, making access and the provision of supplies difficult. The area was fenced by three lines of barbed wire, which did not, in fact, prevent inmates from absconding if they chose to do so.[22] Accommodation was segregated along lines of ethnicity, with the Europeans being housed separately from Samoans, and the Europeans having more facilities (the greater number of toilets and water tanks perhaps reflecting the respective lifestyles of the time in Samoa).[23] Rather than these divisions being based on simply racist categories, as suggested by Akeli,[24] it is evident that the segregation practices implemented at Alia, and also at Makogai in Fiji and Ducos in New Caledonia, were in line with pragmatic social mores of the time to replicate the differing lifestyles of diverse communities. Keeping people with cultural similarities together was an attempt to provide a greater sense of creating a "home from home," as against contemporary ideas that these practices were primarily racially discriminatory, although elements of economic expediency were likely involved in implementing such a system.

Despite the special conditions imposed to ensure the viability of the leprosy station at Alia, the site proved unsuitable for the purpose. The nearby stream dried up, causing severe water shortages, further compounded by the non-delivery of necessary supplies and a shortage of funding.[25] These difficulties were exacerbated by serious defects in the buildings due, apparently, to the rushed construction by builders who were frightened by the prospect of leprosy.[26] This suggests that by that time the fear of contagion had affected public perception, which caused the builders to rush their work. Fear of contagion is also evident in the refusal by Samoan workers to accept appointments at the leprosy station because of the dangers of contamination.[27] These events point to rising stigma, rejection and fear within the public domain towards leprosy, as opposed to the older practice of Samoan families preferring to care for their own sick members.

In the midst of these problems at the leprosy station, German rule ended in 1914 with the commencement of World War One, resulting in the occupation and takeover of the Samoan government by New Zealand. The problems of funding and supplies continued at Alia, and by 1916 the Catholic Bishop threatened the resignation of the sisters if the situation could not be resolved.[28] This led to the closure of Alia by the New Zealand government, and the leprosy station and its nine patients were relocated to the nearby island of Nu'utele in the neighboring district of Aleipata in 1918.[29] Here the problems of transport and accessibility were overcome by supplies being ferried across to the island, rather than having to be carried uphill. The island, now called Leper Island, was fertile and had fresh water, but the problems of funding persisted. That year the worldwide influenza epidemic struck, and Western Samoa lost 22 percent of its population; ironically, those isolated on Nu'utele were unaffected by the outbreak.[30] The move to Nu'utele was popular with patients and the sisters, and by 1921 there were three Samoan and six other leprosy sufferers housed there.[31]

The original establishment of the leprosarium at Alia, with no easily accessible arable land to support the small community, nor adequate finances or facilities to transport food and supplies, contributed to the failure of the leprosarium and poor relationship between staff and leprosy patients, which, it is suggested, affected perceptions of leprosy and increased stigma. This scenario parallels that which existed during the initial years of isolation at Molokai, Hawaii, where the lack of adequate facilities led to a poor relation-

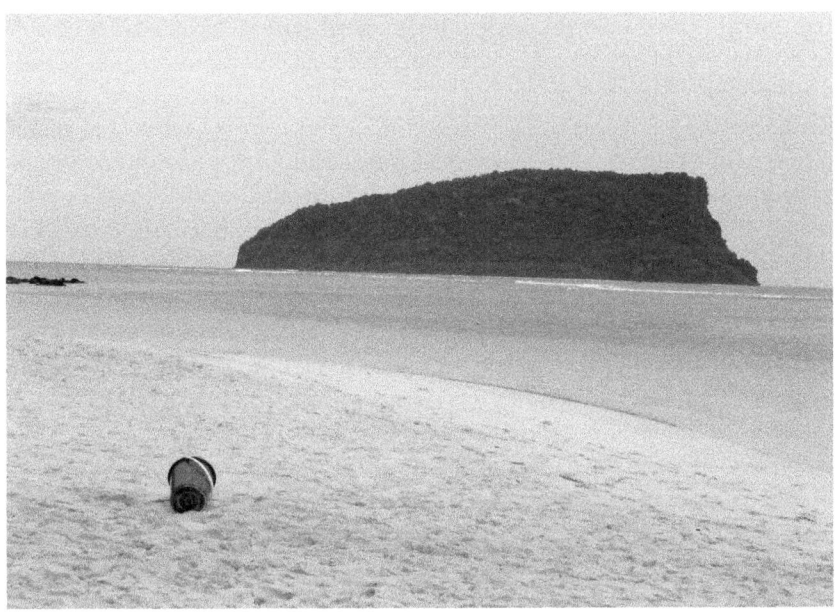

Leper Island, Nu'utele.

ship between staff and patients, in turn increasing fear of isolation and leprosy stigma by others.[32] The abysmal conditions at leprosaria adversely affected public perceptions of leprosy, no doubt resulting in increased stigma associated with the disease. People were fearful not only of the disease but the horror of isolation in poor conditions that would have to be endured. It is suggested this early failed experience of isolation at Alia leprosy station would have contributed to increased leprosy stigma in Samoa.

The rising costs of maintenance, supplies and staffing, which caused the failure of the leprosarium at Alia, continued to beset the new leprosy station at Nu'utele. The New Zealand authorities, with their links to the Fiji government, were aware of the facilities available at the leprosarium by then established at Makogai. In 1920 overtures were made to transfer the long-suffering patients on Nu'utele to Makogai, on the basis that superior medical treatment and facilities would be available to the patients — although, of course, the reduced cost was economically expedient to the Samoan government.[33]

Removal of Leprosy Sufferers to Makogai, Fiji

The Fiji government decided to accept the Samoan patients at Makogai on both medical and humanitarian grounds, as well as the financial benefit that would be derived from sharing the overhead costs on an annual fee basis.[34] In 1922 a total of either twelve or thirteen patients were transferred to Makogai.[35] By this time, the fear and stigma surrounding leprosy was such that the Union Steamship Company would not allow the unfortunate victims of the disease on board; but finally a vessel of Burns Philp Company agreed to take the patients to Makogai aboard the *Maota*.[36] Partitions were erected to isolate the leprosy sufferers from other travelers, and the ship was disinfected after their disembarkation to prevent contagion.[37] This practice was adopted for all vessels in and out of Makogai, especially prior to the time an effective cure became available in the early 1950s. The Samoan leprosy sufferers were the first group of non–Fijian patients received at Makogai.

By this time, the troubled experiences of the leprosaria in Samoa and the eventual removal of the residents to distant Fiji undoubtedly tainted the perception of leprosy in Samoa as highly contagious and doubly feared because of exile from their homeland. This stigma in Samoa appears to have derived mainly from the institutionalization of leprosy, since no substantial evidence that biblical ideas of sin and uncleanliness associated with the stigma were apparent. To what extent the disfiguring physical characteristics of advanced leprosy cases affected Samoan perceptions of stigma is hard to distinguish from the fear of the alien practice of isolation and segregation. The testimonies below suggest that separation from family was the most emotionally painful aspect for those exiled to Makogai to bear.

Following the transfer of the first group of Samoan patients to Makogai in 1922, it is unclear what procedures were initially put in place in Samoa for the detection and containment of leprosy sufferers prior to being transferred to Makogai. Oral histories recorded with Samoan leprosy sufferers who had been isolated at Makogai indicate that by 1944 patients were sequestered in two buildings surrounded by a high fence at the extreme end of the Apia hospital grounds, where they awaited a boat to take them to Makogai, sometimes waiting up to a year.[38]

Sister Marietta, SMSM of Christchurch, the PLF liaison contact for Samoa, had worked previously for forty years as a teacher in the islands, and facilitated my introductions with seven leprosy sufferers in and around Apia and the main island of Upolu, driving me to village homes in the PLF truck. In 2009 in recognition for her service in Samoa, Sister Marietta was invited into the Grand Priory of New Zealand, a branch of the Order of St. Lazarus of Jerusalem.

Five of the interviewees had been born in the 1930s and transported to Makogai between 1944 and 1955. The remaining two interviewees were born in 1941 and 1950, and were diagnosed with leprosy in 1968 and 1957 respectively. The latter two had been isolated and treated at the leprosy ward at

Apia hospital. Two oral history testimonies quoted anonymously here are unrestricted testimonies, but the contributors are related to other interviewees who have time restrictions imposed on the use of their oral histories; thus anonymity protects the privacy and identity of the restricted oral histories.

In contrast to the testimonies of other Pacific Islanders, the Samoan interviews offer detailed and vivid descriptions of the horrendous physical and emotional suffering endured by leprosy sufferers. Generally speaking, interviewees from other islands referred only briefly to the heartbreak of the emotional separation from family; they were often tearful, and it seems that actual words, let alone descriptions, were too painful to recount. The vivid Samoan descriptions may be attributable to the fact that several of the interviewees had siblings who also suffered from leprosy. These individuals had talked about their experiences between themselves and, perhaps having spoken about their earlier traumas, were able to recount detailed descriptions of their memories more easily than others who had not previously discussed their suffering openly. It is also conceivable that the goodwill that existed between Sister Marietta and the interviewees enabled the contributors to speak more freely; or perhaps the English fluency of many Samoans made vocal expression of their experiences easier.

The following extracts of testimonies recount the experiences of leprosy sufferers transported to Makogai from 1944 to the early 1950s, the emotional hardships imposed by a diagnosis of leprosy, their confinement in Apia awaiting transport, and the conditions of the voyage. As mentioned earlier, due to time restrictions imposed by two interviewees on their oral histories, and the close relationship between many of these people, some extracts are quoted anonymously.

Rudy McFarland's (b. 1934) Irish grandfather had married the daughter of a prestigious noble Samoan family, and his father lived the privileged life of a European planter. Aged about fifteen in 1948–49, Rudy was taken by his father to Apia hospital because Rudy had been feeling sick and extremely lethargic, with uncomfortable patches on his skin. Leprosy was diagnosed, and Rudy gave an account of his immediate separation from his father and the conditions awaiting transport to Makogai:

> I went with my father [to the hospital in town] and they talked to my father, and told him all about what I got, and I couldn't come back home again.... They had to isolate me straight away.... So the two of us, my father and me, we were walking right to the back ...of the hospital. When I got there I saw there was a fence. A very high fence, and there was a door, and when I got there, the nurse told my dad that he got to say goodbye to me now and he must never touch me anymore.... This was very hurtful. So I heard this, and I ran to my father and I hang onto him and say, "Oh no, you can't do this to

me, I won't, I won't go into that fence." They had to force me and take me to the fence.... When he comes around to see me, he stands outside, he never comes in ... talks to me from outside ... wire fence, and that is how I was for almost a year, waiting for the ship to go to Makogai.[39]

There were [two other patients] David and Jessie ... just the same as me, also had to stay.... [They] talk to me and tell me not to worry ... because they had been there for quite a while, so we got used to the place. Three of us [waiting], and then another one, then another one, till there was about nine of us ... waiting for the ship.... The nurses ... came with the food, they had to cover themselves up when they come in. In those days the disease was very dreadful to people, and that is how they take care of themselves.... So they just come and give the food and then go.... While we were there, we were lucky. David was, he was training as a teacher when he got sick. So he teaches us, he was very good to myself and other boys, and he taught us a lot — how to write English, because we didn't talk or speak English[40]

When people come over to say goodbye... they have to stand far away, and they come and wave but they can't come near...nobody.... My dad came over, and we were gone; we didn't know we were going to go. So I didn't make the party! There was no idea, no having to watch crying and say goodbye.... So we went to Makogai.... Some of the patients were ...frightening... because

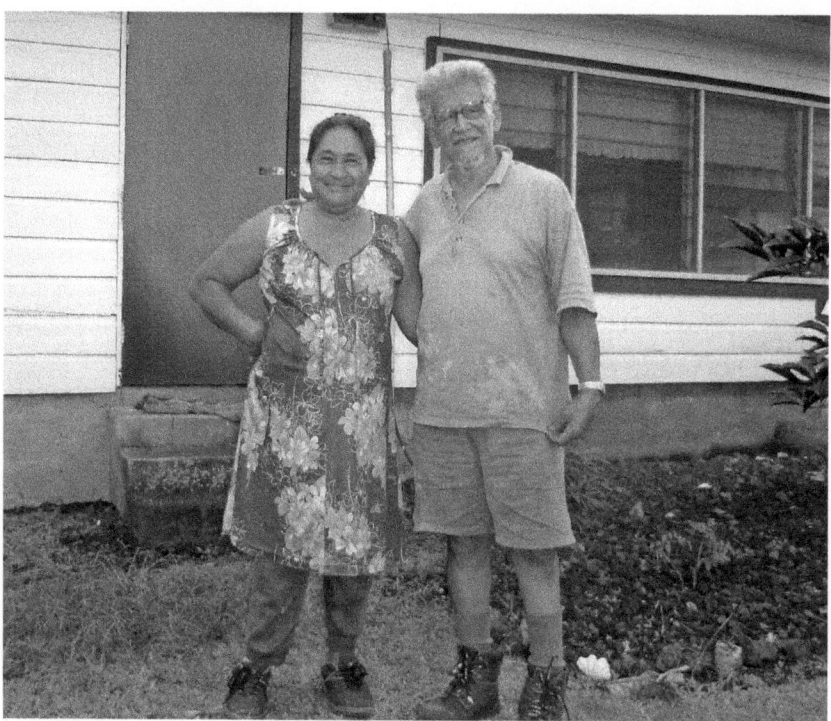

Rudy McFarland and his wife in Samoa.

there was no treatment then. Some people bandaged right from down, up to here.[41]

This testimony indicates the high level of fear associated with the physical conditions wrought by the ravages of leprosy, which it is suggested is the major contributory factor of stigma, although this is not explicit in testimonies. The physical deformities, skin rashes and putrid ulcers caused by leprosy prior to the availability of antibiotics contributed to fear and stigma. The additional fear and anxiety posed by segregation and isolation is highly evident in the above extract, and together these factors constituted stigma.

The anonymous testimonies of another family affected by leprosy supports the anguish of Rudy's account, especially the experiences of children. One child recalled that at the age of five their father was suddenly taken away without any explanation, also recalling a subsequent visit with their mother to Apia hospital and waiting near the fence while the parents talked and cried.[42] About three years later, towards the end of the war, a truck with a large red cross on its side appeared in the village outside their home, and the siblings, seven years of age, were taken crying from their mother to the hospital to await deportation to Makogai. They were isolated at Makogai for up to twelve years, until the mid–1950s. The siblings maintain that they had no symptoms of leprosy before or while at Makogai; in retrospect, they believe they contracted their leprosy — symptoms of which appeared in the 1970s — in Makogai.[43]

One of the siblings recounts the following heart-rending description of their initial isolation at Apia hospital, followed by an account of the conditions endured on their voyage to Makogai:

> [They took] us to the isolation and lock us there.... We just only know we separated from our family, and we didn't see our mother nearly three months. We just lived with other people, some people there, different, they affected by the sickness, and some they still okay like us. So we watch them, we frightened.... We don't understand anything. We just live there without any medicine or any treatment, nothing. They been feeding us, through the wire.... We separated, isolated. Separated from the hospital ... a fence to protect other people ... we were together in one house.... They put food under the fence, and we come and pick it up, the plate.... And always we want to see our mother and then we cry.... There is a pastor, minister, he admitted too ... nothing in his body just like us. [We were there] six months something, nearly a year.... This pastor, he very good.... I think the parson see us all the time everyday.... We want to see our mother, sometimes we cover up under the sheet we cry, and he make us strong.... The pastor taught us a song, it start off a song to our mother. After three months she came around.... She come and sit at the back of the fence, and we sit inside, and we crying.... And we sing the song that the pastor taught us, and she ... she was hiding! ... She said sing

that song again ... and we ask the nurse, can she stay with us. And they say no. So when she go back again, then we cry, cry. We run after her, and they grab us.[44]

Every Wednesday the nurse come and say, put on your shoes ... I take you around to the compound ... for a walk. And then we go every Wednesday, and then we come back. You don't have to touch this, don't have to touch, just walk straight on ... just around the block, outside the hospital. And then suddenly they told us ... you will be taken away with these people. And we say where to, to our mother? He say no! You taken away in a far away place. With our mother? No, no, just only you with this people. How? Taken by the boat. You know we are very innocent, we just jump and the day, we didn't see our mother coming say goodbye to us. They took us again in that big truck, it was to the wharf. And then we take down to the wharf ... then we were put in a small boat and taken to a big yacht ... where they used to put the cattle, they put us there.... We came down the steps down there, one, two, three, four, five, six from Samoa and one old lady from Niue, the same people with us. One man from Niue also was there. And the space they put us in ... very small, and the lady was there when we go down, and we come up and there was smell... it make us sick ... the smell, the stink. When we go there ... all together in one corner, and we held our breath like this.... We eat there, you know sometimes we vomit. I am sorry.... Full of cockroach, full of rats running around. Always squatting in one corner.... Stay there a week — seven days, nine days, something like that.... So then five days, we can't stay there, so we went up to the deck. We take our food up on the deck, we sit there the whole day, whole day until the evening, we hardly go down, because the smell and rats. And the body of this lady, you know, sores, and that is why they smell, without any medicine ... just lying there, all her body is full of sores. It is frightening.[45]

When we come on the deck and he say this island is Makogai, and your father is here also.... Then we saw the nuns come up and they pulled us from the... boat and they took us. We just struggle, we don't know, a lot of people, bandaged all their hands and faces, and some of them swollen, and we frightened. We step back, and the nuns say no, you wait here. And they say you know anybody here, and we say, our father. And then, suddenly, he comes in front of us. Yeah he come and see us one by one. He is okay, nothing in his body. He is just like us.[46]

This testimony provides a vivid description of the awful physical conditions which leprosy sufferers had to endure, personally and caring for each other. Apart from details in medical accounts, these awful physical details are seldom described because of the horrific images that surface, which the interviewees and public at large do not wish to remember or imagine. Thus the physical aspects of leprosy stigma are often sanitized. Another aspect of this testimony indicates the difficulties encountered in the diagnosis of leprosy due to the disparities in symptoms from the less serious pauci-bacillary to most severe multi-bacillary infections, and the problems posed by the wide range of symptoms exhibited. However, the camaraderie that arises, despite the fear of the physical conditions, is evident both in the small group awaiting transfer by boat to Makogai and subsequently on Makogai itself. The shared adversity of living together in isolation appears to have produced strong feelings of empathy and support between leprosy sufferers.

These Samoan testimonies provide unique descriptions of the painful experience of children being wrenched from their families, with little comprehension of the reasons for their separation until in the company of other leprosy sufferers. A total of four of the Samoan interviewees maintained they had been wrongly diagnosed, indicating problems in medical knowledge about leprosy in the islands. Despite this, those isolated at Makogai indicated that they were appreciative of the job training received, so that on their eventual discharge they were able to obtain work and support themselves during their adult lives. Still, other interviewees indicate that the stay at Makogai caused some difficulties reintegrating back into traditional lifestyles.

Samoan Experiences at Makogai and Reintegration Back Home

Upon arrival at Makogai in 1948, Rudy was surprised to find one of his elder brothers, who had earlier moved to Fiji, also isolated because of leprosy. He and his brother shared a home in the European quarters with David, who had been in the Apia leprosy enclosure, and another leprosy sufferer:

> I was treated as European, they didn't take me where the Samoans were, they take me ... another house.... Ernest Wolfgram was there ... but he was very sick, there was no treatment. He died when I was there.... There was another Samoan, part European ... he was very sick, his fingers... he was a very smart man. He was very good, worked out there, do a lot of things. He helps the nuns ... still hard work, and then he came back to Samoa. He was cured.[47]
>
> Chaulmoogra was very painful. [The new medicine made] a very very fast difference.... [In] 1952 I think they started.... Very big changes, because there was a very long hospital ... all the patients in there, some of them lying there, with no legs, no hands, laying, sores all over.... People started to get well, there were patients that had no more sores. Patients who were very sick, they just died, it was too late. But we lucky, I am lucky I got there.[48]
>
> [I stayed] ten years. I find it happy in Makogai. It was a good place. I was going to school.... When I finished school, we get job.... They checked us [for leprosy] every month. When they found out that we are cured, they check us for two years .... I think I was there for eight years, then they start to check me, and then I was normal, and then they check me for another two years. My last test, there was something wrong with it. When I was working, the sis-

ter ... she called me. I went for my test in the morning and when I came in the afternoon she didn't want to look at me, and I know there something wrong. So I went over to her and say what's wrong? She say, sorry Rudy, your test is something wrong. Ah, I feel very bad. I was looking forward to come back home. So I went to my room and I sat there, I think I have to tell you about this. There was a picture of Mary, Mother Mary. I looked up and I saw her and I cried and ask her, this is what I told her, why, why I can't go home? Why, why, why? Please help me. And all of a sudden I feel alright. I stood up, wiped my face and I went back to work. When I went past the lab, the sister call out to me, come, do the test. So they gave me another test.... I came back after work and they say the test is all right now![49]

The huge effect of the arrival of sulphones is evident in this testimony, leading to the diminishment of fear of the disease, especially of those in the early stages of leprosy. It also shows the change in ideas of isolation, since this was no longer seen as a life sentence, but with hope of a full cure and return home.

Rudy recounted his experience of returning from Makogai to his home in Apia around 1958. Arriving unannounced and finding his uncle and father near the docks, he joined his father in a welcome-home drinking spree.[50] At first Rudy did not enjoy beer, but with his father, who was a heavy drinker, he took to regular drinking and smoking, trying to readjust and settle back. After the initial euphoria, he said he cried and was homesick for Makogai and its orderly lifestyle. He continued to drink to drown his unhappiness. Ten years later, in about 1968, he cut his foot, and the reality of living with the after-effects of leprosy hit him.[51] The wound would not heal, and soon he was readmitted to Apia Hospital — also because he said he felt the return of the lethargy associated with his earlier leprosy. This relapse of leprosy would have been one of a huge number of cases worldwide associated with resistance to Dapsone. Rudy appeared unaware that the reappearance of his leprosy was a reaction to his earlier medication, indicating a limited understanding of the treatment of leprosy generally in Samoa. After a year of treatment he was released and took more care of his physical condition.[52]

It was during a later stay at the leprosy ward in the mid–1980s that Rudy met his future wife; they have three children, and grandchildren. All Rudy's siblings had moved overseas many years earlier, and he and his young family lived and worked hard on his father's plantation.[53] He had one leg amputated in the 1990s, and the PLF funded his visits to Twomey hospital in Suva on a number of occasions to have a prosthesis fitted, since the prosthetics laboratory in Apia did not operate effectively, despite being funded by the PLF. It is these later problems associated with anaesthetized limbs (due to the unavailability of medication at the early stages of their disease) which are the plague of leprosy sufferers. These later disabilities often prevent leprosy sufferers from being able to earn an income, and give rise to the erroneous fear that the leprosy is active and contagious. These are the reasons why ignorance about the disease retains ideas of stigma, and why leprosy awareness programs are funded by the PLF in the Pacific.

The late marriage of Rudy, while in his fifties, indicates the level of the difficulties encountered in being accepted back into ordinary life in Samoa. Rudy met his future wife in the 1980s while they were both receiving treatment for leprosy at Apia Hospital. Despite the apparent lessening of stigma towards leprosy in recent years, Rudy said that when he attended the leprosy clinic because of a plantar ulcer on his remaining foot, he tended the ulcer himself, the hospital only providing the dressings. Sister Marietta usually provided dressings on her visits to make life easier. It is difficult to know to what extent the attitude of staff at the hospital was affected by ideas of stigma, making them reluctant to deal with the ulcer and the dressings, or whether a level of internalized stigma by Rudy, as well as his own competency in dressing the ulcer, induced his actions.

Manu Ah Chong (b. 1933) was diagnosed with leprosy at about eleven years of age and waited three months for a boat to Makogai, where he was isolated for nearly fourteen years (from 1944 until 1957). His father, originally

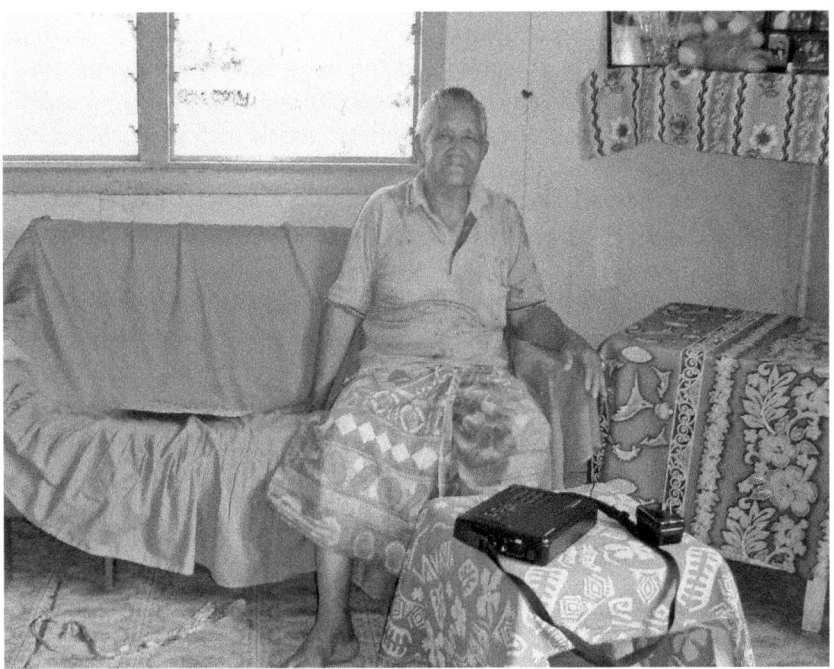

Manu Ah Chong in his home which he built with PLF assistance.

from Canton, China, married a Samoan woman and remained in Samoa. Manu said he learned good English skills and was taught carpentry by a part-German Samoan, Fritz Hydebrand, at Makogai. Stella gives a short account of the exemplary figure of Hydebrand, who, with Ernest Wolfgram, helped make life bearable for others and trained leprosy sufferers in Makogai in the trades around 1954.[54] Sister Marietta facilitated my introduction to Manu and encouraged him to participate. Manu did not speak much about his early life and return home, but said he built his own home, funded partly by the PLF, and said that all his siblings had moved to New Zealand and Australia, although they kept in contact. He said that in earlier times "they can't come in near to us, the people never touch the leper ... very dangerous," although he now believes there is not so much fear of leprosy.[55] The fact that Manu did not marry until 1987, at age 56, supports his suggestion that the stronger earlier stigma relating to leprosy had eased in the last couple of decades. This view is supported by Sister Marietta, who had worked in Samoa for long periods since the 1960s.[56]

The anonymous testimonies of the siblings reveal that they subsequently married and had children, but later separated from their spouses. The testimonies also indicate that, having spent almost their entire childhood under the strict hygienic regime that existed at Makogai, they had problems adapting to the easy traditional Samoan *fale* lifestyle. They felt they needed to continue the Makogai regime of not sharing food and using separate eating utensils.[57] It appears their strict adherence to hygiene and non-sharing of implements made them difficult living companions who ultimately preferred to live alone. Whether this was due to self-stigma and residual fear of contagion, feelings of rejection, or sheer habit is not clear.

All the interviewees who had been interned during their childhood and young adult lives because of leprosy felt a degree of anger about their long segregation, particularly the anonymous siblings, as they considered the leprosy diagnosis to be incorrect and believed their leprosy had been contracted at Makogai.

Another, unrelated, interviewee whose testimony also remains anonymous, and who was born during the same period as the anonymous siblings, was transferred to Makogai much later, in 1955, with suspected leprosy. By 1958 tests confirmed no leprosy bacteria present, and that the symptoms had been due to a condition similar to leprosy, the name of which was not remembered by the interviewee, indicating that the original leprosy diagnosis was incorrect and supporting the notion of misdiagnosis of leprosy in Samoa. Nevertheless, all the interviewees said they were relatively happy living at Makogai because their needs had been met and they received skills that enabled them later to find good jobs, the men usually in the trades and the women as seamstresses, housekeepers or in managerial positions at hostels and hotels.

Leprosy Treatment in Samoa Since the Late 1950s

Following the effective cure obtained with sulphones, by 1958 leprosy sufferers were no longer sent to Makogai but isolated in the leprosy wards set up at the Apia General Hospital. It is unclear when the two *fale*-styled leprosy wards, one for men and the other for women, were established in the rear of the grounds of the hospital, or within the hospital itself. Sister Marietta, the PLF liaison contact, was a mission teacher in Samoa during the 1950s and 1960s and recalled visiting the leprosy wards:

> When we were at St. Mary's College there, I always used to have a group of girls who were interested in coming to visit the people in the leprosy ward at the hospital, Apia hospital ... once a week. It would be our form of service that we would give to others, and they would bring along soap, or toothpaste, or some sweets or something to take.... There was a men's ward and a ladies' ward ... it was right at the back of the hospital. We had to walk all the way, well away from the rest. Open building, which was usual ... could be up to twelve to fifteen in each ward. And then one night a week, I recall seemed to be a Wednesday night, one or other of the sisters of the community would take a film along to show. Take it to the ward and we would all be together and show them a movie. *Were there very serious cases in those days do you think?* Well some of them didn't look too good, we didn't comment too much, because we were teachers.... We just told them not to be touching the patients ... at that time there was a risk that it was contagious. So we used to be careful, and used to say to them afterwards, wash your hands and just don't touch. Yes there were some people who were quite disfigured. It was quite sad.[58]

This testimony indicates a sympathetic attitude towards leprosy sufferers, although tinged with fear of contagion. The location of leprosy patients in the center of Apia receiving regular visits by school children, and possibly visits by their families, would have been a comfort to the patients, and would have reassured the public, as there was no resulting increase in the incidence of leprosy. This situation would have lessened stigma associated with leprosy, marking the end of isolation, which removed ideas of high contagion as well as the threat of separation from loved ones.

As a youngster of six or seven in about 1957, Dick Nansen (b. 1950) had trouble with his eyes and marks on his body, which were diagnosed as leprosy. He was admitted to the leprosy ward at the back of Apia Hospital for one-and-a-half years.[59] He said his older brother Jo had been diagnosed with lep-

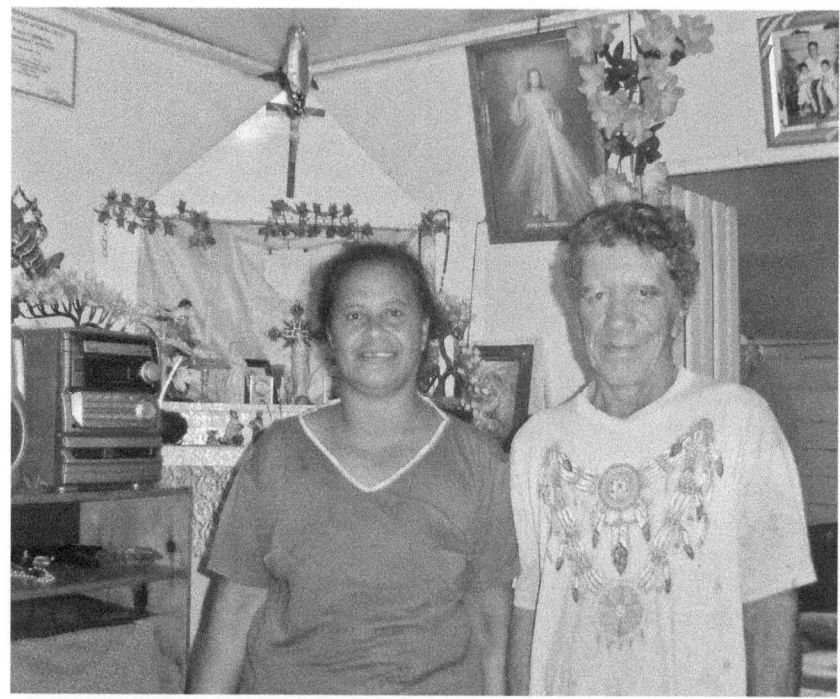

Dick Nansen and wife in their home in Apia.

rosy in about 1950 and isolated at Makogai, but it was not until Jo returned home in the late 1960s that Dick said he even knew he had this brother. Dick spoke proudly of his brother Jo, who was able to speak several languages and obtained a job as a mechanic with Public Works in Samoa, having learned these skills at Makogai. These skills enabled Jo to emigrate to New Zealand, where he raised and supported his own family.[60] The fact that Dick did not know of the existence of his brother Jo until his return from Makogai, despite the fact Dick contracted the disease, indicates a level of stigma, or perhaps shame, prevalent during the 1950s and 1960s.

Dick was an industrious father for his family of eleven children, working on a small plantation near Apia during the mornings to supplement his income. At other times he worked as a builder, having built his own home, with assistance of PLF funds; and he fished in the late afternoons for his family meals, selling any surplus catch at the market. He was provided with a hand sewing machine by the PLF and made the school uniforms for the younger of his eleven children (age twenty-nine down to five years old).[61] The fact that Dick had been in Apia Hospital in the 1950s, and again in the 1980s for recurring problems, but knew nothing about PLF assistance until Sister

3. *Rise and Demise of Stigma* 115

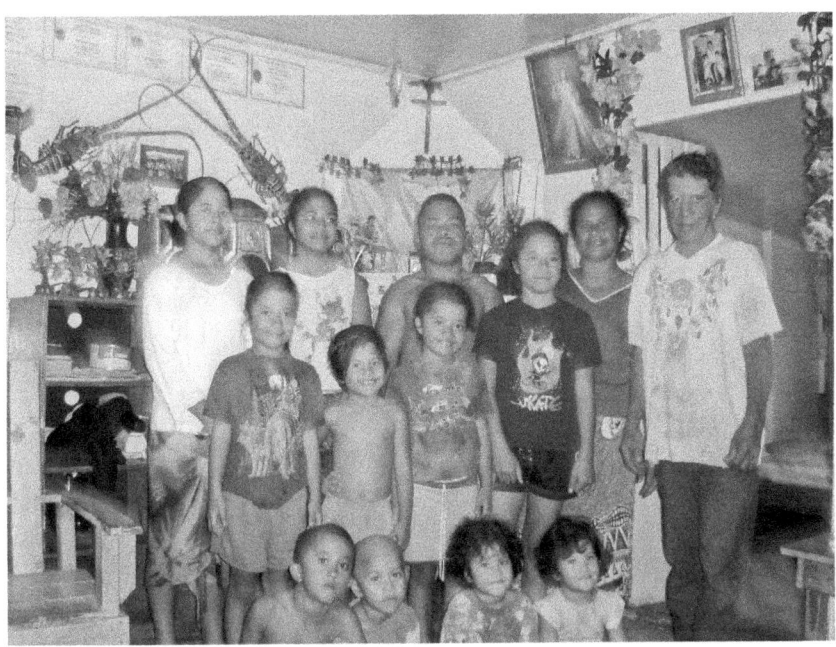

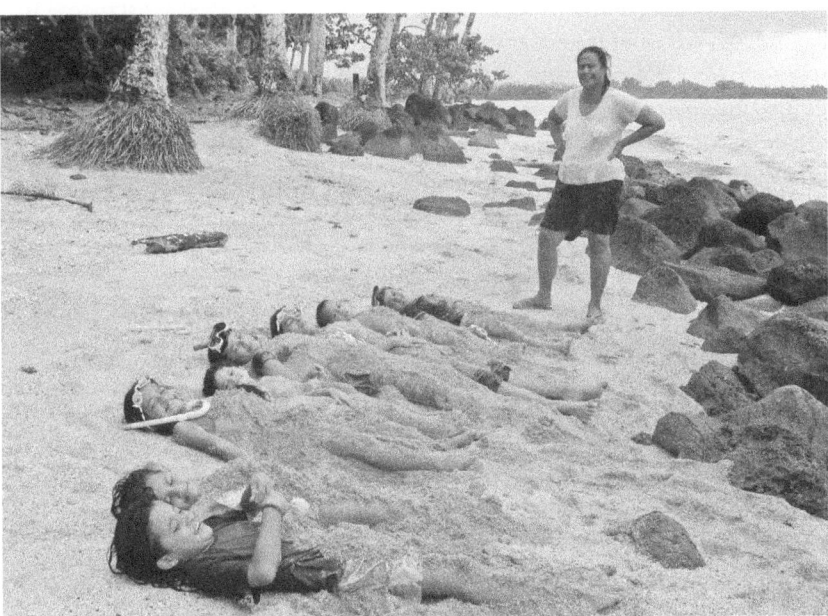

Top: Dick Nansen, extreme right, with his wife on his right and his children and grandchildren in Apia. *Bottom:* Dick Nansen's wife and their children playing at the picnic.

Marietta located him in 1999, is perhaps an indictment of the earlier PLF liaison agents' commitment to helping leprosy sufferers. Dick's family were independent and not looking for assistance, but with their large family, and problems with his eyesight and constant problems with injuries to his hands, the PLF assistance has made an enormous difference to their family.

Prior to 1999 the children had been shy about attending school because the financial requirements of the large family made it difficult for the parents to pay school fees or purchase uniforms.[62] Since these expenses have been met by the PLF, the family has blossomed. Sister Marietta has made it her responsibility in Samoa to pay school fees directly to the schools and at the same time check that the children were attending regularly. The children had recently surprised friends and family by performing extremely well both academically and in sports, art and music.[63] Dick, and his equally hard working wife Fiapotu, who rose at 4 a.m. each morning to iron the children's uniforms and prepare school lunches, mentioned that in the past the children had been teased with "bad words," such as being called lepela children. Fiapotu was particularly angry about this abuse used by a relative towards the family, which affected the self-esteem of her young children.[64] This behavior and attitude indicates that a level of stigma still exists in Samoa, although Fiapotu said most people did not treat her family in this way. With PLF assistance, Dick extended their home and had made furniture, and these improvements, together with the performance of the children at school, were significantly improving their lives. The improved status of the family, especially the children's performance at school, is a huge factor in reintegrating disadvantaged leprosy sufferers back into mainstream communities and enabling them to live normal lives.

Lome Ierone Laulu (b. 1941) Lome lived in a relatively remote village in central Upolu and was diagnosed with leprosy as a young man in 1968.[65] On the day of diagnosis at Apia Hospital he was admitted, and remained in the men's leprosy ward for one year. During this time he met his future wife, Nofo, who had been admitted to the women's leprosy ward earlier. He was happy at the hospital and enjoyed going to the movies every Saturday with the leprosy patients.[66] Both were cured and returned to live and work on Nofo's family taro plantations. They had two children. Taro plantation work is physically grueling labour, especially on the rocky hillsides, and although Lome was a particularly big, strong man, the work caused constant injuries to his feet and later his fingers. His left leg underwent a partial amputation in 1982, at which time Lome was sent to Suva for a prosthesis, as this was unavailable in Apia.

Because of the hard physical work on the plantation the prostheses were often broken, and further injuries occurred, although this seldom stopped

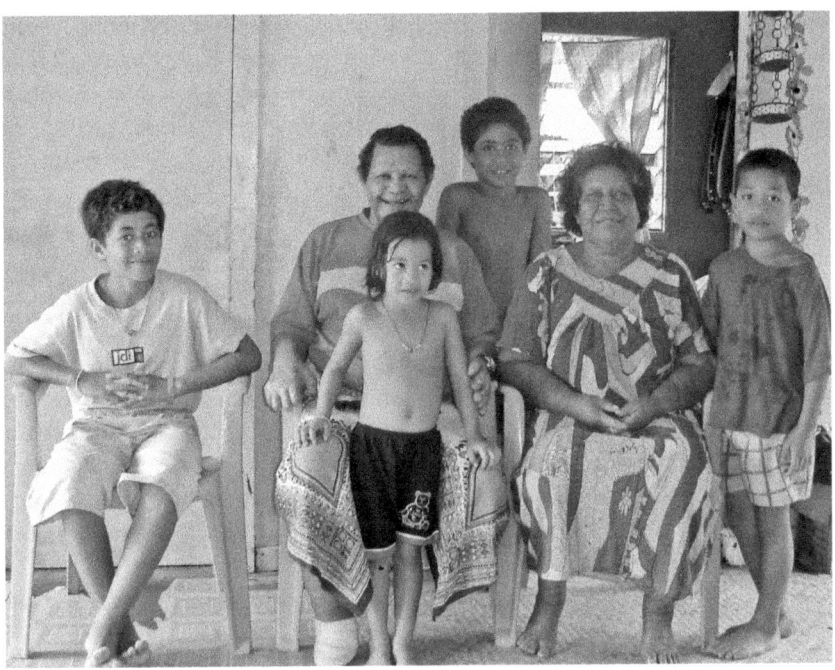

Lome Laulu with his wife and family.

Lome from tending his plantation, often crawling without his prosthesis. Further amputations and replacement prostheses necessitated additional trips to Suva, funded by the PLF. Although Lome greatly appreciated the PLF assistance, he found the medical care inconvenient; he often hid his injuries until they became too serious and required surgery.[67] In fact, the injuries to Lome's legs and fingers were so frequent that he became impatient and said, "I see the bone grow inside, coming up, and that is why I cut it down ... that is why I am going to take the knife and *kwff.*"[68]

Despite Sister Marietta's insistence that rest was needed for his amputations to properly heal, Lome was always impatient to return to work his plantation — because as the family chief he considered it necessary to support the family. Leprosy did not deter him from his work, although his wife's large family, who came to observe the interview and offer information, provided support.

There was no indication that Lome was concerned about stigma regarding his condition, but his impatience and work ethic probably enabled him to ignore attitudes involving stigma. Indicative of this positive attitude was his reply to a question by Sister Marietta after examining his leg. When asked if he needed anything, he replied, "Gramazone"— a weedkiller for his plantation![69] Lome did suggest that a telephone installation would be useful, since he found it difficult to get onto the bus when he occasionally had to go into town, especially when his prostheses were broken. With a phone he could request a relative to come and transport him in their car.[70] Lome's attitude is one of strong-willed independence, despite his circumstances, either ignoring or facing no stigma due to his leprosy.

The testimonies of Dick and Rudy, living in Apia, demonstrate a continuing concern about the lack of public social acceptance, indicating lingering stigmatizing attitudes. This differs enormously from the experience of Lome, who said one should not worry about leprosy because it was the "same as other diseases."[71] Irrespective of the difference in perception of stigma by these interviewees, the assistance of the PLF goes a long way towards providing them with the means to live relatively independent lives. Leprosy sufferers are provided with all necessary medical attention and, where needed, financial assistance, so that their physical disabilities do not prevent them from trying to support themselves and their families. Most importantly, the overall benefits permit the interviewees a level of self-esteem, and their children are not caught in a circle of poverty or disadvantage because of leprosy in the family. This in turn contributes to lowering leprosy stigma.

PLF Assistance in Samoa

Extracts from an interview with Sister Marietta, SMSM, the PLF liaison contact in Samoa, are quoted below to provide an example of the work carried out on the island. The regional SMSM office in Auckland was approached by Michael Gousmett, the manager of the Leprosy Foundation, who in turn asked Sister Marietta to assist with locating leprosy patients in Samoa:

> [In] 1999 I started. It was part-time because I was still teaching some classes, but I didn't have responsibility. Then in 2000 to 2002, three years, I was director of the Catholic Education, so as I moved around all the Catholic schools, I was able to visit the same village and I'd find people. So they interlaced very nicely, the jobs.... I started off with about 500 families that I visited on both islands. No one was looking after them.... Well, there was this doctor at the clinic, but he wasn't going out, and the people weren't going in, for whatever reason.... I started learning more and looking at the records to see where the people were.... I would go into a village ... go to a shop and say, can you tell me where these three people live. "Yeah, that house down there, further down, I don't know that person, but ask the other end of the village"— that sort of thing.[72]
>
> I had only been looking, visiting the people to say, how are you, and what needs they wanted.... I hadn't looked at their medical ... I thought that was all

being taken care of. And not being a nurse, I didn't take too much notice. Anyway, when I took Michael [of PLF] to some of the places, he was aghast at their medical condition.[73]

So bit by bit I found them. When I would go in, I would say what my name was. I'd just say I was a sister I think. "I've come from Apia." You are so-in-so, yes, have you had *mai*— now that means you have got the sickness, but I was not to use the word lepela, which is Samoan ... just to use *mai* [sick].... And they would say, oh yes, he did, or they'd bring him. Where is he? And that is slowly how I got my answers back. Some of the people I visited, some had died, some had shifted out to a new area, to New Zealand or American Samoa, some had gone to a different village — and they could tell me where they were, gone back to live with their mother or their father or something. Some had been healed, and some were still sick, had *mai*. These were ones that had ulcers ... there would be a few people who would come into the clinic to be checked out. Now they might have lesions on their back or on their arm, or they might be itchy.... Just go to your local clinic or your hospital, go and have it checked out with a nurse.... Earlier times, they were often too ashamed ... the lepela family, the leprosy family.... I have noticed over the time I have been working, that is about five years, that it has certainly lessened. For the people themselves, they have the self-confidence to get out and move, like some of them got a new prosthesis, able to walk around. They are not ashamed ... they are accepting.... The Leprosy Foundation are trying to help them, and we only want to help to get them back on their feet again. And we want to build up their family by helping them in the plantations — giving them weedkiller, spraying machines, so they can go and get their own food.[74]

If [the ulcer is] too big, sometimes they need debridement, the white part round the ulcer when it gets too much white skin it has to be removed, cut back. So you need to go to the clinic. I give them the bus fare, $10 here, that will take you there to the clinic or the hospital. Now you have got to go and get that done. Earlier days I used to take them and get it done ... making sure, getting shoes that they need.[75]

One of the methods we have tried over recent time over the last few years is the plaster cast.... I did one of them myself once.... Put it on from the knee down to the foot, so that the person has to keep off the foot ... so that the ulcer is not touching the ground, to keep the weight off.... They still walk around.[76]

Not only does the above testimony demonstrate the continued improvement of the conditions of leprosy patients due to the assistance of the PLF, it indicates that even today the SMSM are prepared to provide physical care to those in need. Sister Marietta — a qualified teacher, not a nurse — was willing to assist in the physical care required to deal with plantar ulcers, which nurses in several island hospitals were reluctant to handle. This testimony also provides insight into the change of attitudes and stigma in Samoan society.

Another reaction towards leprosy demonstrated in Samoa is that sickness sometimes reflected shame upon the family.[77] This is a common reaction where knowledge about health science is limited, and even frequently in Western countries with cases of congenital deformities and hereditary weaknesses. Sister Marietta observed that although the Samoan sick traditionally remained within the family fold, attempts were frequently made to seclude sick members. But once the unfortunate individual was discovered and diagnosed — that is, the public could become aware of the problem — the sick were rejected by their family because of shame of the discovery, followed by attempts to distance themselves from the problem and disease. This description provides a possible explanation why groups of leprosy sufferers in various Pacific islands were often found living together away from their villages. This chain of reactions appears to be highly prevalent in attitudes towards leprosy where ignorance about the disease exists and contributes to stigma.

The stigma of leprosy is evident in the Samoan word for leprosy and leprosy sufferers, "lepela," which also appears to be used as a form of abuse. Despite Samoans having their own word for leprosy, the disease is not referred to by name but as "the sickness" *mai*, because of the taint of stigma invoked by the term "lepela." The testimony of Dick and his wife, and Sister Marietta, indicate that children had suffered sniggering and name-calling as "lepela children" at school.[78] However, the assistance of the PLF has enabled the children of leprosy sufferers to appear well dressed and perform well in class, and the hostile attitude is changing. Sister Marietta has noticed an enormous difference in the general attitude of the public towards the families with leprosy in Apia.[79] This indicates that the assistance of the PLF, by lifting the living standards and status of families with leprosy, has reduced the stigma associated with the disease.

The support of the PLF through Sister Marietta was noticed by other Samoans, one of whom approached Sister Marietta for assistance, saying, "I am a Catholic too ... I would like if you could fix my house up."[80] Upon being told the assistance was given to leprosy sufferers, not to those who were Catholics, he replied he wished he had had leprosy too. This response indicates, again, the enormous benefits leprosy sufferers have derived from the charitable institution set up by Patrick Twomey and effectively administered by the PLF, contributing to the reduction of stigma.

What is also evident in the testimonies of Sister Marietta, Lome and Rudy is that the medical care provided in Samoa, although well served by some doctors and staff, was in many areas deficient. Medical and PLF reports since 1977 identify a range of problems that needed to be addressed in relation to monitoring leprosy patients and carrying out surveillance checks.[81] Leprosy patients appear to have been aware of these inadequacies early on, as is apparent in the comments of Rudy about his return from Makogai, when he noticed people with leprosy who had not been diagnosed and said, "Others never noticed it, but we can just see, and I told my dad, take that boy to the hospital, he has got the sickness."[82]

A prosthetic laboratory had been funded by the PLF in Apia to fit and provide prostheses and special shoes need by amputees. But due to an inadequate service, the PLF regularly transferred patients to Twomey hospital in Suva for assessment and fittings, causing inconvenience to patients, such as Rudy and Lome, who have to leave their homes and plantations for long periods.[83]

In January 2006, on my visit to Samoa, the leprosy clinic door at Apia Hospital was locked, and Sister Marietta had been advised that the clinic had been permanently closed. Leprosy patients were advised to attend the general outpatient clinic, Acute 8. At that time the leprosy specialist was leading a national medical strike against government health policies and was unavailable to be interviewed. When Sister Marietta advised Rudy that the leprosy clinic had been closed, and that leprosy patients should in future attend the outpatient department, Rudy was disturbed. He said:

> People are not happy to go to the outpatients.... We can't go to the outpatients with our sores. People will talk about us. They will say things behind us ... and we can see it.... We rather go in our own clinic and have our dressings there.[84]

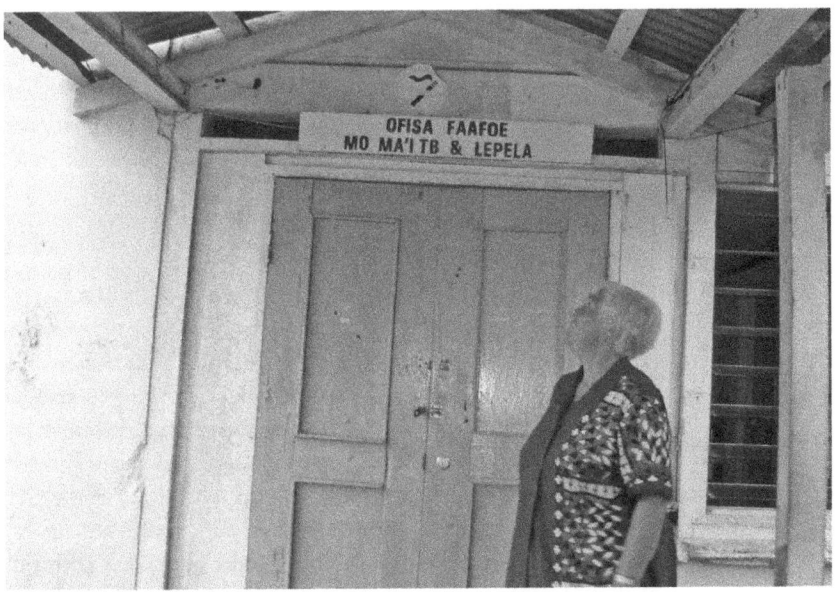

Sister Marietta SMSM at the Leprosy Clinic, at the Apia Hospital, Samoa.

This testimony indicates that because of the past hardships of their lives, despite the courage, endurance and resilience in coping with later problems caused by leprosy, older patients appear to have internalized the public attitudes towards themselves, reflecting an acceptance of stigmatization. Alternatively, stigma is still rife in public attitudes and Rudy does not wish to offend the general public by what he perceives to be his unwanted presence. The fact that the "lepela clinic" (the actual name above the door) had been closed reflects not only the lack of need for the facility, with the current low endemicity rates, but that the fear of contagion from leprosy was decreasing and leprosy was being treated as just another disease. Closure of the clinic can hopefully be seen as a step being taken by the medical fraternity to reduce stigma by having leprosy sufferers attend general hospital wards.

Nevertheless, the transitional period is not easy for many of the older generation of leprosy sufferers. Their comments indicate that they had become accustomed to being treated as subjects of contagion and felt a responsibility not to put others at risk. The look of non-acceptance in the eyes of others was often commented upon during the interviews in many islands, and it is difficult to know whether this "look" exists in reality, as indicated by the leprosy sufferers, or is a reflection of the worry absorbed by the psyche of the leprosy sufferers themselves. Perhaps both contribute to some extent, and the actual truth lies between the two poles and is too subjective to gauge.

The incidence rate of leprosy in Samoa shows that Western Samoa had one of the lowest rates of leprosy per capita in the South Pacific region, being 1.0 per 1,000 population in 1953 and rising to 1.5 per 1,000 population in 1958.[85] This low rate could be attributable to isolation practices commenced on the island very soon after the first cases of leprosy were detected and patients being exiled to Alia, Nu'utele and Makogai; while the slightly increased incidence could have been due to vigilant diagnostic practices. In 1997 Samoa reached the WHO elimination target for prevalence of less than 1:10,000, and case detection has remained at that low level since that time.[86]

As in other Pacific islands, leprosy awareness programs continue to be run by the PLF, and special programs aired on national radio on World Leprosy Day in Samoa. The WHO and PLF provide staff training courses, often run by Dr. Farrugia, so that nurses and laboratory staff are aware of the procedures necessary for the medical treatment of leprosy cases. With the excellent cure effected by MDT, and the low incidence of leprosy in Samoa, few cases present at the hospital; but to avoid stigmatizing effects, especially upon the older patients with physical problems, it is important that staff are aware of the special needs of older cases and receive the training necessary to deal with the variety of problems that do present. At the PLF 2007/2008 AGM, Dr. McMahon reported that leprosy in Samoa had a low incidence but leprosy patients need continuing support because of problems with the country's dysfunctional health service.[87] The visit to Samoa and interviews with leprosy sufferers indicate that the recent level of PLF support has made a huge difference to the quality of the lives of those with leprosy and their families, which in turn has made a dramatic difference in lowering the stigma attached to the disease.

Nevertheless, the long years of stigma endured by older leprosy sufferers, and their physical disabilities that continue to require regular medical care at the leprosy clinic, appears to have caused them to retain the idea that stigma is still perceived by the public. This caused concern regarding the closure of the leprosy clinic in 2006 and the need to attend the general outpatient clinics for treatment. These reactions reflect the difficulties encountered in changing old ideas about leprosy being a disease that is different and has to be treated separately. With the good medication available now, newer cases are not caught in a time warp of old ideas; and as new and old cases are treated in mainstream clinics at hospitals, and the old physical deformities due to late diagnosis cease to occur, leprosy will gradually be perceived as just another disease in Samoa, with the old ideas of stigma dying away.

4

The Loneliness of Isolation—Tonga

Historical Background

The Polynesian Kingdom of Tonga is proud of its ancient history as a major seafaring power in the South Pacific. The ancient dynasty of spiritual and temporal kings, Tui Tonga, ruled Tonga, for a thousand years with their great double canoes plying the southern ocean. The first known European visitors to these islands were the Dutch as early as 1616, followed in 1643 by Abel Tasman, who reported that the Tongans were peaceful, orderly and industrious.[1] Over a century later, during a visit in the 1870s, James Cook named the islands the Friendly Islands, not knowing that plans were in motion to kill him and his crew while they, fortuitously, departed from Tongan shores.[2] The lack of involvement with foreign commercial activities in the Pacific meant the Tongan islands were not targeted for western exploitation, but used as stops to replenish supplies by voyagers, and were naturally of interest to explorers gathering geographical and ethnographical information.[3]

Despite some attacks by Tongans to obtain goods from European ships visiting the islands, the relationship between Tongans and the foreigners remained relatively friendly, mainly because the islanders were preoccupied with battles and challenges between the powerful rival families claiming rights to kingship. Bolstered by the use of foreign firearms, Chief Taufa'ahau Tupou succeeded in the succession battle and established his leadership. In 1828 he told the Wesleyan missionaries, who, through trade and barter had been gaining Tongan conversions to Christianity since their arrival in 1822,[4] that he wished to convert to Christianity.[5] Following the baptism in 1831 of King Taufa'ahau, renamed King George Tupou, nearly half the Tongan population of about 20,000 converted to Christianity.[6] Under the direction of the Roman Catholic Bishop Pompallier, Marist priests of the Society of Mary were sent to "offset the progress of Protestant missionaries in Oceania"[7] and attempted to set up a Catholic mission on another Tongan island in 1842.[8] After initial rivalries and skirmishes, almost precipitating a civil war, both groups were permitted to establish separate missions on different islands, supported by different chiefs; the Wesleyan mission remained closely aligned to Tupou.

Of particular pride to Tongans is the fact that despite rival claims for leadership, their monarchs maintained paramount control over the islands and resisted direct foreign colonization by tactical diplomacy, using missionary influences to counter both local rival claims to overall leadership and prevent Europeans from taking control. Following King Tupou's consolidation as the ruling monarch, he introduced western styled reforms in 1859 to ensure his own personal status, as well as to ensure Tonga's independent status as a participant in treaty negotiations in the South Pacific region.[9] From 1860 to 1890 the Wesleyan missionary Rev. Shirley Waldemar Baker served as Tupou's political adviser and prime minister.

Upon arrival in Tonga in 1860, Baker made use of medical knowledge he had acquired through an English relative who was a doctor.[10] Missionaries were routinely approached by islanders for western medical advice, and frequently the power of their medicines and the recovery of patients were attributed to the perceived superiority of the missionaries' religion over local beliefs, thereby gaining converts to Christianity.[11] Baker's familiarity with dispensing western medicines soon gained him great success and notoriety, as he attended "thirty or forty Tongan patients every day."[12] By 1864 it was alleged that Baker "refused to administer even a single dose of Epsom salts without his fee of a dollar and a half,"[13] indicating a substantial income, whether paid in cash or, as he claimed, in the local currency of barter — particularly when he vaccinated three thousand Tongans against smallpox. Baker was a controversial figure even during his lifetime, being described as "common" and, by the Governor of Fiji in 1880, a "narrow minded, selfish and *ignorant* man"[14] although in later years the Governor grudgingly revised this opinion and even praised Baker's achievements in the interests of Tonga.[15]

In his role as medical adviser, there is a fascinating incident relating to Baker's rise to influence with King Tupou, containing one of the earliest references to leprosy.[16] The King relied on his secretary, David Moss, in his dealings with Europeans, to write letters, draft regulations and act as paymaster and receiver of revenues. According to research undertaken by Rutherford:

> In November 1871 Moss's wife came to Baker seeking treatment for a disease which was causing her hands and fingers to decay. Baker diagnosed leprosy, and Moss was suddenly dropped from the king's retinue. Baker quietly took the vacant place.[17]

It would be interesting to know whether Baker's diagnosis was correct and what medical advice he offered regarding this and any other leprosy cases he may have encountered. It is beyond the scope of this research to investigate archives relating to Baker, and it is speculative whether Baker considered leprosy highly contagious, requiring isolation, and whether as a radical evangelist he might have referred to stigmatizing passages from Leviticus in the Bible to the early Tongan converts to Christianity. Little is known with any certitude about local attitudes that developed towards leprosy during this very early period, but an exclusionary attitude towards leprosy is reflected as early as 1875 in the Constitution of Tonga, Part I, Declaration of Rights, clause 3, relating to entry into Tonga of people from different lands:

> But it shall not be lawful for any one to make any contracts with any Chinese to come and work for him, lest the disease of leprosy be brought to Tonga the same as exists in the Sandwich Islands.*... Any Chinaman wishing to reside in Tonga must first produce a doctor's certificate that he is free from such disease: then it shall be lawful for him to reside in Tonga.[18]

Comments made to the writer as recently as 2006 by Dr. Taniela Lutui, who worked at the Fale'ofa leprosy center in Tonga in the 1970s, indicated that Tongans feared the disease because it was declared unclean in Leviticus and should be isolated.[19] Baker's puritanical interpretations of Wesleyan Christianity, and his dealings in medicine, could possibly have led to ostracizing attitudes towards the unfortunate people who contracted the newly introduced disease. Generally leprosy was reported and perceived at that time in the west as unclean and contagious. In the Pacific Islands disease was often seen to be the result of divine intervention, either wrath or a curse. In the culture of religious conversion and competing claims of superior divinities, evangelical missionaries such as Baker associated leprosy with divine displeasure being wrought upon "disbelieving heathens," and the quotations of Leviticus are likely to be attributable to protestant evangelists who frequently quoted from the Old Testament.

A Tongan stance is evident in the wording of a response regarding the exile of leprosy sufferers in a reply from the premier of Tonga in 1896 to the Samoan government. In attempts to control the spread of leprosy, Samoa sought to establish a joint leprosarium, but Tonga rejected the offer, stating:

> Anyone who is infected with this disease is taken to a town, place or island far away from the people. Furthermore, those with leprosy were disallowed visitation since the area was out of bounds.[20]

These injunctions regarding leprosy came prior to those invoked by the First International Leprosy Conference in 1897 and reflect a Tongan attitude towards leprosy sufferers, which could possibly have stemmed from an extreme evangelical stance taken from Leviticus in the Bible. The Samoan government pursued the idea to establish a joint leprosarium with the Tongans, possibly on Rose Island, but were firmly rejected on the basis that "under no conditions, however stringent, would the Tongan Government permit the landing of a single leper on the shores of Tonga."[21] Moreover, no vessel with leprosy sufferers aboard would be permitted entrance, and the Tongan Government firmly declined "to make any alteration in this most salutary regulation."[22]

Early Incidence of Leprosy

Although leprosy had undoubtedly surfaced in the islands prior to 1900, the first officially diagnosed case of leprosy was not recorded until 1927, and no written or medical records are available for this early period. According to the Tongan doctor Tanelia Lutui, and corroborated by Stella, soon after the first official diagnosis of leprosy in 1927, thirteen leprosy patients were transported to Makogai.[23] The Makogai statistics register from 1911–69 shows that there were eighty-six admissions from Tonga, with sixty-five patients being discharged, twenty patients dying, and one patient remaining in 1969.[24] No further details on these earliest patients are known and archival records were unavailable in Tonga.

Locating archival records in Tonga, as in all Pacific Islands, was extremely difficult due to the humid tropical conditions and their deleterious effects upon paper. The open-style construction of homes and public gathering places, *fale*, which is very suitable for extreme weather conditions and annual tropical storms, offers little protection for the storage of documents. Even offices and government buildings are frequently destroyed by cyclones and typhoons, thereby diminishing the value of paper in Tongan society. Despite being the first Pacific Island with its own independent constitution, Tonga has no public libraries nor a national archive. Government records are held at the Royal Palace, but permission to search these is apparently rarely granted. There was no chance of this writer gaining permission to access these archives, especially in view of the fact that the main center of Nuku'alofa was set ablaze by a civil resistance movement against the monarchy during the time of my visit.

After 1927, and certainly during the period when the older interviewees were diagnosed with leprosy, all those diagnosed were separated from their families—either in an independent hut near their home or isolated in some sort of unit near the hospital—until transport was available to take the leprosy sufferers to Makogai. This policy was still in place as late as the 1950s, as evidenced by the included testimonies of Polutele and Taliai, both of whom waited two years before transportation to Makogai became available in 1954.

Because of the lack of archival material, enormous reliance is placed upon the six oral histories conducted with Tongan leprosy sufferers. References are made to the testimonies in an attempt to trace the recent history of leprosy in Tonga, followed by detailed summaries of their experiences. Details will include isolation either at Makogai or the Fale'ofa leprosy center on the island of Vava'u, the living conditions at these leprosaria and subsequent events following discharge back to their homes. These descriptions demonstrate how the prevailing leprosy stigma impacted upon their lives after discharge and their return to their homes.

The earliest records located relating to leprosy in Tonga to be deposited at Macmillan Brown Library leprosy archives contain lists of patients receiving treatment of DDS twice weekly, through Niu'ui Hospital, Lifuka, on the island of Ha'apai from 1957 to 1965.[25] The local health worker administering the medication and maintaining the records added a comment that the patients "didn't seem to co-operate and [sic] appreciate the help that we try to give them."[26] This could be more a reflection of a health worker unhappily employed than the patients being unappreciative, but the paucity of records prevents any real understanding of this observation.

Since the treatment of leprosy patients with MDT, the incidence of new cases rapidly dropped, and Tonga reached the WHO elimination rate target in 1996, with only three new cases in the ten years to 2006.[27] The incidence being less than 0.1 per 10,000 cases means low visibility of leprosy; and to promote knowledge about the disease in an effort to diminish stigma that still appears to prevail, the PLF continues to sponsor awareness and training programs.[28] It is conceivable that the strict isolation policy adopted from earliest times may have accounted for the low incidence of the disease in Tonga; although, inversely, isolation practices may have contributed to higher stigma in Tonga than neighboring Polynesian islands because of the poor conditions at local leprosaria and/or the removal of affected family members to faraway Makogai. During the visit to Tonga in 2006, attitudes suggesting high stigma associated with leprosy appeared to be prevalent, although gradually declining.

Fale'ofa Leprosy Clinic at Ngu Hospital, Vava'u

At the inaugural meeting of the Tongan Leprosy Patients Trust Committee, on 14 May, 1965, with the effective medication of DDS readily available and negotiations in hand to close the leprosarium at Makogai, it was proposed that a "new leprosarium be established at Vava'u in 1966."[29] Apparently some type of holding facility, details of which were not uncovered, housed the leprosy patients en route to and from Makogai, but these facilities were inadequate for the treatment and support of patients, thereby necessitating the establishment of a new leprosarium. A piece of land a little distance away and behind the Ngu Hospital at Vava'u was fenced off and three buildings erected to form the Fale'ofa leprosy center. One building housed male patients, another was for females and the third building contained cooking and washing facilities. The earliest description of the center is provided by Kulaea Tu'a Leketi, who was diagnosed with leprosy after the birth of her third child in 1970 and admitted to Fale'ofa the same day, remaining there for six years. Kulaea's testimony is through translation by Sister Goretti, a Fijian SMSM who served as PLF liaison contact in Vava'u.

> In the hospital at Fale'ofa there were three men and three women, and she [Kulaea] is the fourth.... The fence was very high. It was difficult to get over. They felt like a slave being there because of the fence, and the fact that they were told that they were completely separated from the world outside.... When they bring their food, their meals, they just put it through this box, there is a box in the fence and they just put it in.... They were not allowed to come in nor were they allowed to get out. Even the doctors came only from the area where they were allowed to come in.... They didn't come in at all to the hospital itself.... There were only two people that as far as she can recall who actually came in, opened the gate and came right into them — the Priest, Father Karle, and Mrs. Mathieson, a European lady.... The lady brought sewing kits and all that and taught them how to sew, some of the patients like that. She bring machines, material, everything.... They were here like Red Cross Society ... brought everything. She asked them what they need, you know shoes and things like that. Every Friday she visited them.[30]

Another corroborating description of Fale'ofa leprosy center is provided by Fusi Takeifanga, a nurse and matron of a ward at Ngu Hospital from 1977 to 2005. Although Fusi did not work or attend patients at Fale'ofa leprosy clinic, she observed some activities associated with the leprosy center:

> Fale'ofa ... two houses, and the other house for the workers.... Kitchen house ... might be they cook their own food. They [hospital] gave the food, and they [patients] do it. They carry the food there, and they do it.... Once a day [a nurse visited] and dish out their medicines.... I saw one of the nurses go, they go and change their uniform, and when they send their food, they go straight away to the other house so somebody will come and take the food out.[31]

Fusi's testimony indicates a limited knowledge about the Fale'ofa clinic, despite working at the adjoining hospital, suggesting minimal contact between hospital staff, leprosy patients and the center since her employment in 1977 until the closure of the center in about 1980. This total exclusion of leprosy patients indicates a high level of stigma. While visiting Ngu Hospital, another staff member suggested that "a professor" visited Fale'ofa in 1979/80 and was

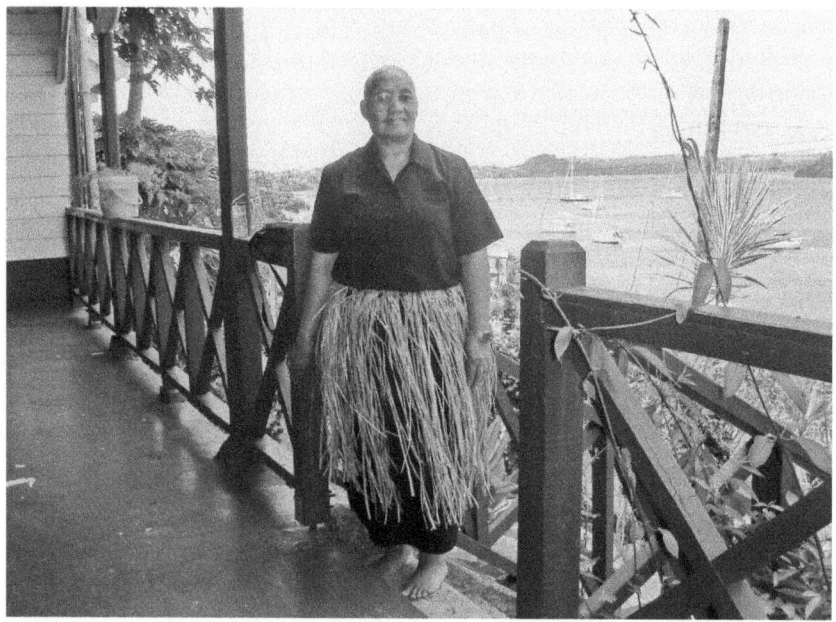

Matron Fusi Takeifanga (now retired) in Vava'u.

so appalled by the conditions that, since patients were no longer infectious, he discharged the patients — much to the horror of others. By 1980/81 the leprosarium was demolished.[32] It is likely the appalling conditions of Fale'ofa leprosarium itself sustained ideas of stigma. The author was shown the oldest leprosy files at Ngu Hospital, the earliest of these files being of six patients treated in 1982, that is, after the closure of Fale'ofa, since patients were treated at the main hospital. No earlier files or documents appear to have been retained at the hospital.

Dr. Taniela Lutui, presently the public health manager at the Tongan Health Society in Auckland, had worked in Tonga in the 1970s and '80s with the late Dr. Tilitili Poluka, the latter being well known for his service to leprosy sufferers in Tonga. Before his death, both Tilitili Poluka and Lutui had hoped to write a history of leprosy in Tonga, but, unfortunately, this never materialized. Head of Public Health, Dr. Malaki Ake, and Dr. Mappa Poluka, son of Tilitili Poluka, recalled notebooks regarding the proposed venture; but despite searches, these documents were not located.[33] Dr. Lutui maintains that "leprosy was epidemic in Tonga as from 1927 to the early to mid–1950s, then, slowly, fewer cases were diagnosed."[34] He commented:

> People were scared to come up to the open because they were scared that they be diagnosed as leprosy and sent away from their families [in] Tonga. Not

only this but the whole family were branded as cursed by God because it says so in the Bible Book of Leviticus, Chapter 13 and 14, shows all signs of skin ailments, including lepers, and what to look for in confirming and diagnoses of leprosy. Diagnosis [sic] were done by Rev Ministers of the Tribes of Israel and the sufferers were declared unclean and had to be isolated from the rest of the Community.[35]

The fact that in 2006 Dr. Lutui could quote directly from Leviticus indicates that the high level of stigma in Tonga was connected with biblical stigma, as suggested previously. Lutui had worked at Ngu Hospital and attended the Fale'ofa leprosy center from 1972 to 1974, and he recalled there had been "four or five sad cases in residence,"[36] as compared to Kulaea's testimony that at the time of her admission in 1970 there were seven residents.[37] Lutui indicated that a high level of stigma persisted during the years of his treatment of leprosy in Tonga:

> When I left six years ago [2000], the strong stigma of the leprosy still exist among our community, because many people still believe that all leprosy sufferers is a curse from God. I tried on many occasion to erase that misunderstanding from healthy population, even with the family of leprosy patients, on seminars and leprosy workshops, but still some people do not believe that leprosy is a communicable disease like any other.[38]

This testimony is totally explicit in connecting the high stigma in Tonga to Old Testament biblical stigma, or conceivably traditional ideas of curses by the supernatural, which falls outside the purview of this research. The fact that local Tongans and even families of leprosy sufferers resisted Dr. Lutui's notion that leprosy is just another communicable disease supports the Japanese findings that the views of the older generation are resistant to change. The testimonies and lifestyles of the leprosy sufferers described below support notions of being treated as outcasts due to the stigma of leprosy in Tonga.

Tongan Experiences at Makogai Leprosarium

Of the six leprosy sufferers interviewed in Tonga, four of these had been residents at Makogai,[39] namely, Polutele Fakatava, Taliai Sanft, Maliakalemeli Nunu, and Manitepi Molimoli, the first two being males and the latter two being females. Polutele was interviewed at Twomey hospital in Fiji, but being a Tongan who was taken to Makogai from Vava'u, relevant portions of his testimony are included here.

The earliest transportee to Makogai was Maliakalemeli, age seventeen, in 1945; she returned to Tonga nine years later in 1954. Taliai and Polutele were on the same steamship to Makogai in 1954, aged 22 and 12 years respectively. Taliai returned to Tonga in 1965, while Polutele chose to remain at Twomey hospital, Suva, Fiji. Manitepi thought she went to Makogai in 1956, returning to Tonga in 1968. Apart from Maliakalemeli, who was briefly married before being sent to Makogai, none of these four interviewees married. Each attributed their single status to having had leprosy and attitudes of stigma attached to the disease. Summaries of these four interviewees will be given first, followed by summaries of three leprosy sufferers who contracted leprosy after Makogai had closed and so remained in Tonga for their leprosy treatment.

Polutele Fakatava (b. 1932) was born in Vava'u, one of seven children, and was featured in the video *Compassionate Exile* when four inmates of Makogai were taken to visit the old leprosarium and recalled their lives in isolation.[40] Short extracts from the documentary were included in descriptions provided earlier regarding Fiji. Polutele recalled that at age eleven he was very sick, but it was not until he was twenty-two that he was diagnosed with leprosy and sent, in 1954, to Makogai, when sulphone medication was available:

> I go to see the doctor in Tonga, and doctor give me medicine but not working. Sometime I getting better and go back to school. My family looked after ... they make one house for me ... we stayed together, eat together, but my family they didn't know I got at that time the leprosy.... Every time I go to doctor they come and check me, give me some medicine, make no difference.... The doctor came ... to Tonga to see me. He not tell me, he tell my father, oh he got the sickness, go Makogai. No medicine in Tonga, go to Makogai. ... My mother crying, somebody tell, that each time when people go to Makogai he go and die there, there is no medicine. I tell my mother, it's alright I will go, yeah, because I know when I get better I will come back and see you and the family.... Only two weeks, the doctor tell me we got six people in Tonga who got the leprosy.... Sometimes [I was very sad], but only in myself. People we came together, younger ones. Some eleven years, some ten years, some fourteen years ... but I am older and I see after, all the family come and tell me, Polu, you look after the kids on the boat. Every night I check the children, ... all the kids crying, all my family crying at that time. We come the big boat, then come the small boat, all my family come.[41]

Polutele's testimony indicates poor diagnosis of leprosy between the years 1943 and 1954 in Tonga, and also demonstrates the difficulty of travel for leprosy patients in order to be transported to Makogai. It appears that although Dapsone was available by 1954, it was not in use yet in Tonga; but according to the earliest records, Dapsone/DDS treatment was provided to leprosy sufferers by 1958.

On arrival in Makogai, Polutele was placed with the serious cases, and the first night two older leprosy sufferers beside him died in succession:

4. The Loneliness of Isolation

I lay down in my bed and see the sister come and cleaned that guy, the smell, and clean the other one and finish all the clothes and put the clothes in one place. When people die and people come and sing the hymn and bring kava and wait for the other day to go and bury. Every day people die, only one day there no place to put the people die. The sister go back and I lie down on the bed, and I know, myself, if this kind of people die like this then one day I will. I say my prayer.... I lay down and look up and I feeling something God gave the life to me, and doctor came and see me and I say, oh, gone .... I sit in my chair and felt God gave life to me at Makogai.[42]

My life is coming, but then I stay there and I help the sister and doctor to look after the patients, the dressing ... and the sisters coming at night time, who clean the patient, help the patient, putting in bed and going to the toilet. I help them very much in Makogai.[43]

Although this description details the horror of the early days at Makogai for new arrivals who had never witnessed the later stages of the ravages of leprosy, Polutele's description confirms to some degree the growing reputation of the leprosarium since the advent of the sulphones, of being an "image of hope" posited by the title of Stella's publication. The dedication and warmth of the care provided by the SMSM sisters eased significantly the isolation and rejection patients might have suffered, although Polutele's testimony shows that nothing could replace the heartbreak of being parted from mothers and loved ones. He stayed at Makogai fourteen years, until the closure in 1969, and offered the following description of his lifestyle in isolation:

Wake up the morning, cut the grass and sweep the village ... go and have your shower and come have your tea. When you go to job, cut the grass or play the house or something like this. If you have problem, go have your medicine. After shower and do your job, half past seven go and have your medicine. You go the hospital and get your medicine from sister. Every village, the sister go and give the medicine half past seven, given the medicine to all the Tongan, Samoan, Fijian, Indian.... Somebody sweep, and in the Tongan [village] we got somebody to cook the food. One week, two or three men cook, next week change cooking.... I learn to carpenter.... Plenty people over there very clever to teach, we go the big workshop over there. Some teaching for the machine, build the houses.[44]

Every afternoon we go and take the clothes for washing, and the women make some food for us. Take the clothes, wash them, bring back. Take food for Tongan women, taro and cassava for the Tongan women. The Fijian feed the Fijian women, the Tongan feed the Tongan women. [Daily routine:] Somebody go in the house, some go and cut the flowers, every people got the job. Some engineer, you got the building and you go in teaching the job over there. One school. They learn the English and Fijian.... I can speak Samoan, I can speak Indian a little bit, I can speak Gilbertese a little bit, I can speak Fijian. Mixed, no problem.... Very happy place, Makogai. Different. Some night we go the Fijian village and drink kava over there, some come to the

> Tongan village and drink kava there and sing a song. Oh, a very nice island, I don't know another island in Fiji like Makogai. Clean and plenty fish, cobs, taro, yams, plenty food over there. Every time we go fishing, plenty of fish over there. We make our own food.... Women cooked their own food. They had a place to cook the food for the patients in the hospital.... In Makogai when we want to eat some food, you go to and get it. No money.[45]

Polutele's testimony confirms that the fertility of the land at Makogai and fishing resources of the island played a huge part towards the success of the leprosarium, contributing to the feeling of usefulness and well being of the whole community. Despite enforced gender segregation, the availability of education to children, teaching job skills to all patients, and the daily tasks involving self sufficiency and independence appeared to motivate those isolated at the leprosarium to be responsible for their own general living conditions, creating their own homes away from home. This life style also provided hope that if and when they were discharged they would have skills to find jobs or take part in work on plantations and gardens, which was the normal island lifestyle. Segregation also meant that young women could retain hope of future marriage. They also received the advantages of an education, which was not always available to girls in the island villages, and certainly not otherwise available to children with leprosy.

The testimonies of several interviewees at Makogai confirmed that the SMSM staff at Makogai encouraged festivities and fun, respecting at the same time the different cultures brought together at Makogai, such as the preparations for the visit by Queen Salote of Tonga. The visit by Queen Salote would have been an important occasion for the Tongans, perhaps indicating a more inclusive attitude towards leprosy sufferers rather than the highly stigmatized Christian views cited by Dr. Lutui. Polutele recalled the Queen's visit and other aspects of living at Makogai:

> Every Christmas day, every Easter, we ... together dance.... Tongan make the Tongan dance, Samoan make the Samoa dance, and Fijian make their dance.... The time when Queen Salote, Queen of Tonga, came to Makogai, only the Tongan make the matting, make for Queen Salote. Bring ... and come and visit the people in Makogai. Make the dancing, Tongan dancing, make the songs.... The Tongan people live together, only the women, only one place. The Tongan men stay one village, Fijian in one village, Samoan one village, Gilbertese one village, Fijian one village, Indians one village. Only the women stayed together.[46]

This testimony demonstrates that different cultural identities were celebrated and encouraged to be retained at Makogai; but everyone contributed towards making life bearable until the time that they might be able to return home. But the harsher realities of living with leprosy at the leprosarium are

4. The Loneliness of Isolation

indicated in the following extracts by Polutele — in participating in medication trials and enduring separation from family. Yet they also demonstrate the sense of camaraderie at Makogai:

> Some time you got the new medicine, the doctor and the sister come in asking, you want to try or not. Up to you.... One sister start telling me, Polu you want to try, and I say I want to.... Nobody want to die, you want to try. It is good everybody can use the medicine ... it was good for me. Pills, not injection, pills, two. Monday and Wednesday, and Saturday I think six months. By the end... changed the skin. Some black in the skin, but by the time you finish it, no more come black.[47]
>
> *So you thought it was better you go to Makogai or better to stay at home?*
> Nobody want to stay in a place like Makogai, I want to stay in my home, but only the sickness. I think you can ask somebody, everybody don't want to stay in Makogai, just the sickness. ... Oh, everybody cry when somebody leave Makogai. Everybody come and gift, people come and make the food, something to take back ... make the party ... sad, but going back to family. Staying on Makogai was like a family, never mind I'm Tongan, Fijian, Indian or Cook Island or Samoan. We stayed there and lived like a family.... Feeling like your brothers are gone ... people very sad to go to Makogai, everyone stayed there was good. Free place, free life. No staying one place, go round the island, go fishing, go sailing, picnic, everything.... Every time you take your smear, you know it is good or not, the smear. You all right, you waiting next month maybe you can go home.[48]

The feeling of being part of a wider family engendered self-respect, as did living in a self-sufficient community like Makogai, which, for many residents, including Polutele, lasted beyond their Makogai days, especially after years of isolation:

> Some people, the family is gone, some places are very hard to go in and keeping home with. Like me, my father and my mother died, and all my brother married, all my sister married, but myself.... They ask me every time I want to go to Tonga, but when I go to Tonga my father and mother are still alive I can do everything I want to, eh.... My family like me to go there, but myself I don't want to go.... My mother and father die, all my brother is married with family and stay with them. [At Twomey hospital] I am working in the workshop. I make some pendants, pins, earrings. Sell them. In the dining room over there somebody come in and buy some. Sometime people from New Zealand come, and I make something for them.[49]
>
> Everyone want to marry, but I am sickness. [If I did marry] my kids and my wife no one to look after, so no good. Sometime my sister tell me why you not get married.... I can't look after.... [Twomey hospital is] very good for old people.... It is better to stay in the hospital, to go home you can't do some things.[50]

Polutele's revealing testimony demonstrates a pragmatic acceptance of his physical condition and approach to life; or, alternatively, it could be interpreted as having internalized a level of self-stigma because he felt unable to find work, marry or support a family. But the high level of stigma evident in Tonga, demonstrated by overt attitudes of exclusion by friends and neighbors of the interviewees, invalidates the suggestion of self-stigma. Polutele feels more useful helping Twomey Hospital staff care for other leprosy sufferers at Makogai rather than returning home. The strong stigma of leprosy in Tonga undoubtedly played a major part in deterring Polutele from returning home, so he chose to stay with his newfound "Makogai family" at Twomey Hospital, Suva.

Polutele's life story demonstrates that although separation from loved ones and isolation at leprosaria was emotionally cruel for leprosy sufferers, if, in fact, the local stigma was so high as to exclude victims of the disease from their home communities, leprosaria provided a home and camaraderie. Additionally, the severe physical disabilities of many leprosy sufferers meant that they could not find work to support themselves, which in turn imposed hardships on their families, so that, again, a leprosarium was the pragmatic residence of choice.

Taliai Sanft (b. 1943) went to Makogai in 1954 and returned to Tonga in 1965. He lived alone in a hut he built for himself on land owned by his parents, a fair distance away from his main family home. The PLF had recently provided funding for the addition of a water tank and toilet. Taliai had successfully established a highly productive plantation around his hut after his return from Makogai. The plantation had spread over a large area from which he supplied produce to family members when requested, and tended the garden at the SMSM home.

He was a very fit, strong, quiet-spoken man who invited us to sit on a fallen tree trunk under a mango tree. There was a mild gale at the time, and the sound of recording was partly blown away by the wind in the trees overhead. Despite my initial suggestion that perhaps the interview would be best conducted in his home, the suggestion was not taken up. As two women visiting a single man, it did not seem appropriate to persist with the suggestion. The weather conditions rendered substantial portions of the interview inaudible, preventing transcription.

Taliai was at school when he first began to feel unwell, with nodules and swellings appearing on his face. He noticed that other children began to avoid him.[51] He was diagnosed with leprosy at age nine, but had to wait two years, until 1954, for the boat to take him and his brother, who also had leprosy, to Makogai. Sister Goretti translated:

> They waited for that boat, and by that time he was told to be separated from his family, so a house was built for these people. *For the other people who were waiting?* No. *All by himself?* Yes, just by himself, none of the family.... About

4. The Loneliness of Isolation   137

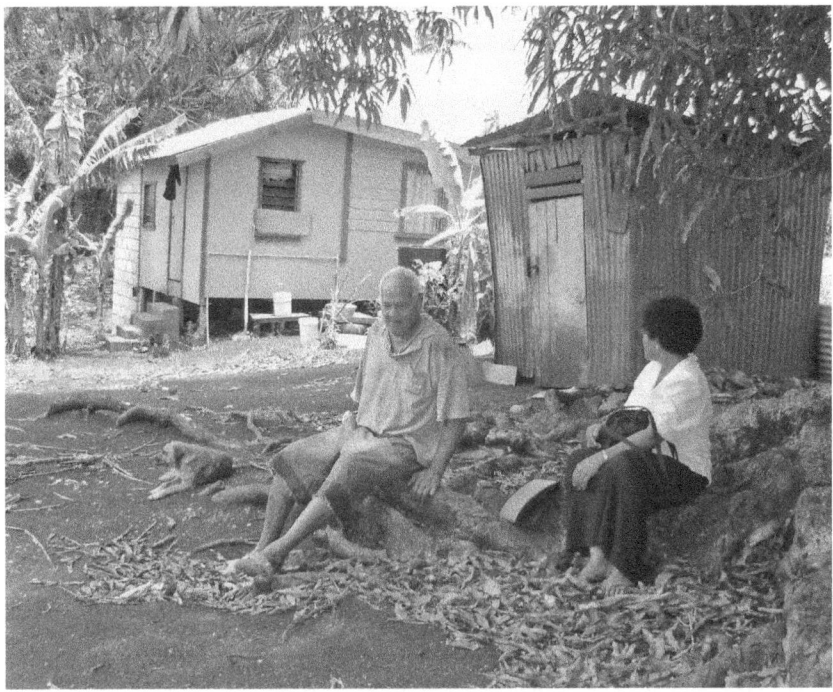

Taliai Sanft and Sister Goretti SMSM sitting on a tree by his old home. In the background stands his new home, built with PLF assistance.

> six people, and it took awhile because they had to wait for the other patients for the boat.... They went together with Polutele and Mani.[52]

Asked if he knew anything about Makogai prior to being transported, he replied:

> They did talk about it and Makogai and the leprosy.... He know that he was going to be separated from his mother.... What he remembers most [is] how he felt it was hard to be separated from his mum and also thinking ... people were scared that they would never come back, that they died there. But when he got there they had this tablet that they could treat it, tablets. Then he said when he arrived there he was very impressed with the place, you know, and he liked it. The only hard thing that he feels that is not seeing his mum.[53]

Taliai was in Makogai eleven years and commented on these years:

> He continued to take the tablets.... It took a long time [to get better].... There were a lot of children in the same position.... He says that he was not the only one. It was a good memory being there.... There is no one being treated different, we all laughed and all concerned when they come to get their tablets, you know, they didn't seem to stand in a queue ... wait ... pull faces ... so even

when they come, even a small complaint like that, they [staff, SMSM] never refused to attend.... Come back from Fiji ... 7th May, 1965 ... stayed in Fiji for two weeks.[54]

The fact that Taliai said the staff at Makogai "never refused to attend" the patients indicates that the treatment in Makogai was different from other times and places when it appears leprosy sufferers might have received assistance begrudgingly, or were even rejected, possibly at Ngu Hospital, Vava'u.

Although parts of the tape are inaudible, notes made at the time and my memory of the interview recall that Taliai indicated he suffered strong rejection on his return home. He had gone to Makogai at the same time as Polutele, who later decided to remain in Fiji rather than face rejection or cause problems for his family by returning to Tonga. Taliai was not permitted to live in his family home, but was allowed to build himself a hut at the end of the plantation.[55] This is in line with biblical injunctions quoted earlier by Dr. Lutui. Taliai would have liked to have married, but it was not possible, he said, because he could not support a wife and family, as his circumstances were such that he could only just support himself. However, his hard work was rewarded by a good plantation, such that his family now asked for the produce; but he said these were not overtures of friendship, simply greed for what they could obtain. It is difficult to assess stigma and whether Taliai had simply been hardened by the earlier stigmatizing attitudes of his family and was unable to perceive or accept that a change of attitude might have occurred over the years. However, a level of self-stigma due to early attitudes of stigma may well have been internalized by Taliai, who continued to keep himself isolated from his relatives and village life around him.

After the death of his parents, his family argued about who would inherit the plantation, but Taliai chose not to associate with his relatives; nor did he socialize with the villagers.[56] He did not attend any village functions, and on the day of the interview, everyone in the village was at a wedding which he did not attend. Taliai appeared to be particularly kindly and at the end of the interview apologized for "wasting our time because he did not speak English," although, in fact, it was apparent he did understand a lot of the conversation, having learned some English at Makogai.[57] Apart from minor problems with his fingers and toes, Taliai had no serious disabilities caused by leprosy. Taliai's solitary lifestyle and comments indicate the high level of stigma associated with leprosy in Vava'u. For a person who had worked hard supporting himself, and even his estranged family, to have remained unmarried and not formed friendships in his village (other than old friends from Makogai) confirms an attitude of high stigma from those around him towards leprosy and victims of disease. It also reaffirms the lasting benefits of camaraderie with those who had been isolated earlier with him.

4. The Loneliness of Isolation

Maliakalemeli Nunu (b. 1928) lives in Sopu, not far from Nuku'alofa on the main island of Tongatapu. Her mother died after the birth of her younger sister, and she was brought up at a local Catholic convent by SMSM sisters until the age of twelve, when her father took her back. But she said she did not want to speak about this brief return home.[58] When she first noticed patches on her face, she suspected leprosy but was not diagnosed at the hospital until two or three years later, when she was seventeen and had returned for another check. She regretted that she had not been sent to Makogai when she first suspected leprosy, as she had been told by the sisters who raised her that Makogai was a place where she would be well cared for.[59] She remembered the names of the sisters who cared for her at the convent, and recalled, through the translator:

> She explaining how Sister Elphemia is like the one who is very close to her like a mother. When she left, she [Sister Elphemia] packed everything she needs ... [for the trip Makogai], and somebody come and told her to wait, she is going to bring a pudding for her. But she said thank you very much to her, I love her, but the boat is about to leave. Many people there, it was a big boat. She loved it. They left on the Tuesday and arrived on the Thursday. She went herself and another lady and her daughter.... It was a boat from Rarotonga ... She stayed in the women's place, she says it was a two-storey house.[60]

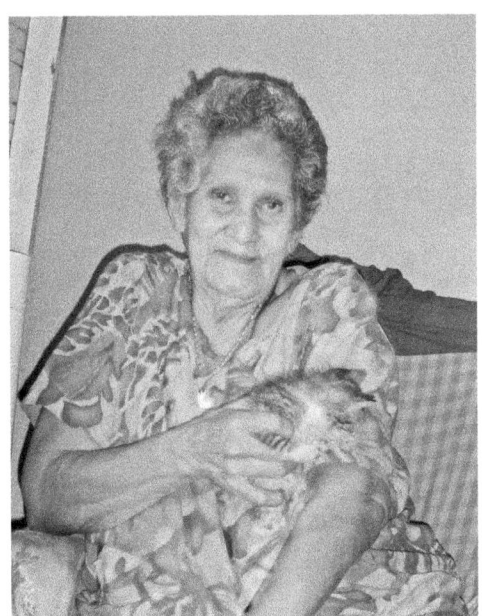

Maliakalemeli Nunu at home with one of her kittens.

Maliakalemeli arrived in Makogai, age seventeen, in 1945 while the leprosy patients were still receiving Chaulmoogra injections, but she did not respond to questions about this treatment. She said how happy she was at Makogai, and how she and her friend tried to feign symptoms in order not to be transferred home.[61] Later in the interview Maliakalemeli mentioned she had been married at age sixteen and had a son prior to going to Makogai.[62] She did not speak about this time of her life, perhaps because it was an unhappy period. Instead, in reply to a question about whether she was sad to leave Tonga, she answered:

> Not very sad about saying goodbye to the family, but [sad] because of not taking her a little bit earlier [to Makogai]. But she was happy to go because she said she would be well taken care of if she goes.[63]

Maliakalemeli is obviously unusual in that she was raised in a convent by SMSM, having lost her mother, so she welcomed being sequestered at Makogai. When pressed to comment on her life, she talked about living at Makogai, confirming the happiness felt at being warmly welcomed:

> It is like a place where she has everything.... She can't find how to explain how to express how she was there at Makogai, she feels at home at everything that they done there. Very happy.... She says she is homesick, homesick coming here [to Tonga].... When they are clear [of leprosy] and she is explaining that if they ask you, how are you, if you say you have pain or something, that mean you can stay.... When they ask, how are you, she says [the translator says Maliakalemeli feels] a little bit pain, and she doesn't want to tell the others. So when they call the names of those, her name wasn't called. She was happy. She is explaining about another person, they were the two that tried to make out things that they would look like they not cured.[64]

This testimony demonstrates a choice to remain at Makogai rather than return home, either because of a better lifestyle at the leprosarium or fear of stigma upon returning home, or both. Maliakalemeli went on to describe the life at Makogai and her return home to Tonga (through the interpreter):

> They used to go to movies, she is explaining the SMSM, doing the movies and there is a little shop.... They don't mix [men and women], they just have their own area and they can see to each other. But ... [laughter] ... they had to go out to the garden and weed, three days a week, and the rest of the days they could do whatever they feel like doing.... She is telling me about when she went to the movie one night, and they came back, and one of the sisters called her, the one doing the blood test, called her and told her, "Do you know you are leaving on Thursday?" ... She accepted that she is coming, but on the other side, she is happy to come and happy to stay. But she would like to come and see her aunty that was still alive here. Because she said if she [the aunt] wasn't still alive, she would make another story so that she would continue staying.[65]

Having been married and had a child prior to her isolation, Maliakalemeli was in favor of the gender segregation at Makogai:

> It is better to separate men from women, but the problem still happened, men can go to the other side. She is explaining ... one of these patients, that he likes her and always wants her to come, but she didn't.... When they come out [back to Tonga] he used to come and see her ... and asks her what does she want. She said, "I don't want anything."[66]

It is unclear how Maliakalemeli picked up the threads of her family life on her return, but by 1986 the LTB built her a home on a piece of family land. While she was in Makogai her husband remarried, and soon after her return home she had another son by a different man but lived with her sister.[67] It is not clear if she remarried, but her home was built on land given to her second son by his father, who in turn gave Maliakalemeli the right to build her home on it. The son had died five years earlier. On the form providing personal details, Maliakalemeli indicated she was a widow but did not name her first husband or the father of her second child. She had several grandchildren, but the separate families were quarreling over rights to the land upon which her home was built.[68] The wife of one of her sons wanted her to leave the land, despite her right to stay. Maliakalemeli lives on her own and still receives assistance from the PLF through Sister Joan Marie SMSM, a nursing sister at the Ma'faanga clinic near central Nuku'alofa. Maliakalemeli often goes for drives and enjoys the outings with Sister Joan Marie visiting other leprosy sufferers, some of whom had been at Makogai. It was difficult to assess through the interpreter the actual stigmatization suffered due to leprosy, but her relatively isolated home and style of living indicate a level of ostracism by her family and local villagers. Her feeling of remaining part of the "Makogai family" has survived over fifty years to the present day, as evidenced by her visiting old Makogai friends with Sister Joan Marie, once again indicating the strong camaraderie that existed between leprosy sufferers.

Village of Longomapu, Vava'u

Two of the interviewees, Manitepi and Kulaea, whose detailed testimonies will follow, lived in the village of Longomapu on the island of Vava'u. Manitepi had been sent to Makogai, and her story is described first, while Kulaea, being a younger woman, had been isolated at Fale'ofa. Longomapu had had many cases of leprosy, for which the village had gained infamy. Fusi, who nursed at Ngu Hospital in Vava'u in the 1970s, recalled an attitude towards those from Longomapu during her school days from the late 1950s:

> When we were in the school, we never eat food from Longomapu.... Not only from the family with the lepers, but all the whole lot in Longomapu.... They just think of the cases of the lepers, it is all dirty and we don't want anything from that.... I think leprosy is a very big problem, most of the people they don't accept, eh, leprosy to mix with them, or eat with them. They are very aware of that.... There was a doctor, Matovo, he told us to bring some food from Longomapu, only this time is good.... By now, in this time it is good, but before, never, never.[69]

Fusi's testimony indicates strong earlier stigmatic attitudes towards the whole village because of the number of leprosy sufferers there, although by that stage most would have been treated and were non-contagious or in Makogai. The explicit mention that "it is all dirty" reflects attitudes incorporating the biblical ideas contained in Leviticus mentioned by Dr. Lutui. However, Fusi's comment that "now... it is good" suggests that attitudes towards leprosy had been changing and improving for the better since about the 1980s or 1990s.

Sister Joan Marie had advised that radio awareness programs were run on the radio annually on Leprosy Day, and slowly the messages were getting through to the general public. But the lives of the older leprosy sufferers interviewed indicated that, compared to other Pacific nations visited, stigma has remained high in Tonga.

Manitepi Molimoli (b. 1936), who went to Makogai in 1956, lives in a home built for her by the PLF in the village of Longmapu. Manitepi appeared to be a strong, reserved woman quite used to solitude, and on our arrival was squatting on mats on the floor of her home, weaving piles of flax and listening to her radio, which was common in Tonga. Manitepi suffered little disability but was troubled by ulcers formed by squatting on the ground in her small home. Sister Goretti commented with surprise when a few villagers who came by wanted to see what was happening and wished to join in weaving with Manitepi. Sister Goretti said that not many years ago villagers would rarely visit Manitepi, and certainly would not join her in weaving. With Sister Goretti translating, Manitepi said:

> She lived here [in Longomapu] all her life, and her younger sister is the only one who went to Tonga and married there and died there, and the rest are still alive, five, and they are still all here in Longomapu.... [Mani] discovered that she had the leprosy when she was eighteen, and the same year she was sent to Fiji.... [Symptoms were] numbness ... especially her hands, she first felt it in the hands. She said she heard of the disease before, and when she was asked to go to the hospital to be examined, the doctor asked her about whether there was any other members of the family had contracted the disease and she said she doesn't know. She was told that she had contracted the leprosy. They started to isolate her to have her own house built. Just here in the village, and then in 1956 she was sent to Makogai. Two years later her brother Sione was sent over, thought that he had leprosy, but it was discovered that he didn't have it, he was free [of leprosy]. But they kept him there for two years just for her sake. Tangioa, who was sent over, her smaller brother, he contracted leprosy [when] he was only eight years old. Tangioa was there for six years, and then he came back.... He also went to Makogai, but for her she was 12 years altogether in Fiji. Sione was there only for two years and came back, and the younger brother was there six years. [Manitepi weeps profusely at the memories but continues talking to Sister Goretti, who encourages her.] She said that

4. The Loneliness of Isolation

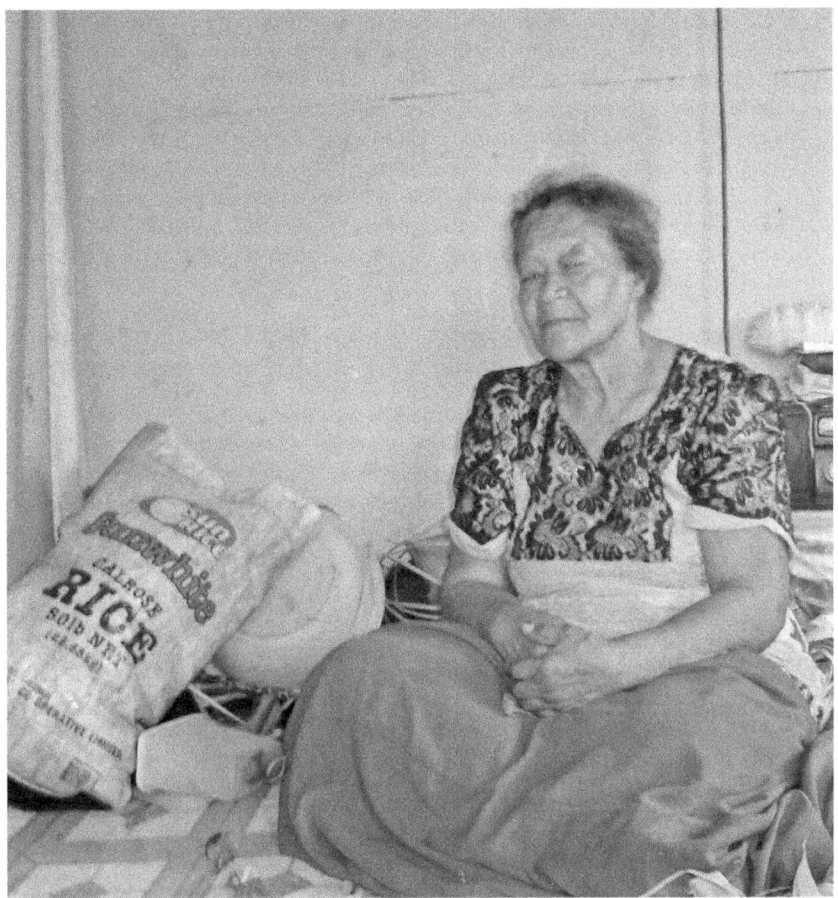

Manitepi Molimoli at her home in village of Longomapu, Vava'u, Tonga.

it's such a sad, sad memory each time she has to talk about it, it comes afresh all this, especially when people feel isolated and people are afraid of her, and how they treated the family.... The whole family feel that isolation. She said that later on there were others, including her relation ... who was sent to Fiji also.[70]

This testimony demonstrates the enormous grief that the separation of family members due to isolation caused, but it appears that the rejection by community members because of the diagnosis of leprosy is the most hurtful aspect of her memory. It is this stigma of having leprosy in her family that has lingered and still causes pain. This pain is in contrast to the memories of life in isolation at Makogai, when the mood of Manitepi completely lifted and she no longer wept while speaking:

> She said when she actually arrived there she was happy, it was a beautiful island and everyone was well looked after and the children... she had good memories being there. It was the leaving that is the hardest. She said when she arrived there, there were other Tongans there already ... also Maliakalemeli. They [the women] had an escort, even going to the movies, it was twice a week. The theater was over the men's side. [Laughter over these memories.] She is talking about in the evenings, at six o'clock they close the gate, close the door, and six o'clock in the morning, it is only then it is opened again.... There was always things to do and there is entertainment and those times just kind of passed.[71]

Manitepi gave her views regarding the enforced gender separation at Makogai, responding to the question whether the men tried to contact the women:

> Yes. She said they [the women] were quite well protected. They protected the women especially. If a man came, but not them. *Does she think that was a good idea, or would she have liked to have been in a Tongan village with men and women?* She says it was done with the men but not with the women.... She said no, for her choice, what she thinks that what they did was good. Yeah, and I think [Sister Goretti SMSM view] that is very strong aim in this culture. They always have to be called in this certain place where they [men and women] are to meet, and there is always an escort there with them. It seems there was a time given that they could go to this certain place at this certain time and then the bell would ring when it's over.[72]

Both Manitepi and Malekalemeli expressed the view that gender segregation at Makogai was in their best interests. Manitepi arrived at Makogai in 1956, and said she was not unhappy at having stayed twelve years at Makogai. She returned to Tonga when she was thirty-one years old. She provided the following account about being discharged and her return to Tonga:

> They were still in Makogai and they heard that they have started building Twomey [hospital], Tamavua, and heard there was a better treatment and they were all going to be sent back. She said that they actually were sent to Suva, they came there, they spent two weeks ... [stayed in Suva at] a place there, in St. Elizabeth's Home. Apparently when they were told that they were going to come home for good, they were given the chance and they were allowed to go and visit their friends or some members of their families in Suva. So they went, and she said she didn't have any family but a friend. Herself and someone from the Solomons, they went to visit her friend. They were together in Makogai and she was happy, obviously, that she went to Nadi, she went to Latoka ... before they actually left. They came [to Tonga] by plane. She said she missed Fiji, she missed Makogai. It seems that it took awhile when she came, she often reminisced back. She said she found it hard to speak in Tongan.[73]

Despite the enormous trauma of being sent away from her family to Fiji, Manitepi was able to talk with affection about her memories of isolation in

Makogai. It is ironic, but likely, that the stigma she faced upon her return to Tonga made life on Makogai seem a happy period in her memory. Manitepi did not marry nor have children, and she said her parents were concerned about what would happen to her when they died. Her parents had adopted two of Manitepi's nephews, so that after the parents died the two boys lived with Manitepi in the small home which had been built for her five years after her return to Longomapu. Although Manitepi had remained very much alone for years, more recently, since the PLF provided her with flax to weave matting, some of the local women came and joined her weaving in her home.

The decrease in stigma could be attributed to several reasons. The annual World Leprosy Day programs on national radio could be affecting public perceptions. Additionally, the fact that the incidence of leprosy had not increased in Longomapu, despite large numbers of leprosy sufferers returning to the village from Makogai in the late 1960s, might eventually be reducing fears of contagion. Sister Goretti was assisted in her work in Longomapu by a local woman who helped maintain regular contact with the leprosy sufferers, and it was suggested that this local involvement had helped change attitudes simply because of the fact that this woman made regular contact with leprosy sufferers without fear of the disease or contracting it. Sister Goretti and the local helper believe that knowledge about MDT since the 1980s had increased and was contributing to a reduction in stigma. Manitepi said through the interpreter, "She reckon those time of darkness are over, people are living in the light. They have come through."[74]

Manitepi's comment was echoed by the local helper, who had been sent to Fiji for special leprosy training, and who undoubtedly was contributing to a lowering of stigma in Longomapu. She said:

> When I came back from Fiji, I saw the people not so afraid of leprosy, because I go to Fiji and I see the doctor, Delaco ... mix together with people with leprosy, drinking kava, eating food.[75]

The testimonies indicate that isolation appears to have confirmed notions of stigma associated with outcasts in the minds of Tongans, and the fact that those returning from Makogai had not reintegrated back into family life meant their isolation was condoned and endorsed within Tongan society. The fear of contagion had not ended with the return of ex-leprosy sufferers, and it was only through years of effort by the PLF and through their liaison contacts, essentially the SMSM, that inroads were eventually being made to reduce the fear of contagion of leprosy, together with ideas that leprosy sufferers should not be treated as outcasts. In Longomapu, where evidence of the containment of leprosy was witnessed by villagers, the long journey to end the stigma of leprosy appears to have begun.

Experience of Isolation at Fale'ofa

Kulaea is the only interviewee who had been isolated at Fale'olfa leprosy clinic in 1970. She had been raised on the main island of Tongatapu but sent to Vava'u for isolation and remained on the island after discharge. Kulaea's story is followed by the experiences of Pepetua, who had been diagnosed with leprosy in Vava'u in 1971 but was not isolated; after her discharge she moved to the main island of Tongatapu, where she was interviewed. The last interviewee is Mele of Vava'u, who was not diagnosed with leprosy until 1985. She was not isolated but treated at Ngu Hospital, Vava'u.

Diagnosed with leprosy in 1970, Kulaea Tu'a Leketi (b. 1947) now lives in the village of Longomapu and is one of the younger leprosy sufferers interviewed. She contracted leprosy about the same time as Pepetua, whose story is detailed next. At age twenty-three, living on Tongatapu after the birth of her third child, Kulaea became unwell. Her symptoms were rashes, red patches, loss of eyebrows and her body feeling tired and heavy.[76]

Dr. Tilitili Poloka diagnosed leprosy, and Kulaea and her family were transferred the same day by boat to Vava'u for her admission to Fale'ofa leprosy center, where she remained for six years.[77] With Sister Goretti interpreting, Kulaea tells the story of her separation from her family and isolation at Fale'ofa:

> She was sent to Fale'ofa, and the husband took the children to Pangai, his family's village. But the family told him to take the children to Longomapu because they are sick. Her husband's family rejected the children but wanted the husband to return back to Pangi. So her husband left the children with Kulaea's sister, her relations in Longomapu, and the husband returned to his family. The eldest [child] was only two years old, and the middle one died, and the baby was only four months. She felt very very sad because of her separation from her family, her husband, her children and the fact that she can't fulfill her responsibilities.[78]
>
> But the members of the family often come to visit her. Just outside the fence, except her husband, he climbed over the fence, spends the whole day hiding from the hospital staff. She said her husband took care of the children even though they were looked after by her family, but he goes over there.... Apparently they had two children while she was in the hospital! From there the family took the baby to Longomapu. They took her to the main hospital to give birth, and then from there she was taken back to the hospital at Fale'ofa.... She said the children were okay because they often bring them over to visit at the hospital, so they knew she was their mother.[79]

Kulaea's account of her husband's visits to Fale'ofa leprosy clinic demonstrates that she was not intimidated by the authorities enforcing her isolation, to the extent that she bore two children while confined. This plucky inde-

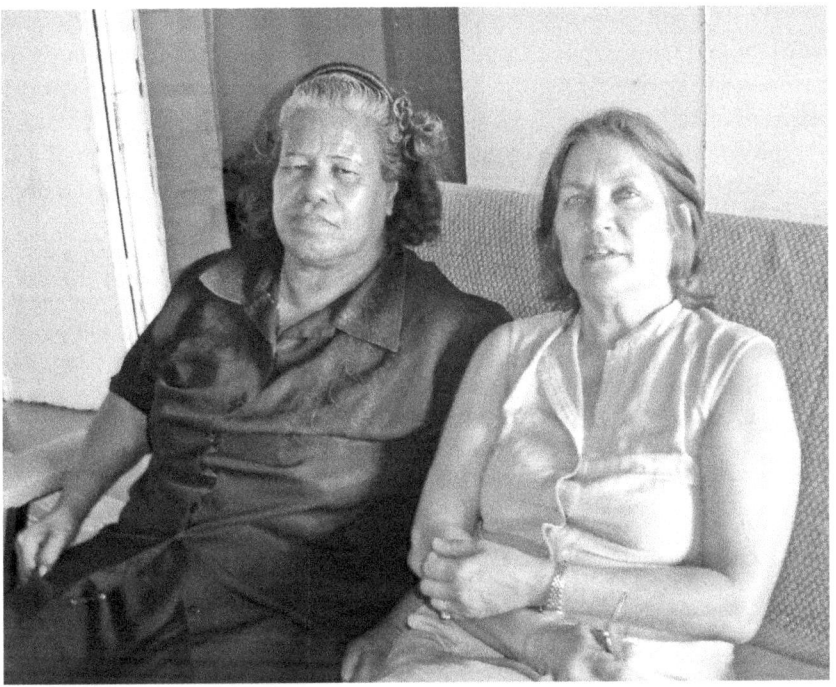

Kulaea Tu'a Leketi and the author.

pendent spirit of Kulaea is demonstrated in the description of her later years, which did not confine her to a solitary life despite the harsh, ostracizing treatment of her in-laws.

After Kulaea's discharge, because her husband lived away with his family, Kulaea remarried another leprosy sufferer, Tofa, brother of interviewee Talaia.[80] They were together for five years, until Tofa died. After his death Kulaea stayed by herself until 2004. At this point her parents-in-law died and the eldest son brought his father to Kulaea, and she and her first husband were reconciled.[81] Kulaea said that during their earlier separation "the children tend to hate their father because they felt he rejected them."[82] However, Kulaea said that the past two years had been the happiest years together, but, sadly, a week prior to the interview, her husband died. Kulaea said her children were happily married, with families. Her third child, daughter Fini, was diagnosed with leprosy at twelve years of age. Fini had been adopted by relations and burned her outer toe. Kulaea noticed that the burn was taking a long time to heal so reported it to the doctor, and "white tablets" were prescribed. Fini was not admitted to the hospital but had regular medical checks and was clear of leprosy.[83]

This demonstrates a strong and responsible attitude on the part of Kulaea, which would have impacted on the attitude of her family, who appeared to have a realistic view of leprosy and the treatment available. Having felt the rejection of her in-laws, Kulaea was fully aware of the strong stigma of leprosy and preferred to live in Longomapu, where she felt more accepted and able to take part in a social life. Nevertheless, she was aware of the general prevalence of fear of leprosy contagion, but still mixed with others:

> She felt that certain people, they still fear the disease and also they look down on them. They don't mix well with them and so they feel as if they, you know, they are being as if tied down.... She said that even the family now, she is with the family since her husband died, she still provides herself with her plate and cup and spoons. Yes, separate ones, you know, just to prevent them [risking contagion]. Because she knows that they don't like her, and even though it is certainly different from that time, the difference is much better, but she still feels that there is still this separation.[84]

Kulaea's comment that she keeps her own set of eating utensils indicates her tactics in order to socialize with communities still afraid of contagion by leprosy. This, in turn, demonstrates the level of ignorance about leprosy and its effective treatment which contributes to the prevalence of stigma and fear that remains associated with the disease. Although these testimonies indicate a growing awareness of leprosy treatment, this is obviously not yet widespread. The PLF continues to support programs to increase leprosy awareness through medical training programs and radio broadcasts on World Leprosy Day, and recently Sister Joan Marie organized a radio broadcast about the life stories of some leprosy sufferers. But stigma in Tonga appears to be harder to eliminate, perhaps, as suggested by Dr. Lutui and findings in this research, because stigma was not restricted to fears of contagion and modern methods of isolation, but also to ingrained biblical ideas that leprosy sufferers should be treated as outcasts.

Since her husband's very recent death, Kulaea lives with one of her grandchildren.[85] She mentioned her gratitude to the PLF for the monthly allowances and the installation of electricity in her home, but went on to say that having a troublesome plantar ulcer, she found laundry tasks difficult and hoped she could be provided with a washing machine. Kulaea's life story depicts the strong stigma that still exists towards leprosy and the lack of public knowledge about modern medical treatment. Kulaea referred to her daughter's medication as "white tablets," not by the name of the medicine, reflecting a lack of explanation by the health department about leprosy and its treatment, sustaining ignorance about the disease. To this end the efforts of the PLF to support regular awareness programs and assist in educating the public about leprosy and its treatment will help lower stigma.

Leprosy Experiences Without Isolation

Diagnosed with leprosy in 1970 in Vava'u, and now living near Nuku'alofa, Pepetua Tu'amelie (b. 1950) was the youngest leprosy sufferer interviewed in Tonga. She was the youngest child of seven, and her mother died after her birth. She was adopted and brought up by an aunt, her mother's sister, on Vava'u. She said there was no leprosy in her own family but they shared a house with another family where there was leprosy.[86] After her marriage and the birth of a child in about 1971, Pepetua noticed a problem with blisters on her fingernails. She was admitted to Ngu Hospital at Vava'u, where the fingers were amputated. But a few months later the problem recurred on her other hand, and it was not until she saw Dr. Tilitili Poluka that she was diagnosed with leprosy and the correct medication prescribed.[87] With an infant child, and her husband working in New Zealand, she was given medication and told to pack and be ready to be isolated; but in the end, much to her relief, no transport arrived to remove her.[88] She saw this as an answer to her prayers but returned to the hospital regularly to continue her medication.[89]

The reason for the lack of isolation for Pepetua is unclear, compared to

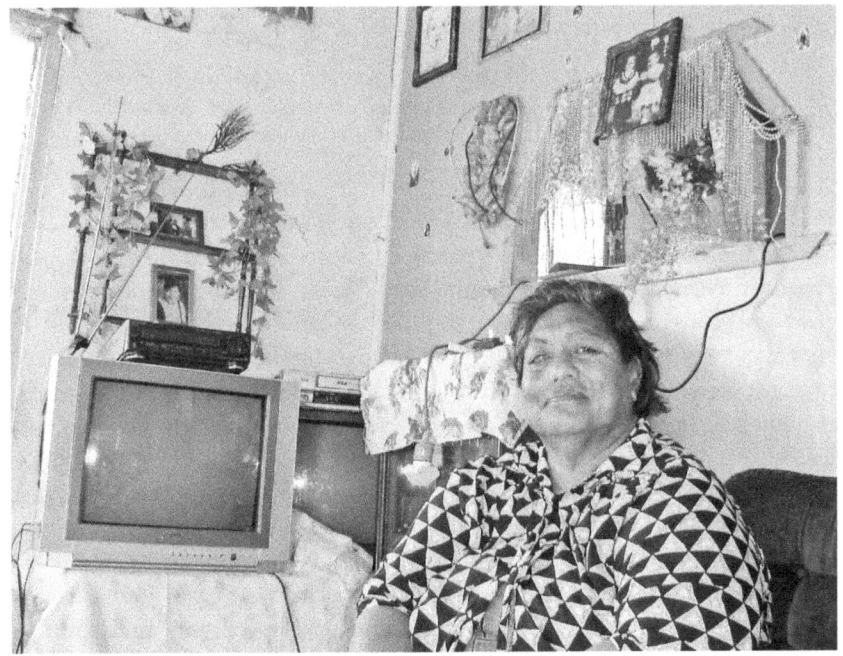

Pepetua Tu'amelie in her home.

seven years' isolation for Kulaea around the same period. The leprosy may have been a less contagious form than that presented by Kulaea, but the interviewees were not aware of the different forms. Pepetua moved to the main island and attended Vaiola Hospital in Nuku'alofa, where she was regularly tested. Nine years later she was declared free of leprosy. Once she was cleared, she bore two more children.[90] Pepetua did not appear to understand her condition but believed she was to have been isolated, and was thankful that her prayers were answered and she was spared separation from her infant. When asked if she knew that leprosy was usually difficult to contract, she said she was unaware of that. She said she "was just hurting," and "she was afraid that her [baby] daughter might catch it."[91] The level of health education and poor communication between health workers and leprosy sufferers in Tonga had done little to reduce the fear and prevalence of stigma of leprosy.

Pepetua remained married and had two more daughters, raising three healthy children; she now had seven grandchildren, with two more on the way.[92] She lived in a home provided by the PLF near a landfill site reclaimed between the sea and a garbage disposal area. It was the only land she could obtain upon which the PLF could build her home. The PLF assistance has made a huge difference to the family, who tried to live a normal life, but Pepetua says she felt the stigma of leprosy from the local community. She says:

> She can tell ... by their looks, that they knew she has got the sickness, they don't want to come near her. She thinks it is fear that they have a chance to catch it. But she can tell [other] people that come with love to her, they see she just normal like one of us.[93]

This comment indicates that stigma is still associated with fear of contagion, but that once it is realized that there is little risk, friendships developed. Pepetua's marriage had lasted despite her sickness, allowing her daughters to grow up in a family atmosphere, depicted in photographs on the walls in Pepetua's home. Her daughters led normal lives, and Pepetua's personal story demonstrates that the cure for leprosy was gradually alleviating the stigma by removing fears of infection that had affected the lives of earlier leprosy sufferers.

Although the evidence is limited to only two interviews, it suggests that the level of stigma was lower in Tongatapu than in Vava'u. The higher stigma apparent on the island of Vava'u may be attributable to the past visibility of the Fale'ofa leprosy center, which has been described as having high fences, near the hospital on Vava'u. The conditions of that leprosarium appear to have contributed to the already fearful reputation of leprosy, containing biblical ideas that leprosy sufferers should be treated as outcasts.

4. The Loneliness of Isolation

Mele Fonoga (b. 1943) is the younger sister of Polutele Fakatava, who was interviewed at Twomey Hospital in Fiji. Mele recalls she was about ten years old when Polutele was transferred to Makogai.[94] Mele was later married, and it was not until the birth of her sixth child, while she was at Ngu Hospital in about 1985, that leprosy was suspected, by which time the Fale'ofa leprosy center had closed. Dr. Delaco, on a visit from Fiji, confirmed the diagnosis. She was given tablets, kept in isolation briefly in a separate room at the hospital, and then sent home.[95] This demonstrates that the treatment of leprosy in Tonga is now included with general health services, which should go a long way towards ending the traditional belief that leprosy sufferers should be excluded from ordinary society.

However, with Mele's past family association with leprosy, her own ideas about leprosy appear ingrained. Despite her experience of inclusion at Ngu Hospital, Mele's attitude is similar to that reported earlier in the Japanese research that the older generation is less likely to accept changing attitudes towards leprosy. To some extent this is what Gussow and Tracey identified as self-stigma, being the internalization of old ideas and attitudes, and the inability to perceive and accept that attitudes of stigma in the public domain and local communities were changing.[96] Mele was becoming forgetful with age, and her memory seemed at times vague and confused, but she worried greatly about public perceptions of having contracted leprosy.[97] She worried about her family, especially her husband. Would she be accepted? Her husband lived and worked on another island. She said she knew about the medicine because the doctor told her, and she felt hopeful, and was happy and thankful.[98] Mele was no doubt affected by the earlier experience of Polutele and the effect of his leprosy on the family in earlier times. Speaking through Sister Goretti, she said:

> Because of the disease, probably the family too was difficult for them to have him [Polutele] around, and also maybe the situation she knows with the people, the reaction is probably very strong.... When he came, the general concern with the feeling was that he wasn't accepted fully, even to the family, because it is so strong. The other children would tease the other grandchildren and all that, and I think [Sister Goretti translating, who knows all the family well] from that he felt it would be better for him not being here. For him and for the family.[99]

> When she [Mele] goes to a meeting, she will notice the faces are a little concerned about her coming. But she has a lot of friends who just come in and out.... People they say to me, Mele, you come, we never forget you .... But sometimes I don't feel like to go, but people come and invite me.... And my daughter say to me you go, and I say no.... I can tell because I pray to the Lord every time I have time. When I finish eating I go to read my Bible and I pray. I said to my daughter, you know you never know how many time I pray,

when I finish eating I pray, when I go to park I pray, every time I walk out ... I pray ... people frightened.[100]

There was a sense of vagueness of specific details in Mele's testimony, but it did indicate a thawing in attitudes towards leprosy, with her old friends assuring her of their continued friendship. Mele's family history prevents her escaping the sense of stigma, despite the reassurances of friends and her daughter's encouragement that she respond to invitations and continue to socialize. When we arrived for the interview, Mele was not home but was visiting nearby friends, although, as described below, this visit caused Mele to express additional concern.

Mele appeared affected by old ideas of the uncleanliness of leprosy. On being complimented about the tidy garden around her home, which had been built with PLF assistance beside her daughter's house, she displayed a sense of paranoia to be viewed as clean by neighbors, as if in response to the taint or pollution of leprosy. She said:

> Foundation (PLF) have done marvelous for these people. And through that way, they [leprosy sufferers] have found dignity. I am so happy because this is one thing I have been wanting them to do, to clean up the compound. You know... every time when I finish and I know they [daughter's family] are still asleep, I go and collect the things [left in the garden] because not [want others] to know.... But when they wake up they know.... [My daughter] says, "Mum, I know you collecting things [weeds and windblown palms, or maybe paper and rubbish] because I see no leaves."[101]

Mele's worry about how the locals and neighbors perceived her family because of leprosy stigma appeared to be of great concern to her. She reiterated her worry about this towards the end of the interview, adding:

> You know Sister [Goretti], ... they still feel that they [leprosy sufferers] are still sick. That is why they [the PLF and Sister Goretti] are still coming.... Everybody come to say the doctor come to see her, don't go there, don't eat from her ... maybe she still has the disease. So when they have a do over here, especially making food, she says don't go there, don't go here. Don't eat the food.[102]

Whether Mele is correct or not about how others interpret Sister Goretti's visits, her testimony demonstrates a level of stigma she perceives by the local community towards leprosy sufferers. She also indicated that other leprosy sufferers experienced the same fears:

> There are three patients now in Vava'u that they just said, don't come. Because they are conscious of their relationship with the people. *And they don't want you [Sister Goretti], being from the Leprosy Foundation, to come?* [Sister Goretti replies directly] I will come. Those ones that I am referring to, they have cut themselves off completely, and she is telling me the same thing now. That she

4. The Loneliness of Isolation   153

would prefer to come up to me instead of me coming to her.... Sometimes I come and ... take her to accompany me to the others.[103]

Mele interjected in English, after Sister Goretti's last comment, "I love to come! See some others."[104] These comments reflect an inconsistency in Mele's responses, due most likely to past family experiences and the strong stigma that existed during the time Polutele was diagnosed. Her confused response to changing attitudes reflects elements of internalization of old attitudes and an inability to accept changes. This is confirmed by Mele's daughter, who recognized a less stigmatized attitude towards leprosy and encouraged Mele to continue socializing in their community. Mele's attitude induced her to voice concerns about her continued connection to leprosy through the visits of PLF liaison agents, yet she wished to accompany Sister Goretti on visits to other leprosy sufferers, acknowledging the easy camaraderie found among leprosy sufferers.

None of the other leprosy sufferers interviewed expressed Mele's concerns about visits by Sister Goretti, arriving in the truck with a very small insignia, "PLF," on the door of the vehicle. The low incidence of leprosy in the island, treatment of new cases at the general hospital, and the rapid cure achieved with MDT medication appear to be contributing to the slow diminishment of the old stigma associated with leprosy. Even Mele's experiences and fears demonstrate that old-fashioned views of treating those who had leprosy as outcasts were changing. This view was expressed earlier by Manitepi in Longomapu, who hoped these enlightened times would lead to the end of the "time of darkness"[105] associated with stigma.

The lack of prevailing knowledge that MDT treatment ended the contagion of leprosy affected Mele's ideas, and she worried that others thought her leprosy was still contagious. This ignorance about leprosy undoubtedly causes fear and stigma, which impacts adversely upon the lives of leprosy sufferers. The interviewees' testimonies do indicate that to varying degrees, leprosy sufferers are still treated as outcasts in Tongan society; but a softening attitude is evident in the responses of Manitepi, who believed that the old ideas were dying out and was able to enjoy the company of visitors.

The social disorder and protests that reached their height during the time of my visit to Tonga in November 2006 stemmed from discontent with the prevailing governance by the monarchy in Tonga, objecting to outdated attitudes and policies which are unacceptable in the twenty-first century to a large numbers of Tongans. With the changing social climate in Tonga, and the continued perseverance with education about leprosy through the annual radio broadcasts on World Leprosy Day, it is likely that the diminishment of stigma will continue and new cases of leprosy should no longer face stigma. The policy of treating leprosy cases in general hospitals with MDT, as in the case of Kulaea's daughter, would reduce public ideas of exclusion and separate treatment of leprosy sufferers, further hastening the end of stigmatizing attitudes towards leprosy.

5

The Benefits of Leprosaria — Vanuatu

Historical Background

A Melanesian archipelago became known as the New Hebrides from the time it was mapped and named by James Cook in 1774 until independence was gained from Britain and France in 1980, when it was renamed Vanuatu. The northern islands had first been discovered by the Europeans in 1606, by the Spanish explorer Quiros, but within weeks the climate, sickness and hostility of the local people forced the Spanish to withdraw.[1] It was not until 1768 that another European, the French mariner Louis de Bougainville, landed on the small western island of Ambae (formerly known as Aoba, Oba or Opa), naming it the Isle of Lepers because of a widespread scaly fungal condition on the skin of the inhabitants, which was widely prevalent at that time.[2]

With the discovery of sandalwood in 1825, the resource was exploited by western traders to sustain trade with China from the 1840s; but after the sandalwood trade petered out, many local kanaka people were lured away by the attractions of European goods and adventure. The indigenous kanaka (later called Ni-Vanuatu) were increasingly used as cheap labor in the sugar cane fields in Queensland, Australia and Fiji, or the coconut plantations in Western Samoa and nickel mines in New Caledonia.[3] To satisfy the colonial demands for this cheap but able work force, the crews of European ships virtually kidnapped kanaka recruits, the practice becoming known as "blackbirding," which lasted into the late 19th century. Apart from ill feelings caused by blackbirding, the movements of islanders through the region in unhygienic conditions on overcrowded ships contributed to epidemics being spread through the South Pacific, including diseases such as leprosy.[4]

The earliest European missionaries arrived in the southern islands of the archipelago, the first being John Williams of the London Missionary Society at Erromanga, in 1839, then John Geddie of the Presbyterian Mission on Aneityum in 1848. Williams was soon killed, whereas Geddie was able to establish a base, often using Polynesians from Samoa to help establish friendly links throughout the islands.[3] The Presbyterian Mission extended their work towards the northern islands, attending also to the needs of the sick, as it was recognized through earlier experiences that medical knowledge was helpful as a means to influence local people to adopt Christianity.[6] The Anglican Melanesian Mission, through Bishop Selwyn in New Zealand, made the first exploratory voyage to the New Hebrides in 1847 and met Geddie of the Presbyterian Mission on Aneityum. An agreement was reached in 1881 whereby the Melanesian Mission operated in the northernmost islands of Banks and Torres, and in Pentecost, Maewo and Ambae; while the Presbyterians operated on other islands.[7] By 1867 the Melanesian Mission ship *Southern Cross* was plying regularly between New Zealand, the New Hebrides and the Solomon Islands; along with their different brands of evangelism, the missions offered medical care.[8]

The Presbyterian Mission based in Australia and New Zealand continued to send medical missionaries to the islands and in 1893 the first general hospital was built on Ambrym, with further "cottage hospitals" on other islands.[9] The London Missionary Society and Melanesian Mission built their stations on different islands, and the missions cooperated with each other in terms of medical care. However, the management and running of these ad hoc health services was impeded because Melanesian society was extremely fragmented, with very different dialects and languages throughout the islands. Only a few people were even able to converse with neighboring islanders.[10] Disease and injury were believed by the Melanesians to be caused by sorcery, and were treated by traditional kastom herbs and rituals, but the effective remedies and care offered at the missions was welcomed.[11]

With rival colonialist interests in the islands, by 1887 an Anglo-French Joint Naval Commission was established, which in 1906 culminated in the formation of the Anglo-French Condominium of New Hebrides, whereby dual British and French administrative systems operated in the islands, including parallel health services. In 1938 regulations were passed for the provision of public health services by the Condominium government, a role which until then had been fully funded by the Presbyterian, Catholic and Anglican Melanesian missions, who now received government assistance, as the responsibility for preventative and curative medicine was undertaken by the French and British.[12] Prior to this, in 1937 the Melanesian Mission established the Godden Memorial Hospital at Lolowai on Ambae, named in honor of the first missionary to Lolowai, Charles Godden, who was murdered in 1906. A leprosarium was subsequently set up here in the 1950s.[13] An indigenous oral account, as retold by Anna Tevi, a nurse who trained at Godden Memorial Hospital, indicates that Godden was killed as revenge for earlier European atrocities.[14] With honor satisfied, according to local oral accounts, the relationship between the islanders and westerners on Ambae and the other northern islands improved.

Oral history testimonies were collected from Sister Betty Pyatt, and Dr. Bruce Mackereth and his wife and nurse, Catherine, all now retired and living on the North Island of New Zealand, who were the medical staff in charge of the St. Barnabas leprosarium in Lolowai, Vanuatu, from the 1950s to the 1970s. Their testimonies describe events leading to up to the establishment of the leprosarium and the conditions at the hospital. Oral histories with local residents at that time in Lolowai corroborate the testimonies and add further information about life at the leprosarium until the mid–1970s. Few sources are available from this time until about 2000, being the period leading up to independence of Vanuatu in 1980 and the early years of independence. However, since 2000 the PLF consultant leprologist, Dr. Roland Farrugia, initiated a program to re-trace and assist leprosy sufferers in Vanuatu, which his testimony included here describes. Extracts of oral histories with seven leprosy sufferers resident on the island of Espiritu Santo narrate their experiences of living with leprosy. Interestingly, they denote a lower level of leprosy stigma evident in Vanuatu.

Earliest Accounts of Leprosy

Leprosy is believed to have been encountered in the Melanesian islands some time prior to the mid–19th century, before the advent of European settlers and sandalwood traders in Melanesia.[15] But it was not until over a hundred years later that the first case of leprosy was officially recorded in Vanuatu, in 1883,[16] and about another seventy years before the central leprosarium was established at what was originally referred to as the "Isle of Lepers" at the eastern bay of Lolowai on the island of Ambae.

An early account of a medical officer adopting special methods of care for leprosy patients was Dr. J. Campbell Nicholson, at what came to be known as the Paton Presbyterian Hospital on the southern island of Tanna in 1909. His methods prevailed until his departure in 1917.[17] In line with accepted medical practice of the time, Nicholson attempted to control the spread of leprosy through isolation. His reports include the observation that wives without leprosy accompanied their husbands with leprosy into isolation, and when the husbands died, if they had not contracted the disease, the wives bathed, took new clothes and crossed the river to return to their former lives. Nicholson noted that husbands never accompanied wives with leprosy into segregated areas.[18] The series of *Live* publications, which are a history of the formation of the Presbyterian Church in Vanuatu, contain these references to Nicholson's work with leprosy. Further details may be available in the original Presbyterian archives at the Australian offices of the Presbyterian Church of Vanuatu in Sydney, where the author, Rev. Graham Miller, conducted his research.[19]

Another early account of leprosy is reported by Dr. Bowie of the Presbyterian Mission on Ambrym, where a young married woman convert to Christianity, Rebecca, was found in 1909 to have contracted leprosy.[20] Dr. Bowie suggested that she and her husband return to their home village of Wilir because "leprosy was no bar to tribal social life"; so Rebecca and her husband reportedly did this, and "by the time of her death the church had been planted in Wilir."[21] This suggests that leprosy in Ambrym was treated as any other disease by the kanaka, with little evidence of stigma by the local villages. Some idea of isolation is evident on the part of Dr. Bowie, although the report indicates that Dr. Bowie visited Rebecca at the village of Wilir and provided another Christian helper to aid Rebecca in her Christian endeavors. Apparently, for two years prior to her death Rebecca attended church regularly, sitting just outside the door.[22] This casual attitude, albeit with a degree of segregation, does not demonstrate total horror or rejection of those with the disease, but does suggests a low level of stigma. The testimonies collected in this research suggest a similar level of distancing of leprosy sufferers in the past from ordinary society, but without a heightened sense of leprosy stigma. The awful physical conditions of putrescence in advanced leprosy cases no doubt led to this segregation.

In 1942, upon learning of the results of the leprosy survey by Dr. R. Innes in 1937–39, which reported a high incidence of leprosy in the Solomon Islands, Patrick Twomey in New Zealand made contact with the Melanesian Mission in Honiara, and funding was provided for medical care in Melanesia.[23] The LTB also provided financial support to the Presbyterian Mission and Catholic Church, as it was recognized as unrealistic that medical officers would be available exclusively for leprosy, and the provision of funds to general medical teams would ensure that support was extended to those suffering from leprosy.[24]

With the cooperation of the South Pacific Commission, Twomey organized LTB funding for a leprosy survey to be conducted in the islands of Vanuatu in 1948–51, carried out by Dr. Jean Davies.[25] Davies' survey, carried out with remarkable fortitude and endurance in reaching the islands, let alone the villagers, was a feat in itself, confirmed that leprosy cases were relatively few but very scattered, making the provision of medical care difficult and expensive.[26] In 1951 it was reported that there were about one hundred cases of leprosy, with the greatest concentration being in the northern islands.[27] In the report by Lonie, this figure represented a prevalent rate of leprosy of 2.6 per 1,000 population, whereas by 1958 the rate rose to 3.6 per 1,000.[28] This increase in the prevalence and spread of leprosy in the northern islands was attributed to a lack of fear of leprosy, but might also be due to greater diligence and penetration by the health services to detect leprosy sufferers.[29] Nonetheless, this attitude confirms the earlier report of Dr. Bowie in 1909 that villagers did not fear leprosy and that no strict exclusion was evident, which indicates a low level of associated stigma, if any, despite long contact with various Christian missionaries.[30] A small isolation colony for leprosy had been established on North East Malekula, but by 1950 it was considered unsuitable for the remaining twelve patients and a decision was made that the only viable lazarette was at Lolowai.[31]

Melanesian Mission and Establishment of Leprosarium at Lolowai

The Godden Memorial Hospital at Lolowai had been served by nurses through the Anglican Melanesian Mission, with the support of visiting medical officers. With the proposed larger numbers of leprosy patients to be sent to Lolowai, it was decided a leprosarium would be annexed to the hospital. The testimony of Sister Betty Pyatt of the Melanesian Mission, quoted at length below, describes her work as matron at Lolowai hospital commencing in 1949, giving details of the provision of health care in the northern islands and particularly the establishment and running of the St. Barnabas leprosarium at Lolowai.

Sister Pyatt's account, together with that of Dr. Bruce Mackereth, the doctor stationed at Lolowai in 1962, and his wife and nurse, Catherine, provide an original comprehensive account of the establishment and operation of St. Barnabas, which was built on a small plateau on an elevation behind Godden Memorial Hospital. Upon completion of her training as a nurse, and completion of various courses (such as Plunket and mid-wifery) at various hospitals around New Zealand, Betty Pyatt boarded the *Southern Cross* to take up a post at Godden Memorial Hospital, Lolowai, in 1949. Several years later, Catherine qualified as a nurse and married Dr. Bruce Mackereth, and they had two young sons. He applied for and obtained the appointment as medical superintendent at Lolowai Hospital in 1962, where subsequently their two younger sons were born.

Pyatt recalls her training in New Zealand to become a nurse in Melanesia:

> I graduated in 1943 with this idea that I was going to be a nurse in Melanesia. And my feeling was I had to get as many certificates as possible, so I just went from one study to another. Later in Christchurch ... an elderly deaconess ... asked me what sort of preparation I had for Melanesia, and when I recited off the various certificates I had gained, her face got graver and graver and she said, "But what about the preparation for missionary work?" And I think that was the first time I'd really ever sort of come across this idea that I was a missionary because I was going to be a nurse in Melanesia.[32]

The training preparation for her appointment at the Lolowai hospital, and her surprise at being reminded that she was a Melanesian Mission Sister, indicates that nursing was her first priority, although undoubtedly she wished to serve the Church.[33] The testimony does not support a proposition that Sister Pyatt was heading to Melanesia specifically to save souls, although the Church was all important to her. Her goal was to take up the position of matron at the hospital, a post for which she had been extensively trained, to help the sick in this earthly life, as opposed to the suggestions that nuns and missionary sisters working with leprosy merely prepared the patients for the afterlife.[34]

Age twenty-eight, Sister Pyatt boarded the *Southern Cross* bound for Lolowai; coincidentally onboard also were Patrick Twomey of the LTB and his assistant, Noeline Harris (née Kiely).[35] Twomey was on one of his many journeys around the South Pacific, this time to the Solomon Islands to update his knowledge of the position and conditions relating to leprosy care, and to disburse funding to various religious missions, including the Melanesian Mission. Betty Pyatt recalls arriving at Lolowai and observing the leprosy facilities:

> I found that there were five lepers in leaf houses round the bay ... and remember walking around the bay with Mr. Twomey. He was very serious about this, telling me what could happen.... They [the LTB] hadn't been there before, but this was what Mr. Twomey was touring for, to investigate to see where he could work.[36]

The previous matron of Lolowai hospital who had run the hospital during the difficulties of World War Two was on sick leave, never to return, and Betty Pyatt simply had to take over. There was a young inexperienced assistant medical practitioner, trained on a special three-year course in Fiji, but because he had never worked with a doctor after graduation, he lacked the confidence to perform most medical duties.[37] Initially, Pyatt worked alone, with one European trained assistant. The following extracts provide descriptions of the hospital and working conditions, and the setting up of local medical clinics on the islands:

> When I first went there we had two 12-bed wards, a four-bed ward and a maternity ward of about twelve. Then we put up a hut and that was another

ward. At first we did all the work, I always had an assistant sister. There were always two of us at least, sometimes three. They came from everywhere — England, Australia and New Zealand — more from New Zealand. I seemed to be the one that stayed.[38]

So that first two-and-a-half years I spent mostly at the hospital I didn't really go out to the villages at all, and I worked very hard with no days off. And being on call 24 hours a day, I very much wanted to see some of the local people helping with some of this work.[39] At the end of two-and-a-half years I was more than ready for leave; I had had chronic dysentery for awhile and was a shadow of my former self, but there had been nobody to relieve me.... A sister ... heard of my plight and ... offered to relieve me. So she went to Lolowai, and it was the most wonderful thing really because she was a person who had seen the work in the Solomons ... the training school ... and she got everything going. By the time I returned after three months leave, there was the place just as I had wanted it, with locals who were going to be trained ... and you really felt as though you were going to be able to pass on your work.... I was always very, very grateful to her. But that first leave really was very necessary. I regained my strength and had a good think about things. And, in fact, what she had accomplished while I was away is more than what I had intended doing when I returned, and so it was lovely to go back.[40]

I remember once after we'd started nurse training, sitting on the grass with this [Melanesian] woman and another elderly woman. One of the nurses of our team [who] we'd been a bit worried about, passed by, and my eyes must have followed this nurse across the grass because Veve Maria, which was this woman's name, said to me, "You're worried about her aren't you?" And I said, "Yes I am a bit." And she asked me to express what my worry was. She and the other woman, to my surprise, suddenly burst into gales of laughter and even stretched back on the grass and came back to a sitting position again. And I said, "What's wrong?" And they said, "You white people want to make everybody the same, we look upon people as being individuals much more than you do." It was really quite a lesson, and I found that I could learn a lot from the philosophy of some of those elderly Melanesian people and I found, that really very interesting.[41]

This recollection that "white people want to make everybody the same" is reminiscent of the observation by Silla in Mali, Africa, and used as the title of his book *People Are Not the Same*. Both observations perhaps indicate that in places where European medicine had not been available, or where local medicine and healers could not effect cures or healing of certain conditions, the people had little choice but to be accepting of what were unavoidable health problems that imposed physical handicaps on the unfortunate victims. At the same time, Betty Pyatt's interest in the different philosophy of the Melanesians displays empathy rather than Christian indifference to local attitudes. Her description of the methods employed to provide health care in the islands also displays an empathetic understanding of island life:

> We also started to go out to villages more and thought that this should be part of the nurses training. So you took a nurse with you out to the village, because we were training them not for hospital work but for village work. So we would do long walks. I remember being put down at the other end of our island, which is about 28 miles long, and walking back to Lolowai and taking about ten days. You would do medical work in each of the villages you passed through. I had a… I've forgotten what you call it, but it was a slide and film strip projector to which you put a pressure lamp, a kerosene pressure lamp, and that was the light. Of course it depended if you'd managed to get the pressure lamp going without clogging up the mantle as to how good your slides were. We would do medical work in the afternoon, then show slides of medical things, like hookworm and malaria and all these things we wanted to prevent. Then I had film strips of bible stories and things like that. And this was before the days when they didn't know anything about cinema and pictures or anything, so this was absolutely amazing. They'd have had me go on all night, but you can imagine after walking all day through the bush and doing medical work in the afternoon, we needed our sleep. But I got to know a lot of people really very well and I loved the villages.[42]
>
> At first we didn't have penicillin because we didn't have a fridge and in those days the penicillin needed refrigeration…. We then got a kerosene fridge so we could have penicillin, but then of course it started to change and all the other antibiotics started to come in tablet form or capsule form, so it was really very different.[43]

Pyatt had no special training regarding leprosy, but her meeting with Patrick Twomey stood her in good stead to take on the new responsibility. Leprosy patients kept arriving and needed to be accommodated. The following extracts provide a description of the leprosy patients at Lolowai, building the St. Barnabas leprosarium, conditions at the leprosarium and her final departure twenty-five years later in 1974.[44]

> The little group [of leprosy sufferers] started to grow as more people came in. At that time there were no real drugs; Chaulmoogra oil wasn't really any good, horrible stuff…. We got up to about fifteen [leprosy sufferers], and we'd started another little leaf place right over the hill.[45]
>
> We just dressed their sores, that's about all really…. They didn't really understand anesthesia, their anesthetic limbs, very well and how they had to protect them. We would have to be very careful about that and teaching them those things. But it was so easy, when they had fires on the ground, to put their foot on a fire and that sort of thing. And of course some of those did arrest and go no further; that seemed to be something quite natural that happened.[46]
>
> There were very few text books even on it [leprosy]…. About 1952 the Leper Trust Board sent us the text book on leprosy. It was the first one really printed, and there were articles by all the known leprologists then in Africa and India…. They [the LTB] were very much in contact with us and letting us have literature and that sort of thing…. One of our excitements was, when we

did get this book, how many of our own observations were accepted.... Then we started to use the first sulphone drugs in 1955.[47]

This testimony indicates the late arrival and use of sulphones for leprosy in Vanuatu was not until the mid–1950s. However, in terms of isolation of patients at Vanuatu, the treatment arrived fairly soon after their admission to the Lolowai leprosarium. This appears to have reduced the fears associated with isolation at a leprosarium, as compared to the other Pacific Islands visited, where segregation and isolation were implemented early in the twentieth century and isolation was seen as a life sentence. This difference has affected perceptions of leprosy stigma in the Pacific, with negligible signs that leprosaria led to an increased fear of leprosy or caused stigma in Vanuatu. Betty Pyatt describes how they learned from experience to care for leprosy sufferers at Lolowai:

> We had a British medical officer who would come, and he would sort of really not know as much about it [leprosy] as we did. I can't remember the name of the leprologist in India, but I wrote to him a couple of times. He was very good, he would write back; and he had a lovely expression at the end — always said "keep on keeping on!"[48]
>
> In 1951 I think it was, I did a tour of the Banks and Torres islands with the bishop and I was horrified to see how much sickness there was.... There were people covered in horrible ulcers. So when we returned to Lolowai, I had a talk to the bishop with my colleague and we decided that the only thing ever going to help those people was to open clinics there. That meant we had to train people for them. So we started training the nurses.... Yaws was very distinctive really. I don't think I've ever coupled them together.... I've forgotten what year it was the World Health came in and simply went round the group and injected everybody ... gave penicillin to everybody, not just those who were affected.... Yaws just disappeared. By the time I had nurses in training in the 1970s I was having to show them pictures of yaws in case it came back.[49]

This extract indicates the general condition of people with diseases in remote regions, not just leprosy, and the lack of medical care or support available.

> In 1956 we had a new bishop who was very enthusiastic, and he was doing the Banks islands. To my horror I got a radio message from him to say that he'd found 25 lepers in isolation on one of the islands and he was sending the boat back with them the following day. Where were we going to put 25 lepers? We had a girls' school over the hill [Torgil Girls School and St. Patrick's Boys School], what is now St. Patrick's college ... they were 15 and 16 year-olds, and they all came over and built coconut leaf houses almost overnight. And it was into the coconut leaf houses that we admitted these people. I wrote out to Christchurch [the LTB] ... but I better start at the beginning. The condominium had always been going to build a leprosarium but it never did, and so we decided we had to do something.... By that time we would have had about forty [leprosy patients].[50]

This testimony confirms that advanced cases of leprosy were subject to segregation in Melanesian villages. Whether these sufferers segregated themselves by choice to support each other or due to rejection is unknown, and inevitably, individual circumstances would differ. A level of fear is evident with leprosy, as with any serious disease, but there did not appear to be the same level of fear of contagion that contributed to higher levels of stigma in other Pacific islands. To what extent patients suffering from other debilitating and festering infections, unrelated to leprosy, were also rejected or chose to leave their homes because of the unpleasant affects upon their families is unknown.

In other South Pacific nations the awful physical mutilations and odor emanating from leprosy sufferers had given rise to rejection and segregation, and even the clubbing of the unfortunate victims in Fiji. In these other islands, fear of the mutilations caused by leprosy had subsequently been heightened by the fear of the idea of contagion and permanent isolation from villages and families in the early 1900s. In Vanuatu the introduction of isolation didn't come until the 1950s; and with the availability of sulphone treatment only a few years after the establishment of the leprosarium, stigma did not appear to arise in connection with ideas of contagion or a life sentence of isolation. Nevertheless, leprosy did cause despair for those contracting the disease:

> Those 25 lepers that the bishop found had been all, sort of, sent away to the bush.... They were from all the different islands in the Banks islands, so they'd obviously got together.... They were just there ... looking after themselves.... They weren't too bad, I mean, their village life is a very primitive one, they would just build themselves leaf houses in the bush.... *I mean their skin condition?* Oh yes, some of them were bad.... *Do you have any knowledge of what they used to do for themselves?* Umm, well there were a lot of suicides connected with it, but otherwise it was just almost plain common sense looking after yourself.[51]

Although Betty Pyatt had heard about suicides by leprosy sufferers, no suicides occurred at Lolowai. The above testimony again confirms that leprosy sufferers did face segregation and isolation in their homes and villages, driving some to despair and sometimes even suicide, as had occurred on other Pacific islands and elsewhere. Whether this segregation was through rejection, or they left their homes because the advanced conditions of leprosy adversely affected their own families is unknown, but it is likely both factors were involved in local segregation of leprosy sufferers. In such circumstances, transfer and admission into a leprosarium offered superior medical assistance, comfort and the opportunities for friendships. In Lolowai, the arrival of the group of leprosy sufferers instigated the setting up of a local leprosarium by Betty Pyatt:

5. The Benefits of Leprosaria

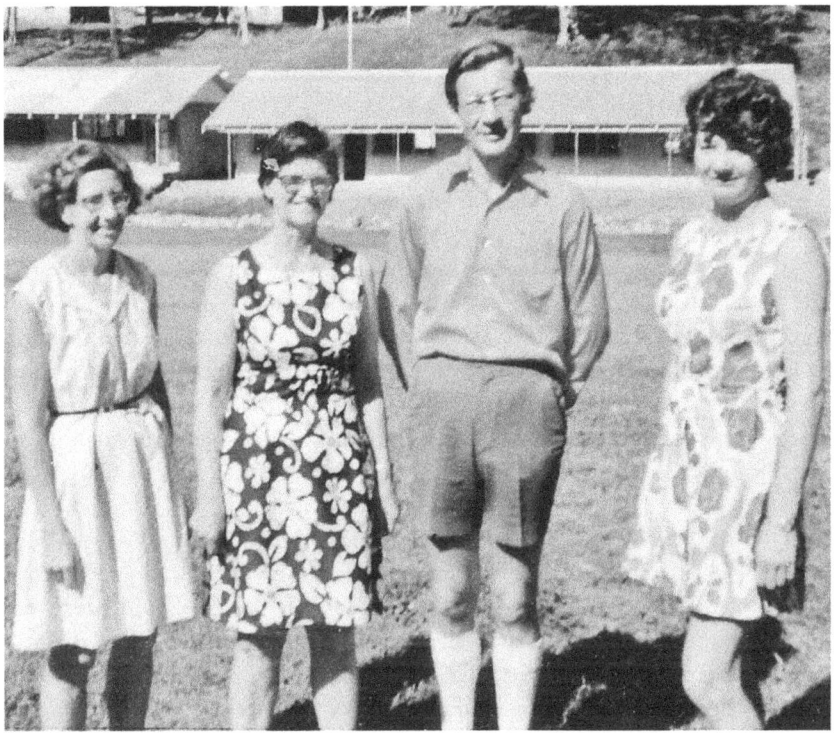

Mr. Clegg, leprologist, visits Lolowai in 1973. Left to right: Ms. Salt, school supervisor, Betty Pyatt, Mr. Clegg, Ms. Coleman, teacher.

I wrote out to Christchurch, and they just wrote back and said build a leprosarium. We started from scratch, and I still remember my colleague and I sitting around the kitchen table with a graph and working out the houses, and exactly the lengths of wood we would need, so that when it came they could put it up quite easily.... The early churches in New Zealand were built with eight-by-one batons — you know, up, down and across — and it seemed to be an easy way for our materials. So we had all our buildings done with eight-by-one batons. Well, we had to send our orders out, and then when they came back we didn't allow the builders to have any saws at all because they had to find the right place for the lengths of timber, but they were very good.... We chose a site ... I hadn't realised how flat it was because it was all covered in bush ... on a plateau behind the hospital.... The bush was cleared and it was a vast area, and so half of it was kept for a playing field, and that became the local football ground.... The leprosarium was at the other side, and they could watch. They couldn't really participate because kicking balls was pretty tough on anesthetic feet and that sort of thing.[52]

Gradually the fitter lepers themselves put it up. They did very well because some of them were fairly new cases who didn't have anesthesia.... An English priest helped a lot in supervising them, David Salt. They [homes for patients] just seemed to go up quite quickly really because they were quite plain houses. They didn't have windows, they had shutters because of the hurricanes.[53]

Setting up this leprosarium was obviously quite different to that established by the Fijian government at Makogai—which was on a planned basis rather than an "as needs" basis. Although segregation was imposed in Vanuatu, it was not enforced by strict rules, high fences or any form of official government control, as was the case in leprosaria in nearby New Caledonia. The highly fenced local leprosaria in Samoa and Tonga, with strict isolation, appear to have contributed to fear of leprosy, but these restraints were not implemented at Vanuatu. Moreover, St. Barnabas leprosarium was constructed along simple lines, like most other island buildings, and was certainly not situated in old prisons or places that had been used for outcasts of society, as in New Caledonia.

It is suggested that this relatively casual method of creating a leprosarium averted the fear and build up of stigma associated with ostracization of leprosy sufferers. Additionally, it avoided ideas that leprosaria in remote places were intended to contain highly contagious individuals who posed a danger to ordinary society. The location of St. Barnabas leprosarium—being built near an ordinary hospital, with access to arable land, a pleasurable beach and the sea for fishing—did not introduce undue fear into the local community with regards to the risk of contagion from leprosy. The fact, of course, that the Lolowai leprosarium was built in the 1950s makes an enormous difference, since earlier leprosaria were established well before an effective cure was available. Although it took some time for leprosy patients to be free from active leprosy, it was an enormous benefit that the majority of patients were admitted to St. Barnabas after sulphones were available.

Betty Pyatt recalls the formal recognition of the establishment of the leprosarium by some French inspectors visiting the leprosarium:

> The Condominium was always considering [building a leprosarium], and it rather solved something that I never quite understood.... In the early 1960s a boat arrived on our beach, and two French doctors got off it. They were really quite rude. They shook hands, and all they said was "St. Barnabas." And so we took them up the hill, and they walked around very quickly, didn't talk to us at all. But as they went down the hill I could hear one saying in French to the other "*sufficant.*" I thought perhaps somebody had reported that it wasn't very good or something, but I could see now what they were saying was they didn't need to build a leprosarium because there was enough. And do you know, it's taken all those years to find that out, because they were really very rude, the way they didn't attempt to communicate with us—whether they

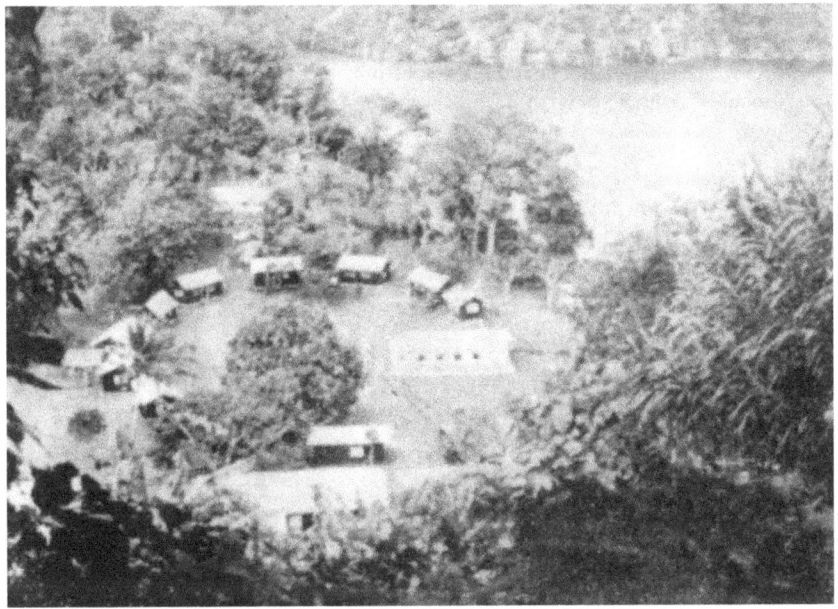

St. Barnabas leprosarium at Lolowai, huts for patients.

couldn't speak English or not. But I could've spoken a bit of French, but they didn't care. They didn't take any notice, but they just went right around the whole place and then back and got into their boat. But that's all I heard — "It's sufficient."[54]

Conditions at St. Barnabas Leprosarium at Lolowai

The location of the leprosarium behind the main Lolowai hospital has been described, but the following adds further details about the conditions for leprosy patients:

> The lepers had their gardens ... they'd grow a lot of their own food. Behind St. Barnabas [unfenced] was a track down to a lovely beach, and we called it the *Ome Quatatui*, which is small beach. But it wasn't all that small, and they loved it down there. They had their canoes, and they did everything down there. They'd go fishing in their canoes, and that was lovely having that beach for them. And they ended up by doing kastom dancing and that sort of thing. We didn't have...[a nurse resident] in the leprosarium, but our nurses in training had time ... rostered... up there. There was a dispensary and a nurse rostered [who] would work about 9 till 5. Some of them [patients] had babies ... Hannah had one [baby]. I used to go up most mornings to see how things were.[55]

> One of the lepers, Alfred Bani, had been a teacher. So when we had some younger lepers, he was able to have school in the leprosarium, and we ended up by having a good classroom once we opened St. Barnabas. There were probably about 10 children.... Some of them weren't really children, they were 16, 17 year olds.[56]

This description demonstrates the benefits of larger leprosaria for patients, as opposed to simply being segregated and living in small groups away from their villages. Although segregation at the leprosaria often involved several years of more distant separation from their families, the patients had access to special care and effective treatment, as well as the opportunities for wider friendships and schooling for the children. By the 1960s, St. Barnabas leprosarium had the benefit of a resident doctor, who performed surgery to relieve some of the problems associated with leprosy. Betty Pyatt went on to describe some of the later activities:

> When Bruce [Dr. Mackereth arrived 1962] came, he started to go to islands outside our usual area, and so we ended up by having lepers from all over Vanuatu .... Once Bruce came and started to do a lot of research, it grew up to a hundred people.[57]
>
> There was one boy who I was very upset about.... He was about fifteen and had lepromatous leprosy, but he was responding to drugs. And then he was poisoned by crab ... because there's a crab that is a poisonous crab if it's eaten something else. The patients sort of go paralyzed, and it's very seldom they recover, and I think even today they can die of it.... I was really upset about that. I think I can actually say nobody died from leprosy.[58]
>
> We did have quite a number of lepromatous patients, and they could be quite sick. It really was a worry at the time when they started to react so badly to sulphones, and, of course, afterwards, after I left. I suppose they started to build up resistance to it, and that's why they're now on the three different medicines. When the drugs really started to work and ... the World Health started to come into it ... we had a little doctor, I think it must've been after Bruce left, we had a little doctor, Doctor Bravo from Spain. He was one of the most enthusiastic little men I've ever known, and he was so enthusiastic about them picking up the very, very first signs of leprosy. And he had our nurses enthusiastic too, it sort of rubbed off on them. They went back to where they opened all these clinics. We had 15 clinics ... and now that's what happens. Most of them are found in the village clinics, sent to doctor for diagnosis and then sent back to their villages for treatment, which is just marvellous. Marvellous because when I think of the problems those people had being isolated from their villages and families in the early days — that was the worst part of the leprosy really.[59]

The enthusiasm, not only of Dr. Bravo, but obviously Betty Pyatt and her staff no doubt contributed to an efficient program to detect, treat and control leprosy. The role played by Dr. Mackereth from 1962 to 1971 as medical superintendent at Lolowai and in pursuance of health programs in the northern islands demonstrates the manner in which compliance with leprosy treatment was accepted by villages.

The Mackereths and their two young sons were in Dunedin, New Zealand, when they originally learned that a medical officer was required at Lolowai. Dr. Mackereth applied for the post, which he subsequently obtained. Catherine Mackereth already knew about Betty Pyatt's work in Lolowai through the Melanesian Mission literature, and was excited about the possibility of living and working at Lolowai. After nine months training in Sydney in February 1962, which included tropical medicine, hygiene and public health issues for sanitation, the young family set out for Lolowai.

Bruce Mackereth's observations of the conditions at the hospital indicate high praise for Betty Pyatt's work.[60] He recognized her as the driving force behind the training of nurses and dressers (male nurses). He considered this the most important and effective change in providing health care because the trainees went out and staffed dispensaries where sick patients could be treated locally on islands which previously had no medical facilities, and only a small proportion of these sick patients needed to be sent to the hospital. He said that medical consultations were free but medicines were paid for, although those who could not pay would send a relative to work at the hospital or in the gardens. Among the leprosy patients at St. Barnabas he found only one misdiagnosis:

> I got an interpreter in to talk to him and found out that he'd dislocated his shoulder, and the village people had tried to put it in. They'd obviously fractured his humerus, and it had set at a much better position, which was actually an old-fashioned treatment for a dislocated shoulder that couldn't be reduced. So he had a perfectly functional arm, but ... when they fractured his humerus they pranged one of the nerves going down the arm and he got paralysis.... They thought the paralysis was leprosy, so he ended up in a leprosarium.[61]

By the time Dr. Mackereth arrived, the treatment of Dapsone for leprosy was well established in high dosages, but a small percentage of patients could not tolerate the medication, as it produced a "sensitivity rash."[62] This was a violent skin reaction which was serious and had to be managed in the hospital with steroids. In these cases Dapsone was discontinued and an alternative anti-leprosy drug used. He explained that this was the reason why treatment for leprosy began in the leprosarium. The following extracts provide additional details relating to patients at the leprosarium:

> We tried to keep down the number of people in the leprosarium, those that didn't actually have leprosy. But sometimes if both the parents had leprosy you had to have the children. I mean, you didn't have much choice, so there

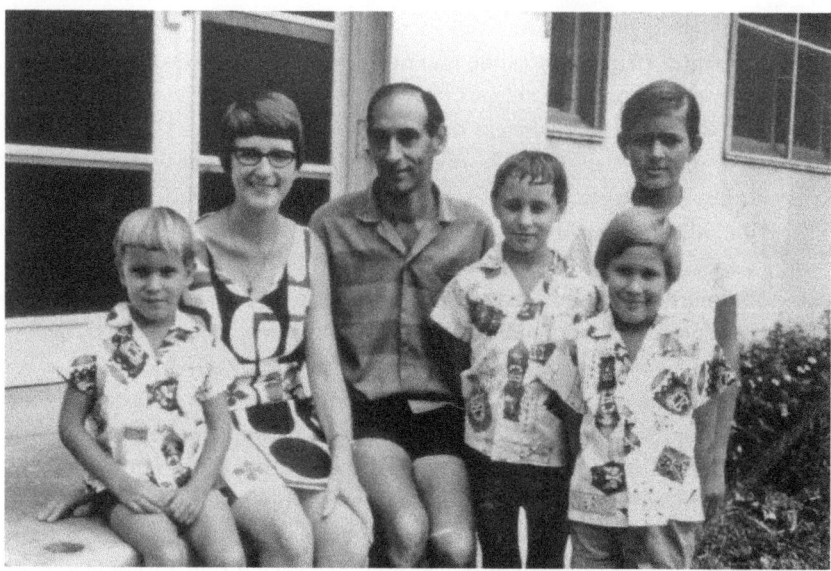

Mackereth family (left to right): Graham, Catherine, Bruce, Daniel, Anthony (at rear) and Simon.

were a few children around that didn't actually have it, but we tried to minimize this.... The Melanesians attached very little stigma to leprosy. The problem came with some Europeans who wouldn't carry them on their ships and things like this, and even government ones [ships], but there was a difficulty in striking a balance between irrational fear and spreading infection.[63]

This testimony confirms the difference in attitude between Europeans and Melanesians — the Europeans demonstrating stronger fears of contagion and stigma towards leprosy, while the Melanesians were happy to bring their families to the leprosarium. Nevertheless, it is apparent that the pragmatic attitudes of Pyatt and the Mackereths at the Lolowai leprosarium made an impact on leprosy patients and the surrounding communities, as the following testimonies demonstrate (the testimony of Catherine Mackereth is shown in italics):

> *Some people stayed years! The head man up there — what was his name?* Alfred, who was a schoolteacher ... he ran the school in the leprosarium.... I'm not sure there was any desire to go back, and nor was anyone particularly keen on sending him back ... because from the earlier years, the [patients] would have stayed a long time because there wasn't a proper cure, so it would have been a kind of idea that people did stay. *At one stage one of our nurses contracted leprosy, she was from Vila.* She was sent to us with leprosy, wasn't she? *Yes, so she was able to be the nurse for the leprosarium.* She was a PMH [Paton Memorial Hospital] trained nurse, trained at the Presbyterian hospital. She was sent to

5. The Benefits of Leprosaria   171

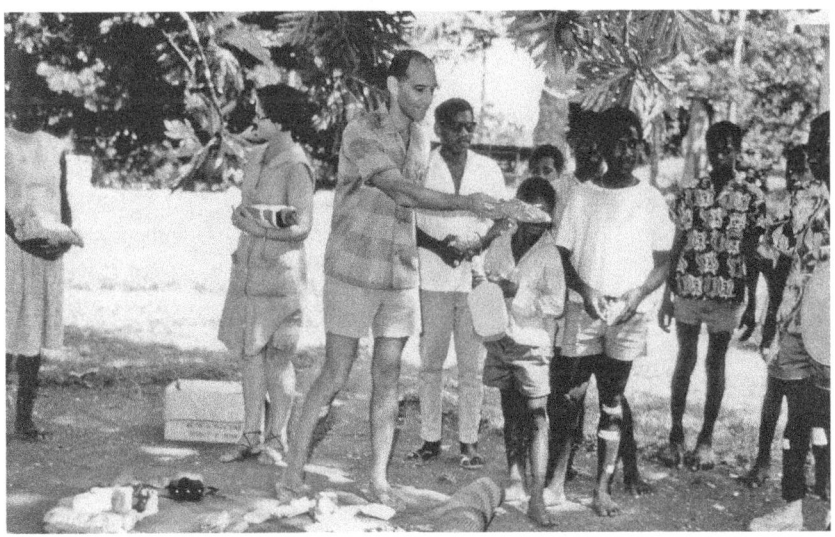

Bruce Makereth giving presents to leprosy patients, 1970.

us with leprosy, so we made her the nurse for the leprosarium. *She was lovely....* There were no Europeans [with leprosy at leprosarium].[64]

This testimony indicates that leprosy sufferers were sometimes content to remain at the leprosarium and were happy to provide assistance and help others in the same position. This is a feature common to many leprosaria around the world still today, such as in Raoul Follereau in Ducos, New Caledonia, and Twomey Memorial Hospital in Suva, Fiji. But once St. Barnabas leprosarium in Lolowai was closed, no leprosaria remained in Vanuatu, and patients were treated at clinics or in a ward at the general hospital. No sources were found to provide details regarding this interim period.

Dr. Mackereth spent a great deal of time traveling to other northern islands and walking to villages to examine patients. He describes how surveys were carried out:

> I did a lot of surveys, and the people all lined up for me to check them, and they were very cooperative about this. They were nice and easy to examine because they didn't wear all that number of clothing, and also the women weren't really worried about their breasts, even if they had them covered. You could just line them up out in the field and go along the line. We found a lot of leprosy, but people knew a lot. I think there was enormous value of going to all these places. There's an enormous difference between asking people to come to the leprosarium than telling them to go to the leprosarium. If I went out to the village, they normally came. So I made a point of going around the various islands.[65]

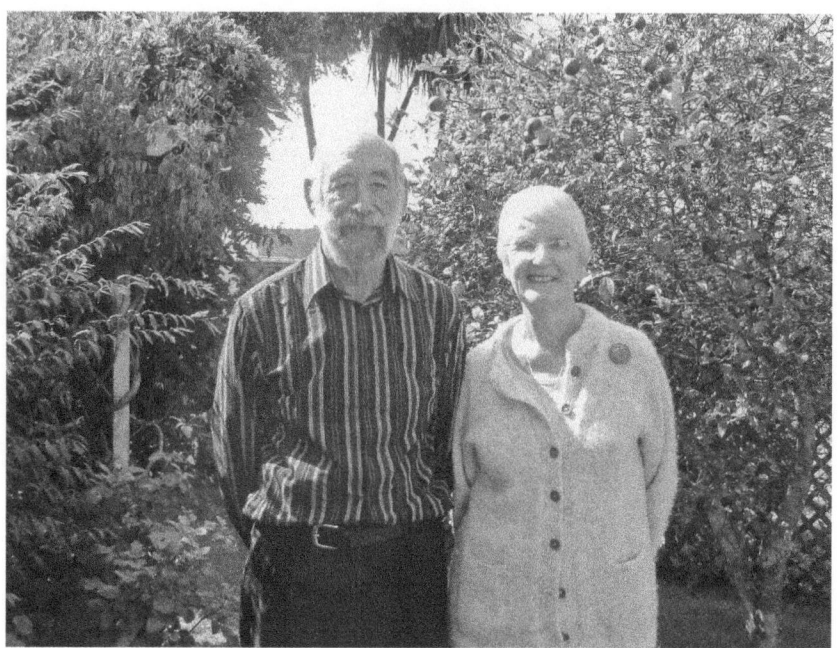

Dr. Bruce and wife Catherine Mackereth, now retired at their home in New Zealand.

I got the impression that in the ten years we were there, it [leprosy] got largely controlled.... I did sort of an epidemiological study on each patient. I had a little sheet to fill in with questions if any of their relatives had leprosy.... There were certain patterns that became very apparent. There seemed to be a strong hereditary factor about susceptibility to leprosy. For instance, it was very unusual for a spouse to be affected, and when a spouse was, it was a different form of leprosy.... Whereas within a family you'd find most of the children infected, or parents and children infected, and it tended to be the same form of leprosy.... You find clusters in a family, and if they were blood relatives it would tend to be the same form. But if they weren't blood relatives, like a spouse, they usually didn't get it at all, and if they did it was a different form. To my mind that indicates that there's a strong genetic tendency towards susceptibility. The other thing is that Melanesians in general don't have a great deal of physical contact.... You don't see them sitting on a seat close together touching; they squat on the ground separate. Except on one island, Mota Lava. There you saw them sitting on seats, all touching each other in a row, and they had by far the worst [leprosy] problems. I went [to Mota Lava, Banks Islands] a number of times.[66]

The approach of Dr. Mackereth towards patients, making a point of visiting villages and asking the sick to accompany him for treatment, is indicative of the whole difference in approach towards leprosy on Vanuatu, which avoided introducing ideas of stigma. Although Dr. Mackereth did suggest some problems were encountered conveying patients to Lolowai, his policy of asking patients to accompany him to the leprosaria avoided this problem, as the patients frequently traveled with him. Thus, leprosy patients were just another group of patients needing hospital treatment, and since sulphones were available, an effective cure could be administered. Leprosy, certainly in less advanced stages, appears to have been viewed in the same way as any other serious ailment that required hospitalization and temporary removal from village homes. This testimony also demonstrates the lifestyles of Melanesians, with a possible explanation offered for the higher incidence of leprosy in the northern islands — because of their closer proximity in their daily lifestyle, sitting close together, as opposed to non-contact groups in the south.

Leaving Lolowai

On the news of the death of her father, Betty Pyatt returned suddenly to New Zealand, but she returned later to Lolowai following Independence in 1980, with Catherine Mackereth. Betty describes her feelings about having left Lolowai:

> I left when my father died [in 1974]. And I almost needed a reason for leaving, but I could see that things were changing. They were already starting to be discharged, and when I went back six years later there were no lepers there at all.... Catherine [Mackereth] and I went back in 1980. They had a big party ... at Lolowai itself, around the bay from hospital. We had a big service first in the church, and then we went out and had this party, and I really learned something that day.... We [had not said] ... goodbye, and that was the whole theme of the whole thing, they hadn't said goodbye. That really showed me how necessary it was to finish something, and I was sitting there with tears streaming down my face because I realised I hadn't said goodbye.[67]
>
> When I went back ... I stopped still because half way up the hill there was still the fallen tree on the side of the path.... If I walked up that hill and there was someone sitting on that tree trunk, it would mean that they wanted to talk. And somehow it all came back to me when I was walking up that hill all those years later.... A lot of it was stories from their villages that they'd heard. They were worried about ... what was happening to his wife and if she was playing around with somebody else and all this sort of thing. It was really, really hard for them being isolated from their families.[68]
>
> Over the time I was there, 25 years, the whole place developed. There were all sorts of training programmes for Melanesians, teacher training started. Schools were opened everywhere. I just feel so fortunate to be associated with it all, over that development period. It was wonderful.... [It had been] a natural development, I think, that the expats came to train the Melanesians, and then the Melanesians could take over.[69]

Bruce Mackereth had fallen ill while working at Lolowai in 1972 and was admitted to the hospital at Port Vila, where it was considered best that he return to New Zealand for the sake of his health. In the long term they decided it was also best for the education of their four sons.

Supporting Accounts of Conditions at Lolowai Leprosarium

Working under Betty Pyatt at Lolowai hospital, Anna Tevi was one of the first local nurses trained, and she worked at Lolowai. Her mother was from the island of Pentecost and her father an Australian aboriginal, from the blackbirding days, she said. Anna went to Lolowai in 1958 to work at the hospital and became one of the first group of Melanesian nurses to be trained. Her testimony sheds more light on some of the benefits available to leprosy patients at a leprosarium:

> [I was a] 1962 graduate, and then I took a baby born with deformity hair lip and cleft palate to New Zealand.... Baby of the leprosy, the two parents they both leprosy and they married and they took them down to leper colony at Lolowai. Then we look after them, and when she delivered the baby we took straight away to hospital, not living with the parents.... Sister Pyatt took me along ... before she went down to Wellington, because her parents lived down there. ... The baby was only six months when I took her to New Zealand.... She had treatment in Middlemore Hospital in Auckland. So when I first took her down there, the doctor ask me, they think that I was the mother. I said no, sorry, I am a nurse from Lolowai Hospital, they choose me to take the child over. Then I have to look after her for six months there.... I stayed and helped. I was a nurse, they give me a room, they give me uniform, and I joined them. I was really happy.[70]

Anna Tevi said the child was returned to the parents. She led a normal life and is now married with three children living in Port Vila; they still visit each other. This is an example of the huge benefits some leprosy sufferers were able to receive at leprosaria because of the special funding provided by the PLF.

Jean Woi Tarisesei, now working in Port Vila as a women's community program coordinator, was the daughter of the local baker at Lolowai and lived a day's walk from the hospital. At the age of eight or nine in the late 1950s she regularly visited Lolowai and played with children in the leprosarium, although she said this was not really allowed.[71] On feast days, everyone in Lolowai mixed together, sitting and talking, even people from the leprosarium, although those from St. Barnabas cooked and ate their food separately.[72] This

5. The Benefits of Leprosaria 175

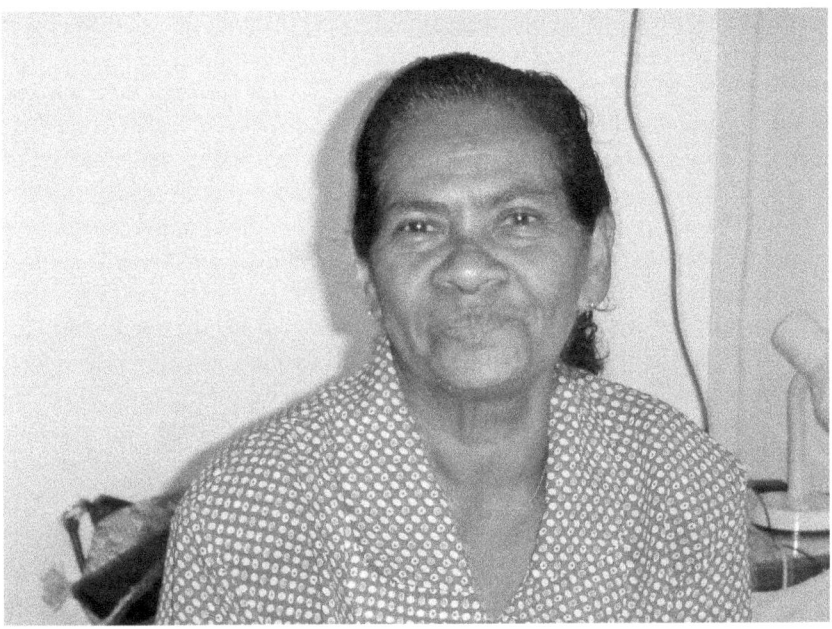

Nurse Anna Tevi. Now retired, she was trained by Betty Pyatt in Port Vila.

confirms that the manner of segregation of leprosy sufferers at the leprosarium did not contribute to increased fears of leprosy in the neighborhood; this is in direct contrast with the Fale'ofa leprosy clinic in Tonga, and Ducos in New Caledonia, which had high fences and strict isolation within a restricted area, or distant islands like Makogai. However, some concern about contagion was evident as food was not shared with those suffering from leprosy.

The sad plight of those contracting leprosy was also confirmed by Jean Woi Tarisesi's testimony, which indicated that family rejection was felt by some patients. Jean said she knew one patient had committed suicide by hanging himself off the cliffs.[73] Although sympathy was evident for their plight, she believed there was no real fear of leprosy or mixing with those known to have the disease. She was familiar with the routine at St. Barnabas, the daily visit by nurses, self-sufficient gardens tended by the patients, their schools, and many of the names of patients.

Betty Pyatt's testimony indicates she was aware of suicides among those with leprosy who were not at Lolowai, but did not provide any details.[74] She indicated that fear and anguish, separation from loved ones, and worry about what may be going on back home contributed to despair. The Ministry of Health leprosy officer, Russell Tamata, recalled a cave near his childhood home where he said leprosy sufferers were banished. He maintained that family members never saw these people again, although Tamata said that food was left regularly at the cave. It was only when the food stopped being collected that families realized their relatives had perished.[75] This indicates that isolation in the villages was more complete than isolation at Lolowai leprosarium, and that the leprosarium provided benefits which, in fact, led to the reduction of stigma of leprosy.

Dr. Frank Spooner, medical practitioner in Port Vila, praised the achievements of Betty Pyatt and the Mackereths, and added that Betty Pyatt had been awarded an MBE.[76] Dr. Spooner had been the relief doctor at Lolowai hospital for four weeks in 1966, then again as locum for five weeks in 1970. In 1972–3 he was appointed the medical superintendent at Lolowai, at which time he recalls there were about twelve maternity beds, twenty beds for tuberculosis patients and about fourteen beds for general patients. He thought there would have been between 150 and 200 leprosy patients in residence at St. Barnabas.[77] Dr. Spooner indicated that St. Barnabas leprosarium was closed around 1974–75, as leprosy patients were treated at their place of diagnosis rather than being segregated at leprosaria. This testimony indicates that leprosy sufferers were treated as ordinary patients as early as the mid-1970s, preventing a possible rise in stigma.

Incidence of Leprosy and PLF Assistance

Reports by WHO leprologist Lopez-Bravo indicated that in 1976 there were 272 cases of leprosy registered and that twenty-eight new cases were registered the same year.[78] A rehabilitation department had been established at the main hospital in Port Vila, although no qualified staff was available. The lack of being able to provide adequate facilities was blamed on the ferment prior to independence from Britain and France in 1980, and the complexities involved in merging the two administrative departments.[79] In 1981 Lopez-Bravo reported that 258 cases remained on the leprosy register, of which only ninety-six cases needed to be regularly followed up, but that the difficulty of recruiting senior medical staff for leprosy control impeded adequate surveillance.[80] The PLF continued to grant assistance to the Vanuatu Health Department, and provided shoes and orthopaedic aids to patients.[81]

Dr. Roland Farrugia, who had first worked with leprosy at the Ducos leprosarium in New Caledonia in the 1970s and retired as WHO leprologist in 2001, accepted the position of consultant leprologist with the PLF for the South Pacific region. Together with Tony Whitley, the voluntary PLF liaison contact for Vanuatu, who lived in Espiritu Santo, they embarked on a program to investigate and update the position regarding leprosy sufferers in Vanuatu.

5. The Benefits of Leprosaria

Tony Whitley said that the PLF had been on the verge of ending support to the Vanuatu department of health, as no facilities were available to leprosy patients, until Roland Farrugia took on the direct role as leprosy consultant.[82] Dr. Farrugia obtained the old medical database from which he initiated searches to locate and identify leprosy patients still alive in the country. Contact was made with Tony Whitley in 2002, and together they put into place a plan, described by Dr. Farrugia:

> The breakthrough came when we started using a core of intermediary people, go-betweens, if you want, using people with little or no education at all. But multiply that by their number and the fact that they were mobile, available, and were paid a very reasonable price, those people could do at once the job of 60 or 100 consultants doing the same thing. So we started using those people.... They were called here in this country volunteers.... We had the good fortune of being provided by the Minister of Health with a full list, database of the recent patients for decades. Again and again those patients had been registered and nothing had ever happened, nobody knew whether they were alive or dead or disappeared.... The database was not the best, but it had anyway the enormous advantage of being [in existence].... Santo is a good example because of the problems of the terrain. It's a very difficult island; there are no roads at all, two-thirds on the coast and very little in between. I mean they [patients] are across the island.... So what we did was, taking that database, divide the island theoretically into different parts, and provide a group or team of volunteers with a copy of the list of patients by village and establish an itinerary with the volunteers. We just asked them to go to the villages from the part that had been offered, and start asking about the patients. Firstly, would be to take the list of people one by one and ask if they were alive or dead, so we would know they were dead, they had disappeared, they were not there anymore, or they were there. [From] the date of registration ... there was [a gap] of seventy, eighty years.[83]

This time lapse suggests that the original databases were lists that had probably been compiled by Sister Pyatt and Dr. Mackereth, as were most other leprosy surveys conducted during the 1950s and 1960s. Dr. Farrugia describes how his survey to update the position was conducted using local Melanesian helpers:

> I would take a team of volunteers somewhere — either the hospital in Santo or go somewhere and have them gathered, all of them at the same place. That place could be anything, under a tree or whatever, and give on-the-spot medical education to those volunteers. So of course it had to be very basic, but it proved quite useful and quite valid. I would tell them and I would try to show them what a skin lesion would be, and would talk to them about the basic tests, touch, pain. I would show them how to test a degree of paralysis of muscles in the face, in the hands and in the feet, extremely basic. So I would give them a lecture, but of course the lecture would have to be adapted to

their level of education, it was very basic.... Sometimes it had to be interpreted, go through an interpreter and given anywhere. I remember giving that kind of teaching in a hut with a family cooking dinner.[84]

The conditions described by Dr. Farrugia reflect the conditions under which these oral history interviews were often conducted, and also demonstrate that despite the limitations of language and the use of interpreters, Melanesians were quick to understand and undertake the action required:

Well, the list started shrinking of course very quickly.... Some of those people ... needed [treatment] for plantar ulcers. Plantar ulcers in leprosy are really a plague. It's often missed in recurrence. The plantar ulcer is an infection which is characterized by a hole in the flesh, in the sole of the foot, and that happens because of the insensitivity of the foot. People keep putting the same pressure, which is high because of the weight of the body, exactly on the same spot. We all do that because we all walk roughly on three points — the heel and the two heads of the metatarsals, the first and the fifth — but we change our weight, it happens sometimes in the same day. We don't realize it, but as we walk we must feel some tiredness or whatever and we change [pressure points] and we don't even realize it. Leprosy patients don't have any sensitivity; therefore they will keep walking on exactly the same muscles, and it's a well known fact that when you put an enormous pressure on the tissues you create damage to those tissues. And actually you end up with a blister and a hole. For years and years and years they could have bandages and dressings, cleaning or whatever, that won't do a thing as long as they walk, it won't do a thing.[85]

So what we do now, we do cure those plantar ulcers by putting the foot in a plaster cast for weeks so that it heals.... In Vanuatu, which is humid and hot, if they have the plaster cast when they go back home, of course it is very difficult, they walk on difficult terrain on the stones.... But we try as much as possible ... to keep them in hospital, and that's best for them of course, they have a bed where they are treated, they are fed and so on, and they are at rest completely.[86]

The number of new cases has dwindled seriously in Vanuatu, to such an extent that for a few years, let's say from 1998 to 2002 or '03, there were no [new leprosy] cases reported. I have my doubts about the real results; there must be cases that will never be diagnosed and people who will eventually die in the bush and absolutely nobody to diagnose their disease.... Sometimes they hide and they eventually die but create a lot of damage by disseminating their bacilli. But anyway, for a few years the numbers of active cases went down so much that we had no new cases reported. And now for the last three years we have the odd new case appearing, one, two. Yes it is probably lower than New Caledonia, and it is surprising because the level of resources is totally different. That would probably be the level [of] stigma to it and people coming forward.... You have differences between the provinces, between the islands. You have places where the stigma is strong ... in Ambrym, in Pentecost.[87]

Dr. Farrugia indicates that, despite the high level of resources available in nearby New Caledonia, the incidence of leprosy in Vanuatu is much lower. Additionally, he suggests that although stigma in Vanuatu is lower than in New Caledonia and other South Pacific islands visited by this writer, there was a level of stigma and fear in Vanuatu which varied in intensity on the different islands. The oral histories with earlier medical staff, and the more recent testimonies of leprosy sufferers in Vanuatu, tend to suggest a low level of stigma (if indeed stigma is the correct term) and fear associated with leprosy.

Testimonies of Leprosy Sufferers

Of the seven leprosy sufferers spoken to on the island of Espiritu Santo in July 2008, four were males (Rere Abana, Charlie Vuti, Rocky Andrew and Bialoloso Varu) and three were females (Mary Alma Namtaktak, Emrere Vira, and Vearu Stephen).[88] All four men had been married, and had three, seven, eight and nine children respectively. Of the two older women, Mary Alma had married and adopted a child, while Emrere had one child but had not married. The third woman, Vearu, the niece of Emrere, is a younger married woman with four children who was only diagnosed with leprosy in 2004 after the birth of her last child. This suggests that males with leprosy were not ostracized and were able to marry and have families, but the older women might have faced some exclusion. However, the women lived with and were cared for by their extended families, indicating little or no stigma towards leprosy sufferers.

Of the seven people spoken to, only two were able to provide their year of birth with any certainty. Since the presence of the American troops during World War Two had a huge effect on life in Santo, the simplest way to ascertain an idea of age was to ask whether they were born after the war, or if born before the war what were they doing at that time (e.g., a child or working adult). Although the testimonies offer enormous insights into the lives of leprosy sufferers in Vanuatu, arriving and questioning the interviewees in their homes immediately after introductions in the space of an hour or so, surrounded by family and relatives interjecting and enjoying the stories, inevitably left gaps in gaining a full understanding of their individual situations. Speaking through an interpreter, who sometimes had trouble translating my questions into a form understandable to the interviewee, increased the limitations because of cultural differences in questioning the status quo, which often puzzled the interviewees. Nevertheless, the friendly cooperation and helpful responses indicate that the work of the PLF is welcomed and much appreciated locally. This goodwill flowed on and was even extended to a complete stranger — myself— a foreigner coming into their homes and asking personal questions.

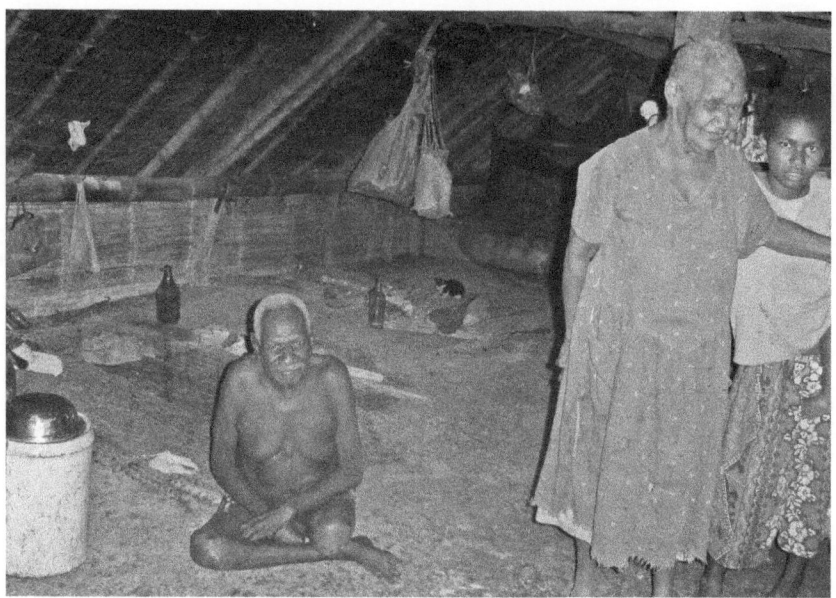

Bialoloso Varu, within his traditional dark Melanesian home.

Memories of Lolowai

Four of the seven interviewees had been to St. Barnabas leprosarium at Lolowai — namely, Rere, Bialoloso, Emrere and Mary Alma. Charlie Vuti said his mother had leprosy and went to Lolowai, although he said he knew nothing about her experiences. His own leprosy had been treated locally soon after diagnosis and effectively, although he was now troubled by an ulcer under one foot, which Dr. Farrugia routinely checked.

Bialoloso Varu recalled, without any prompts, his memory of Dr. Bruce Mackereth walking into his village and checking all the inhabitants, and said that he then went with Dr. Mackereth to Lolowai on "big fella ship, the *Selwyn*.[89] Another member of Bialoloso's family, who was present at the interview, said he was also taken to Lolowai but returned after tests for leprosy proved negative. Bialoloso stayed at Lolowai seven years, on three separate visits. He recalled that leaving home the first time was difficult, but other times it was okay.[90] Initially he had to take six tablets every Thursday, but then the dosage was decreased to two tablets every Thursday and he felt better. He said many other villagers went on the same voyage as him on the *Selwyn* to Lolowai.[91] This ease of travel, as compared to travel to Makogai by Pacific islanders described earlier, would have prevented heightened ideas of contagion associated with leprosy stigma in Vanuatu.

5. The Benefits of Leprosaria

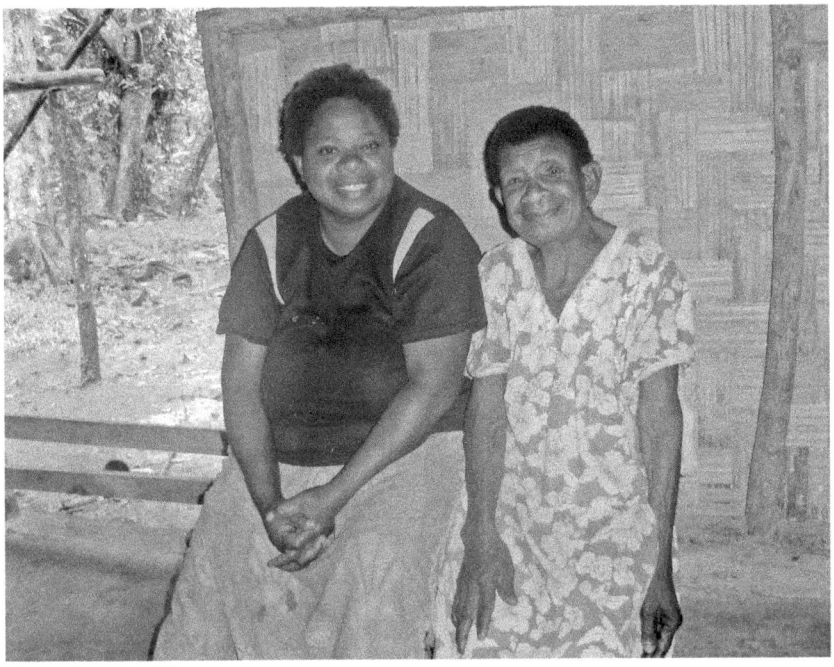

Emrere Vira (right) with Vearu Stephen.

Emrere Vira had stayed three months at Lolowai, but having no idea of when she was born or when she went, dates and times are sketchy. She said her brother had been to Lolowai earlier and returned, but neither of "his arms or legs worked" and he died soon after he returned home.[92] She confirmed men and women lived separately at St. Barnabas and added that she did not "feel ashamed, they made her feel good." When asked if she feared going away to Lolowai, she replied with a giggle that she was very frightened of going on the ship to Lolowai and back again. This indicates that life at the leprosarium was accepted and not feared, nor was there any strong leprosy stigma.

Mary Alma Namtaktak did not think any of her family had leprosy, but both Betty Pyatt and Dr. Mackereth indicated that Mota Lava, one of the Banks Islands which was Mary Alma's home, had the highest incidence of leprosy, so undoubtedly she had been in contact with the disease. Mary Alma suffered a facial disfigurement which she believed was caused by falling out of bed when she was a child, soon after which she was diagnosed with leprosy. She was at Lolowai for one year and remembered Betty Pyatt, the Mackereths and nurse Anna Tevi.[93] She said the women patients helped keep the houses clean and washed the sheets. Women lived on one side and men on the other, while married couples lived together.[94]

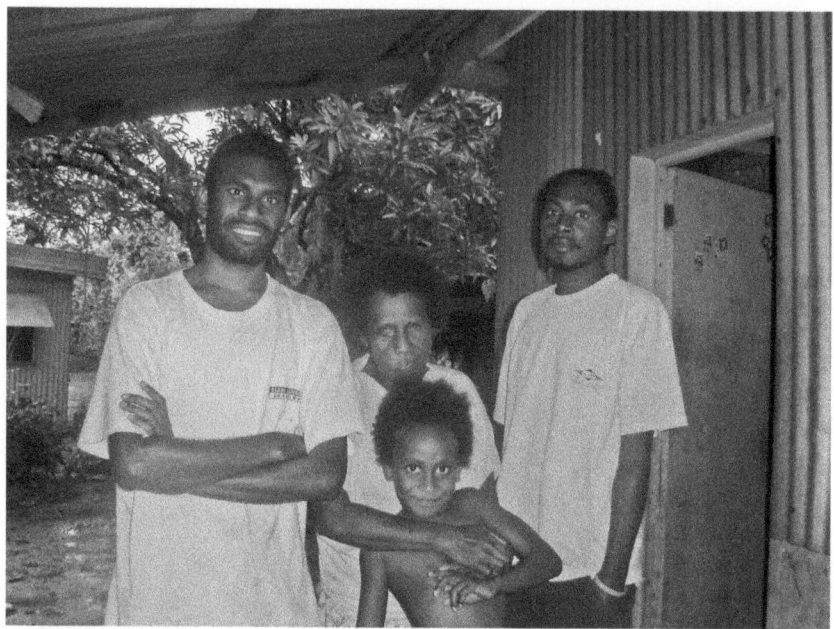

Mary Alma Namtaktak (center rear) and nephews in Santo, 2008.

These descriptions of conditions at the leprosarium corroborate earlier testimonies. The testimonies indicate that women were not locked in their living quarters at night, as in Makogai; nor were there strict rules relating to concern of contagion by having "clean areas" that were off limits to patients or sterilizing items touched by patients before use by others. This more relaxed attitude towards the risks of contagion is confirmed by Betty Pyatt's comments relating to lack of fear of leprosy by relatives and visitors to St. Barnabas, so much so that she regularly had to remind visitors not to sit on the beds of patients. This, nevertheless, indicates that hygiene remained an important part of the regime at the leprosarium. The earlier comments of Jean Woi Tarisesei confirm that simple measures to restrict the possibility of contagion were adhered to, and that leprosy patients did not share their food and utensils with others.

It was difficult to ascertain the interviewees' feelings about their separation from their families and going to Lolowai, and whether they thought they would ever return home; but the fact that they did return would have impacted on local perceptions of leprosy and reduced fear in others about being sent to the leprosarium. Translations of my questions by an interpreter into the direct style of Bislama, a form of pidgin English, evoked responses which simply confirmed the sentiment posed in the style of the interpreted question.

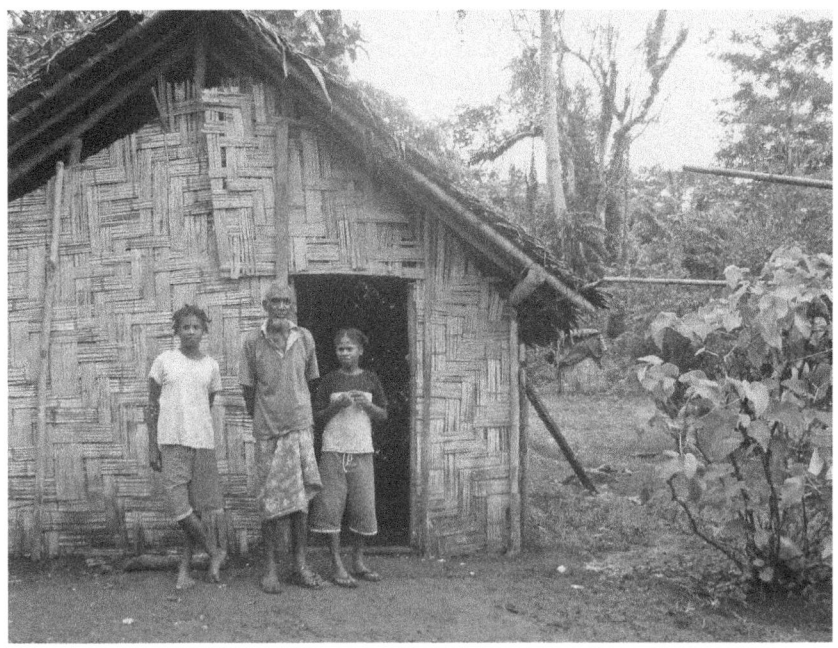

Rere Abana and his granddaugthers outside their home.

The responses tended to confirm an impression of acceptance that being sent to Lolowai was for the best. However, the responses tend to reflect their present views, with the wisdom of hindsight, rather than the feelings actually felt at that time. Although all four of these interviewees "agreed" with the proposition when asked whether they had been afraid, they went on to say they had been well treated. The only person who admitted real fear was Emrere, a shy, elderly lady whose fear of the sea appeared to be greater than fear of segregation at Lolowai. No evidence of any level of stigma appeared to be associated with isolation at Lolowai leprosarium.

Rere Abana offered the most detailed description of the leprosarium, where he was taken after World War Two as a grown man, married and with children. He remembered Betty Pyatt and Oscar, a popular man with leprosy who worked at the leprosarium. Rere's recollections include:

> Fresh meat and running water were available.... Patients cooked their own food. There was a river by the hill ... had to climb the hill to go to the garden. He didn't like that [climbing the hill]. There was a man from Pentecost, Oscar, with a tractor.... There were three houses. A shelter house, tin house, tin roof [with] bamboo, cane walls ... [they slept in] a long shelter, dormitory. He totally lost hope just after drinking the medicine. The medicine was so strong, he thought he would die there, he wouldn't come back. He

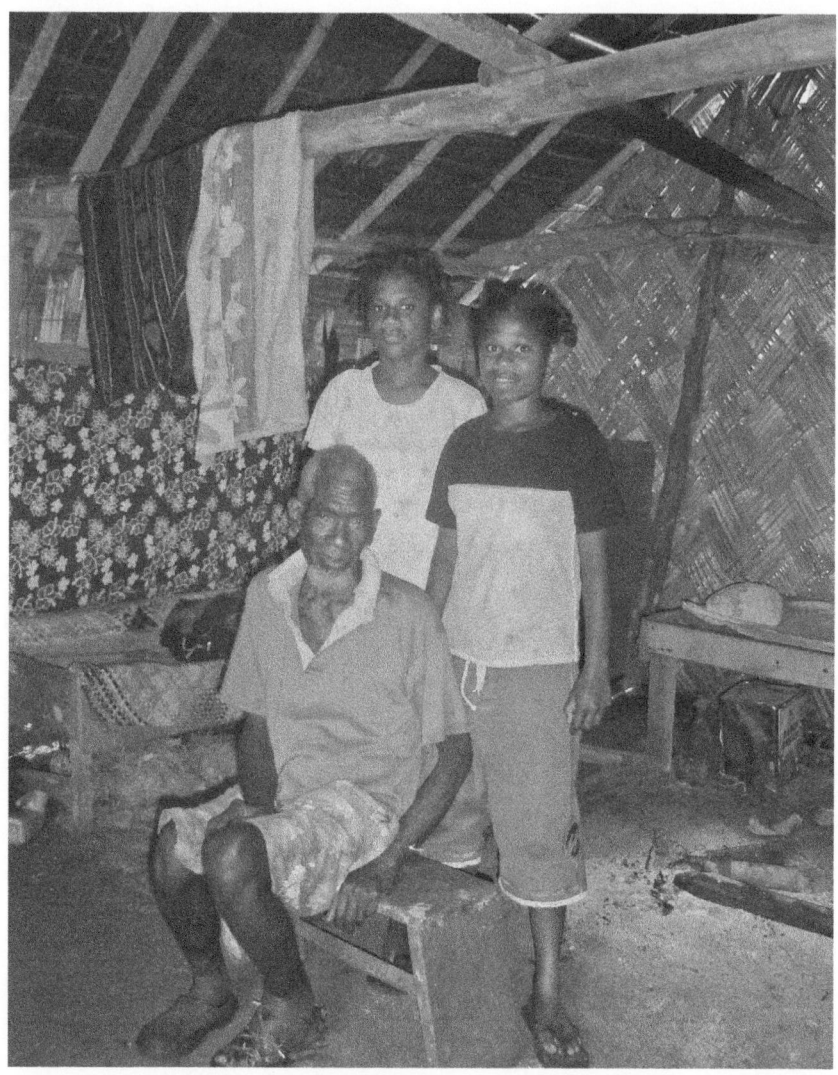

Rere Abana and granddaughters inside their home.

[said he] went [to Lolowai] by plane ... with Lindsay, another patient, by plane.[95]

One of his aunts [had leprosy] long time ago. She couldn't walk any more. They tried some of the kastom medicine, but it didn't work, but it turned out leprosy because the kastom medicine didn't work on her. *So how did they know she had leprosy?* They just look at her, she doesn't work and she doesn't move, they have been doing a lot of kastom medicine to her and they believe that it is just leprosy and she dies. Looking back they figured that she had leprosy.

She never went to Lolowai? No ... it was a scary thing, between themselves, the kids and the family. Only her husband was closer to her, he looked after her. The others were afraid of her. They know that it is a sickness.... They just scared of it. Only her husband was really taking care of her.[96]

Rere's testimony demonstrates perhaps a typical Ni-Vanuatu family attitude towards leprosy prior to admission to the leprosarium. There was some fear within the family, and as the disease progressed only one family member continued to care for the victim, while most other family members avoided contact. This is a different scenario to the earlier incidents of leprosy sufferers being excluded from their families and living together in groups. The interviews with all seven leprosy sufferers in Santo confirmed the general view that in contemporary times there were no ideas of leprosy stigma, although the condition still provoked fear and ongoing physical difficulties for some of the older leprosy sufferers.

The following cases demonstrate that there had been a lack of early diagnosis of leprosy since the 1980s, but the renewed assistance of the PLF in the 2000s, through Dr. Farrugia and the PLF liaison contacts in Vanuatu, was of enormous importance in preventing a resurgence of leprosy in the islands. In particular, the PLF assistance provided the means for patients who had disabilities and were unable to live a normal lifestyle because of leprosy to earn an income.

Experiences Living at Home with Leprosy

In all cases, the victims of leprosy lived with their families, with no apparent exclusion, although, as mentioned, the disabilities of the interviewees were not as severe as those seen in advanced cases of leprosy. Bearing in mind the limitations of coming to any conclusion with such a small sample of interviewees, the lack of severity may indicate that since the 1950s, when the effective treatment became available, leprosy sufferers in Vanuatu were well served medically, and the incidence of leprosy contained.

Rocky Andrew (born 1947) had contact with leprosy after his arrival in Santo in the 1970s from his home in Vermele, when he began to live with a family from Tahiti, of whom the wife had leprosy.[97] It was not until many years later that he felt unwell. For the last seven years he has regularly attended the hospital for an irregular heartbeat and other health problems, but leprosy was not diagnosed until 2000.[98] The extent of his disability suggests that leprosy had been present long before the diagnosis. Being the main breadwinner for his family of eight children, Rocky appeared the most disadvantaged by his claw hands and troublesome toe infection, as these prevented him work-

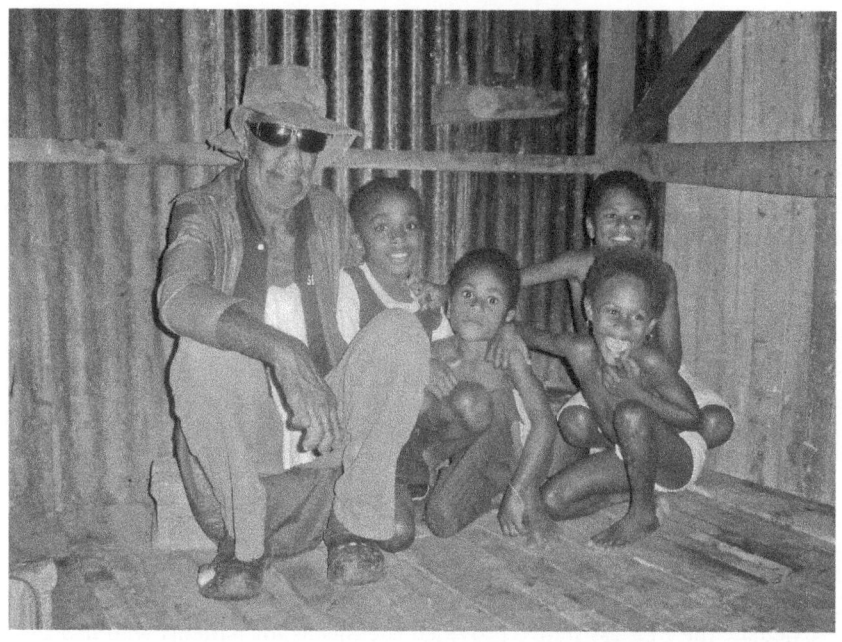

Rocky Andrew at home with his family in 2008.

ing.⁹⁹ However, as part of the PLF micro projects to aid leprosy sufferers, Rocky was to be given funds to set up a copra heating hut so that he could earn an income to support himself and his family. In the past, Charlie Vuti, who also contracted leprosy as an older man, had likewise received funds to set up a successful copra heating hut, which is a hut where coconuts were heated to produce coconut oil and copra.¹⁰⁰ The hut was also hired out for use by villagers, thereby supplementing the income.

Vearu Stephens (born 1975), a young married woman with four children, said that she had attended the hospital with early problems of numbness in her leg and foot, but it was not until she was seen by Dr. Farrugia in 2004 that leprosy was diagnosed.¹⁰¹ Vearu had a dropped foot, which made it difficult for her to walk and work in the gardens (a term used in Vanuatu for subsistence farming). She was unhappy that her dropped foot prevented her from working to help support her family.¹⁰² The PLF liaison present at the interview assured her that the schooling expenses of her children would be provided to help their situation. This PLF assistance ensures that leprosy sufferers and their families are not disadvantaged by the disease and prevents ideas of stigma which could arise because of the low status and poverty that leprosy victims would otherwise face.

Apart from Rocky and Mary Alma, who contracted leprosy from contact

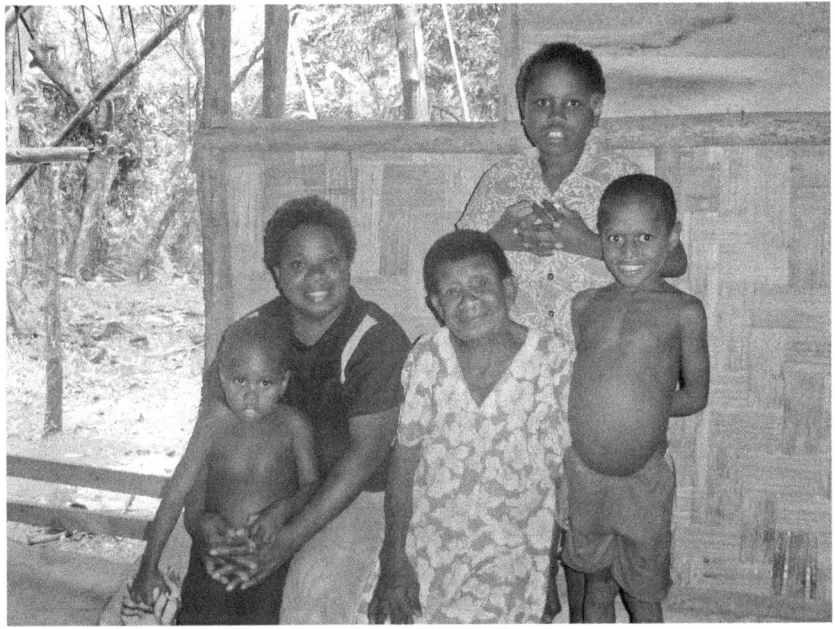

Vearu Stephen (left) and her children with Emrere Vira.

with other leprosy sufferers, all the other interviewees had family members, either a parent, aunt, uncle or sibling, who had had leprosy. None of the interviewees could provide details of the form of leprosy they contracted, nor did they know the different forms of leprosy. Their knowledge of leprosy was personal and through family experience.

Of the interviewees, Bialoloso was the most severely incapacitated due to the amputation of one leg at the knee in about 1999. His injury was caused by stepping accidentally on the hot ashes of a fire lit on the ground in his home, which is the usual way to warm the village homes in the cool evenings and provide light, as there was no electricity in his village. Even interviewing Bialoloso on a rainy afternoon was problematic, because the darkness in the high-roofed thatched Melanesian homes, with no windows, made it difficult to read and complete the personal details and oral history consent form. After his leg amputation, Bialoloso had hoped he would obtain an artificial limb from the specialist Fijian leprosy hospital; but, unfortunately, when the amputation was performed in 2000 the site of the amputation was such that his leg was unsuitable for the fitting of a prosthesis.[103] The testimony of Bialoloso suggests that although leprosy patients were treated in the general hospital, since the closure of the leprosarium, the medical treatment offered was not sufficiently specialized to meet the needs of leprosy patients.

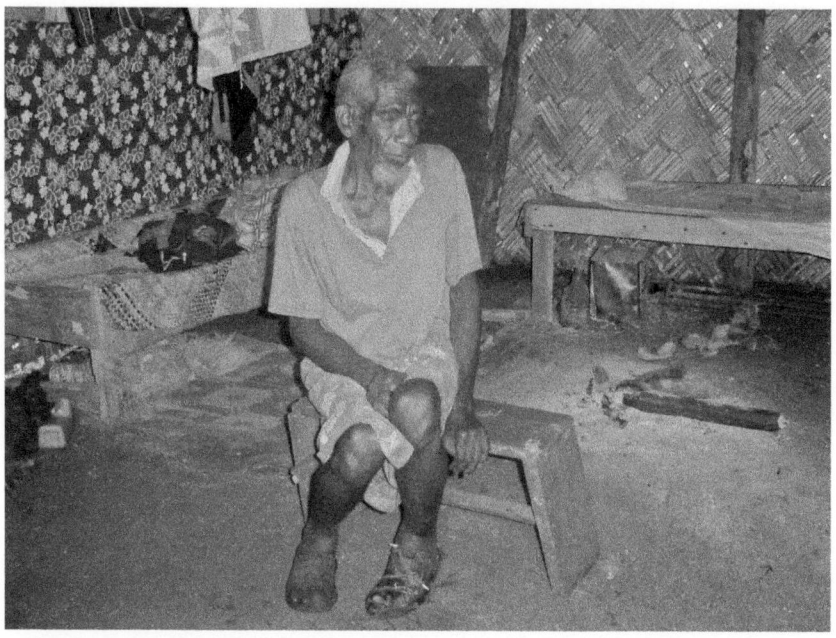

Rere Abana in his traditional styled home. Behind him is the usual lit fire on the ground to provide heat and light.

Additionally, the experiences of Rocky and Vearu indicate that until Dr. Farrugia directly intervened in leprosy control with his vigilance campaigns in Vanuatu as the PLF consultant, leprosy patients such as these two people had slipped through the system undiagnosed, despite the best efforts of the PLF and the availability of effective treatment in Vanuatu. This indicates that the medical service provided for leprosy sufferers is deficient in Vanuatu, and the assistance of the PLF makes an enormous difference to the lives of leprosy sufferers and ensures that they are not unduly disadvantaged.

Several of the interviewees mentioned trying traditional kastom medicines as well as western remedies. Although details were not obtained from Betty Pyatt and the Mackereths regarding local traditional beliefs and health practices applied to leprosy, it is likely that these were encountered. Bruce Mackereth indicated that he avoided commenting on "leaf medicine" when it was observed, and instead relied on results of the western treatment offered to convince and obtain compliance. As recently as 2006, when speaking to a young female relative of the newly appointed Bishop James Ligo at the Melanesian Mission in Port Vila, she mentioned that she had married a childhood friend who contracted leprosy as a teenager. After noticing a spot on one arm and a thigh, he spent a couple of years at St. Barnabas Hospital during 1970-71. After he had been cured, they were married, but in 1992 he suddenly disappeared, abandoning his wife "because of witchcraft."[104] Despite the lack of detail, the statements confirm a lack of stigma because leprosy did not put an end to the prospects of marriage. However, it also shows that neither rational explanations nor superstitious beliefs fully explain or reveal the personal suffering imposed by leprosy, although other personal circumstances might have attributed to the disappearance, rather than the view suggested that leprosy and witchcraft had been the cause of the disappearance. Certainly local attitudes and practices towards diseases in Vanuatu were influenced by traditional beliefs in black magic and sorcery, but the benefits being derived from European methods of hygiene and the basic preventative measures offering medical relief were recognized and had gone a long way towards changing local attitudes.

My questions relating to how each leprosy sufferer felt regarding the afflictions imposed by leprosy, such as isolation and separation from family, appeared somewhat puzzling to the interviewees; their replies indicated there was little choice but to accept the conditions imposed by their plight, even living at the leprosarium in earlier times. Despite the limitations imposed through the use of an interpreter, this acceptance does not necessarily suggest a sense of disempowerment or enforced isolation, but perhaps a willingness to undergo anything that might offer a cure or relief of their suffering.

The low incidence of leprosy in Vanuatu falls within the WHO elimination rate goal to 2005, indicating that leprosy has been well controlled in the islands. In addition, the oral history testimonies confirm Dr. Furrugia's observations that stigma in Melanesia was nowhere near the level of the stigma he had witnessed towards leprosy in other countries. A low level of stigma, if that can be used as an accurate description, is evident in the fear or even revulsion of the physical disabilities caused by leprosy, and it exists in Vanuatu. This is evidenced by Rocky Andrew's experiences on his visits to the hospital in Luganville, Santo. Through the interpreter, his wife had said he regularly visited the hospital for dressings required for ulcers on his feet:

> His wife was saying that when he does go to the hospital, people do run away from him.... He will go to the hospital, just now for this. He will sit there and wait for an hour, and they won't want to attend to him.... So he says he uses his own money to go to the pharmacy to buy bandages and all of these things to dress his sores. And he says, if he feels shameful, he wants to go to the bush.[105]

This suggests that although leprosy treatment is now available in general hospitals rather than being treated separately as outcasts of society thereby creating stigma, there is a need for specialist treatment of leprosy patients at the hospital to avoid situations in which patients are dealt with by inexperienced staff. Feelings of rejection are aroused when nursing staff display reluctance or disgust in dealing with unsightly infected toes and/or plantar ulcers, which are a plague with leprosy. The PLF assistance to leprosy sufferers and training of medical staff at the hospital is provided to actively prevent such situations that contribute to leprosy stigma. The direct PLF assistance to leprosy sufferers in Santo helps to maintain a normal standard of living, which in turn prevents a rise in stigma towards people with the disease and their families.

Cause of stigma due to fear of mutilating physical deformity is thus evident to varying degrees in the interviewees' testimonies, but not to the extent that caused patients to become outcasts from their families. There was evidence that earlier advanced cases had been segregated within families, with their essential daily needs provided by one family member; but this does not necessarily indicate specific leprosy stigma, but a devolution of duties in any family to provide care for a seriously sick family member.

Nevertheless, the reluctance and perhaps revulsion felt by current nursing staff in general hospitals to treat the ulcerated wounds of leprosy patients in Vanuatu was evident also in Samoa and New Caledonia. The provision of specially trained nurses and staff to deal with leprosy patients would avoid this stigmatizing attitude by staff who are unfamiliar with the causes of these ulcerations. Rather than being caused by dirt, neglect and infection, the problems are caused by anaesthetized nerves and normal repetitive actions in daily life that contributed to the ugly wounds and infections. This scenario demonstrates and confirms how ignorance is considered to be the most stigmatizing element that causes leprosy stigma. All the leprosy sufferers interviewed in Vanuatu lived with their families and were included in family activities, with no mention even of separate eating utensils or excluding them from ordinary routines.

Conclusion

The oral histories included in this account reveal a rich new dimension with which to understand the lives of leprosy sufferers in the South Pacific. Often told between tears of sadness or tears of joy, these sufferers relate the frightening experience of receiving a diagnosis of leprosy and the variety of ways the disease impacted on their family and their own later lives. The unexpected discovery while undertaking this research was learning that those who suffered tragic separation from their family and were isolated at the distant island of Makogai in fact found camaraderie. At the leprosarium they were taught a means to earn a livelihood for the future. This is a remarkable finding, contrary to the usual perception that leprosaria signify isolation and despair.

Isolation and camaraderie are normally a total contradiction in terms. The fact that while isolated from society the residents at Makogai and some other leprosaria actually formed lifetime friendships and camaraderie is something that the interviewees still cherish. Their memories of these times are clouded with mixed emotions of initial fear of a life in exile that was gradually overcome with gratitude for the level of care they received. Many of the leprosy sufferers recall those days as some of the happiest times of their lives because of the warmth of the friendships that continue into the present day. Within these accounts of the lives of the interviewees are revelations of how government health policies and staff dealing with leprosy patients affected their lives at the time of diagnosis, and (after treatment) cure and discharge. It is these details which reveal the levels of stigma each interviewee has had to deal with during their lives.

This research finds that from the nineteenth century until the early twentieth century little can be definitely said about the attitudes of the indigenous people towards leprosy in New Caledonia, Samoa, Tonga and Vanuatu because no written sources are available. However, it can be concluded that high stigma existed in Fiji because of the practice of clubbing the unfortunate victims, and it is likely stigma was associated with fear of leprosy from the earliest times of its incidence in the South Pacific. It is also feasible to suggest that the experiences recounted in the 1940s and 1950s in the New Hebrides (Vanuatu) is a scenario that could have existed in the other Pacific islands prior to the implementation of isolation policies for leprosy sufferers towards the turn of and during the early twentieth century. In Vanuatu family members who contracted leprosy appear to have sometimes been cared for by their relatives either until death intervened or the manifestations of the disease became such that segregation occurred.

Such an example is provided by Bialoloso in Espiritu Santo, Vanuatu, who recalled an aunt with leprosy that lived isolated in their home, cared for only by her husband. Alternatively, leprosy sufferers were found living in groups in the bush, caring for each other, in the 1950s. These people would have either been cast out, or left home voluntarily because they felt rejected or wished to protect their families from contagion or any associated stigma from neighbors. The reason for segregation of leprosy sufferers would be the offensive odor and unsightly putrid mutilation caused by leprosy, which is a prime constituent of the fear that causes stigma. The Fijian practice of clubbing victims, albeit on the grounds of being mercy killings, implies that the gross physical condition and suffering caused by leprosy gave rise to the practice which, in turn, contributed to horror and stigma towards the disease. It is therefore reasonable to conclude that varying levels of fear and stigma existed prior to the introduction of isolation by the colonial health authorities. Nevertheless, it is clearly evident that western ideas of the contagion of leprosy and the policy of removal and isolation to distant places, especially leprosaria with poor conditions, exacerbated and heightened fears of leprosy.

The three factors identified in the introduction that past researchers have suggested gave rise to leprosy stigma will be directly addressed. These are that (1) biblical teachings by Christians and missionaries suggested that leprosy sufferers should be treated as outcasts of society; (2) heightened fears were induced by the western policy of isolating leprosy sufferers at leprosaria; and (3) the fearful mutilating and debilitating effects of the disease were increased by ideas of contagion which, over time, added a dimension of self-stigma.

Minimal Biblical and Missionary Causes of Stigma

Apart from in Tonga and possibly Samoa, there is no evidence that Christian missionaries or European settlers specifically connected old biblical ideas of sin and uncleanliness with leprosy, which exaggerated notions of stigma towards the disease. Evidence indicates that fears introduced by Europeans were in connection with the heightened fear of contagion due to the identification of the bacillus by Hansen, and the subsequent adoption of isolation practices.

In Tonga the nineteenth-century injunctions against leprosy invoked in the first Tongan constitution might have been influenced by early missionaries, which appear to have given rise to strong biblical notions of stigma, such as those contained in Leviticus in the Old Testament. This official stance created a pervading stigma, evidenced in the interviews and testified to by Dr. Lutui, which is only very recently diminishing. In Samoa the policy of segregation and isolation endorsed in the early twentieth century by the colonial government was in line with guidelines of the First International Leprosy Conference in Berlin in 1897; but as late as the 1980s the Fijian leprologist Dr. Daulaco suggested that religious leaders in Samoa should stop associating biblical ideas of stigma with leprosy. This evidence indicates that in Samoa and Tonga some early biblical teachings did contribute to heightened levels of leprosy stigma.

There was no evidence in the testimonies of the leprosy sufferers who had been at the three central leprosaria (at Makogai in Fiji, Ducos in New Caledonia, and Lolowai in Vanuatu) that the staff who were either Catholic sisters of the SMSM, Cluny Order, or the Anglicans of the Melanesian Mission had increased leprosy stigma by quoting biblical texts or teachings that held leprosy to be sinful or unclean; nor that the victims should be cast out of their homes and villages. But as Christians, the patients were often aware of the biblical references to leprosy. In fact, ideas of segregation of leprosy sufferers to avoid contagion appeared compatible with their own isolation at leprosaria. However, with the availability of medication that destroys the leprosy-causing bacilli and renders patients non-contagious, old stigmatizing attitudes appear outdated and are fortunately fading.

Leprosaria and Stigma

In terms of leprosaria themselves causing fear and thereby creating stigma, this research suggests that the level of stigma, if any, varies according to the conditions of individual leprosaria. The fact that leprosy sufferers had earlier banded together of their own accord, helping each other to deal with their physical afflictions and finding succor and friendships living together, indicates that at a basic level leprosaria extended these facilities by providing larger, more comfortable surroundings, qualified doctors, nurses and efficient medical care. Moreover, leprosaria became places where medical observations and laboratory research was undertaken to ease the suffering of patients.

Conclusion

The gradual formation of St. Barnabas leprosarium at Lolowai during the 1940s and 1950s is an example of the emergence of a leprosarium that did not attract heightened fear and corresponding leprosy stigma. The removal of groups of people with advanced leprosy, who were caring for themselves in the outback islands in Vanuatu without any medical facilities, to a hospital where facilities were available was an extension of their own isolation, but with vastly improved conditions. However, this leprosarium was set up much later than the other South Pacific leprosaria, and within a decade sulphone treatment became available, which killed the leprosy bacilli as well as prevented heightened fears of contagion. The visits of medical staff, particularly Pyatt and the Mackereths, and their personal encouragement to patients to receive medical care at St. Barnabas — rather than compulsive removal of individuals living in their homes to Lolowai for treatment — avoided stigma. Additionally, this personal approach prevented ideas of enforced isolation and stigma associated with the institutional care of leprosy. The efficient medical care, and informal and friendly conditions, at St. Barnabas that other inhabitants at Lolowai observed (with no fences around the leprosarium) contributed to the overall lack of stigma in Vanuatu from the 1950s to the present day.

Conversely, the original removal of Fijian leprosy sufferers to Makogai did impact on ideas of high contagion and fear, but the excellent level of care and facilities available at Makogai somewhat compensated for the separation from family caused by segregation. The large number of resident leprosy sufferers of all ages and at different stages of leprosy meant that individuals were able to live as a community and form friendships without fear of being the source of contagion. The testimonies of Wati Moria and Susau Fatiakawa in Fiji, who said, after diagnosis, that they wanted to go to Makogai to end their solitary isolation near their homes and join children of similar age in order to be able to socialize again, indicates the benefits of leprosaria perceived at the time by leprosy sufferers. The photographs of leprosy sufferers going about their daily lives and celebrating special events in Stella's account of life at Makogai demonstrate the ordinary lifestyles that were successfully developed at Makogai; large numbers of residents appeared fit and otherwise healthy, either fishing, working on plantations, cycling or playing sport.[1]

The strict measures of hygiene to prevent contagion, especially prior to the availability of sulphones, both in everyday living at Makogai between staff and patients, as well as the problem of securing transport from Pacific islands to Makogai, did contribute to fears of contagion and stigma. However, the lack of any increase in the incidence of leprosy and the regular number of discharges of leprosy patients from Makogai right from the earliest times appear to have helped diminish the fear of total banishment and stigma associated with contagion.

With the advent and level of cure offered by sulphones, the rise of patient discharges from Makogai, without any increase in the incidence of leprosy, contributed to the enormous difference in perceptions of leprosy. A good level of general knowledge about leprosy is evident in Fiji, with a corresponding low level of stigma. The visibility of Twomey Memorial Hospital near Suva, and the excellent facilities it provides for leprosy sufferers in the South Pacific, combined with the lowered incidence of leprosy, has helped leprosy to be seen as just another communicable disease in Fiji. The residents at Twomey Hospital demonstrate the strong friendships and sense of camaraderie that had originated while isolated at Makogai. Not only did this camaraderie exist with the residents at Twomey, but it extended to those living with their families in Suva who enjoyed returning to meet old friends and reminisce with nostalgia about the carefree days and deeply caring lifestyle at Makogai.

The Raoul Follereau leprosarium at Ducos in New Caledonia provided for the needs of leprosy sufferers, although the strict isolation enforced on residents from the time of the first leprosy station at Belep in 1892, and the location of the leprosaria at former prison sites until the 1980s, appear to have consolidated ideas of leprosy and the unfortunate victims as outcasts of society. These conditions heightened the stigma associated with early cases of leprosy. The strict stance on segregation and its rigorous enforcement, together with the higher incidence of the disease among the large population of poor white settlers and mixed-race population residing near the industrial center of Noumea has contributed to a higher level of stigma persisting in New Caledonia. This fear of exile was translated into fear of diagnosis and of the medical authorities. Some leprosy sufferers remained hidden, causing the risk of continued dispersal of bacilli and spread of contagion.

Only one long-term resident at Ducos was interviewed, but this testimony, together with some of the accounts published in the memoirs of other residents, indicate that lifelong friendships were formed and strong communities arose at that leprosarium. Leprosy sufferers built their own homes in the grounds of the leprosarium, married and raised families, but remained segregated from ordinary society. By 2006 only a few elderly leprosy sufferers remained at Ducos. Because of the long years of isolation, they had no family to return to, and so remained dependent on the leprosarium. In recent times, all new cases of leprosy are treated at the central Territorial Hospital at nearby Noumea; and with the effectiveness of the MDT cure, the stigma associated with leprosy is diminishing.

The poor amenities at smaller leprosaria in Tonga and Samoa in the early and mid-twentieth century had the effect of increasing stigma in those islands. The first leprosy station at Alia in Samoa may have raised fear and stigma because of the removal of leprosy sufferers from their families to a remote area with inadequate facilities, but no records were found for the period from 1912 until the patients were removed to Makogai in 1922. The conditions relating to the removal of patients from Alia to Nu'utele and later to Makogai is unknown. The later leprosy wards at the general hospital in Apia, Samoa, and also at the Fale'ofa leprosy station in Vava'u, Tonga, were surrounded by high fences and the leprosy sufferers were held in poor conditions. These conditions were visible to the public and resulted in heightened fear of contagion, as well as fear of being isolated in such conditions, giving rise to increased leprosy stigma. The fences around the old wards in Apia Hospital were removed at least a decade before the Fale'ofa clinic was demolished in 1980, so it is not surprising that a higher level of stigma has persisted in Tonga. The current level of PLF assistance in Samoa and Tonga ensures that leprosy sufferers are able to either earn a living or maintain a normal island lifestyle. This in turn helps reduce stigma because the families of leprosy sufferers are not totally disadvantaged or perceived to be socially inferior.

The continued residence of leprosy sufferers in the existing leprosaria in Suva, Fiji, and Ducos, New Caledonia, indicate that these institutions offer some elderly residents a quality of life and level of comfort and camaraderie that they could not otherwise attain, even if they had families, relatives or friends with whom they could live. Residents in Twomey Hospital described how some of their physical disabilities, which could not be prevented due to medication being available too late to prevent nerve damage, made them prefer to remain at leprosaria rather than reside with their families. Living in simple Fijian homes with a leg amputation, where wheelchairs cannot be maneuvered, meant that when their prosthesis had to be removed, they had to crawl along the floor. Leprosy sufferers found that the facilities at leprosaria offered a lifestyle more conducive to a life with a measure of independence and dignity. For those who had lost contact with their families or were rejected, Twomey Hospital and Ducos provided a home, especially the interviewee at Ducos who was grateful to be able to reside at Raoul Follereau Center, as he had lost contact with relatives after about seventy years of isolation.

Stigma and Self Stigma

The leprosy sufferers who were institutionalized for long periods tend to be somewhat sensitized to stigma, to the extent of having internalized their own perception of public attitudes towards themselves. They are tolerant of stigma in the public domain and prefer to live either alone or quietly with their own families, keeping the company of others who understand leprosy or have had similar experiences.

Examples of this attitude are the Tongan interviewees who had been isolated at Makogai, all of whom lived alone due to the higher stigma prevelant in Tonga. In contrast, also in Tonga, leprosy stigma differs depending on individual attitudes and personalities. Kulaea had an outgoing, pragmatic personality and did not succumb to the stigma in Tonga. She had been isolated at Fale'ofa clinic and rejected by her husband's family, but hid her husband when he managed to enter Fale'ofa and bore him children while in isolation. After her discharge, despite rejection by her in-laws, she ignored local taboos and took another partner, but after his death and the death of her in-laws, she was reunited with her husband. She cared for her children and encouraged them to be checked for leprosy regularly. Despite the stigma of leprosy in Tonga, Kulaea lived a social life, albeit carrying her own eating utensils.

In contrast, Mele, who contracted leprosy in the 1980s in Tonga, but whose elder sibling had experienced isolation and removal to Makogai in the 1950s, was hesitant to continue socializing with neighbors because she felt stigmatized, despite her daughter's and friends' encouragement to continue her visits. Mele's sensitive response reflects the findings of the Japanese research which concluded that older victims of leprosy were less able to accept changing attitudes and the lower stigma associated with leprosy. At the same time, despite Mele's fears, the overtures of continuing friendship indicate a lowering of stigma. This softening attitude towards leprosy in Tonga is also evident in the village of Longomapu, as voiced by Manitepi that the "time of darkness was over."

In Samoa a similar personal contrast is evident with the testimony of Lome, who worked on his hilly plantation despite amputations to both legs, crawling when his prosthesis broke on the rocky terrain and attending himself to trimming any of his bones that became exposed through injury. He took the view that leprosy was just another disease, ignoring stigma or any suggestion that he should stop physical labor on his farm. Alternatively, Rudy who worked equally hard on his plantation near Apia, was nervous at the prospect of having to attend a general hospital ward for treatment of his plantar ulcers because he felt that other patients would object to his presence. He preferred being treated at the separate leprosy clinic, which had closed, where nurses were accustomed to dealing with the problems presented by leprosy patients. This apprehensive view towards being tended by general rather than specialized hospital staff is shared by Rocky Andrew in Vanuatu, who, despite the apparent lack of stigma in those islands, indicated that nurses at Santo hospital were unhappy and often unwilling to treat his ulcers.

These physical problems caused by leprosy give rise to the most common form of stigma prevalent in the South Pacific islands. However, the increased and efficient surveillance of leprosy through the work of the PLF consultant leprologist and of specialized training for medical staff in the South Pacific region, together with the efficacy of MDT treatment, are resulting in fewer physical disabilities and lessened fear of the disease. Where earlier nerve damage has caused physical disabilities, the medical care and support available to older cases continues to be provided through the PLF, and the absence of visible physical deformity is diminishing remaining stigmatizing attitudes. This is evident in a question by a Samoan witnessing the support offered by the PLF through Sister Marietta to a local leprosy sufferer, who asked if he too could receive assistance because he was a Catholic. This question reflects either unawareness of leprosy or an absence of old stigmatizing attitudes towards leprosy sufferers.

The work of the PLF through their liaison contacts, especially in Tonga and Samoa, has improved the living conditions of leprosy sufferers and their families. In Tonga, where stigma was more pervasive, several of the older leprosy sufferers had not married nor had children, so continued to live alone with PLF assistance. In contrast, by the 1980s in Samoa even older leprosy sufferers had married, often later in life, and had families. With PLF funding of school fees, the children were achieving well at school, and the public perception towards these families had correspondingly improved, thereby reducing overall stigmatizing attitudes.

In Vanuatu only two female leprosy sufferers interviewed had not married, but had children and lived with their extended families, and little if any stigma appeared to exist towards leprosy. In Fiji the presence of elderly leprosy sufferers at Twomey Hospital demonstrates the ambivalence of leprosy; that is, the old signs and deformities of the disease were visible at the hospital in Suva, but the public had more understanding of the disease and did not feel at risk of contagion because there was more knowledge and publicity about leprosy. The quality of specialist services available at Twomey Hospital, and its role as the medical training center for leprosy in the South Pacific region, have made Fijians aware of the modern treatment available for leprosy, resulting in reduced fear.

The WHO aim of eliminating leprosy by achieving the low incidence of less than one case of leprosy within a population of 10,000 has been achieved in the South Pacific islands visited, except in New Caledonia (as of 2006, but the incidence has now fallen below the WHO goal). The general low incidence of leprosy, and the free availability of medication that prevents later physical manifestations which have long been associated with leprosy, have resulted in a marked decrease in stigma. It is envisaged and hoped that stigma will be totally eliminated when the mode of transmission of contagion is eventually definitively known and internationally publicized, so that leprosy becomes simply another disease treated in general hospitals by specialist staff.

Appendix

The Betty Pyatt Letter

Godden Memorial Hospital,
Lolowai,
NEW HEBRIDES
(undated: c. 1964)

Dear Margaret and Dudley

This hospital was started in 1936 with Sister McKenzie from Australia in charge. The first patients were nursed in the Sister's bathroom, but it was not long before the present men's ward and the middle building, now called the Dispensary were opened. The women's ward followed soon afterwards known as the "main block." One of the disadvantages is that each is 15 foot wide which makes only a 3 foot passage between the beds, resulting in the wards always looking cramped and making it impossible to wheel trolleys, etc., down the middle. In fact, these wards have never been used as proper wards in that the staff has to go backwards and forwards to the Dispensary for all needs.

A small isolation of 4 beds was added just before the war and after the war 3 army buildings brought over from Santo, were erected. Two were wooden huts which have since been replaced, and the other, a Qansett Hutt, is, much to our shame, still being used for a tuberculosis ward. It is in very bad condition.

In 1959 the British Government started taking an interest in this hospital and has since then either subsidized or completely paid for all buildings with the exception of a Classroom provided by N.Z. "Corso" and a 6 bed female Tuberculosis ward provided by the Mission.

The bed state at present stands at, 14 maternity, 23 tuberculosis and a "bunk house" for 5 ambulatory tuberculosis men, and 20 general beds. There should be 24 general beds but 4 of them are taken up with the orphan babes. Just completed are:- ablutions blocks, laundry, hospital office/duty room and pharmacy. Also a building is the Mothercraft house given to us by N.Z Corso. Next in the plan are the theatre, sterilizing room, outpatients and X-ray with Laboratory. The Government has already given us the go ahead for these buildings but we need another builder badly. The Government is interested in replacing all the old buildings with a virtually new hospital. The policy of the British Government in the New Hebrides seems to be to subsidize existing services rather than start those of their own, while the French Government subsidizes very little, if at all, and tries to make provision for educational and medical work itself.

Up till 1951 the hospital was staffed with dresser and nurse aids but there was very little classroom teaching. In 1951 we started a definite 2 year course for Dressers and 3 year for nurses and insisted, for the nurses, on an examination set by the British Medical Officer. This examination, however, has not been official, and our trainees have had no official standing although they have done very good work. From the end of 1965 the examination will be an official British Government one, and the Presbyterian hospital in Vila and ours here are the two chosen training schools. The French, as yet, have shown little interest in training programmes for Melanesians. They rely on Sisters of a Religious Order to staff their hospitals in Vila and Santo.

This training programme has always been a difficult one to work out, because we have had girls of a low standard educationally, who have had to be prepared to go to their, often, remote islands, where they are the only medical personnel. Only one island in the Banks group has a tele-radio, and shipping is most irregular. Sometimes the people in the Torres Islands, for example, do not see a boat for four months. So the syllabus has to be simple, yet has to prepare trainees for procedures which no nurse in our countries would be allowed to do.

The northern New Hebrides forms the Southern Archdeaconry of the Melanesia Mission and in the past there were European Missionaries on many of these islands. About 1936 centralization at Lolowai was started and now there are no Europeans outside Lolowai, employed by the Mission. The Melanesians, themselves, are taking over more and more with Europeans touring to be able to advise and help where necessary. At Lolowai here the Mission is lucky in owning a good section of the land which forms the north east tip of the island. There are 5 stations:- Vureas Senior School where there are about 150 picked boys and girls, Lolowai itself which is headquarters and where there is now a Junior Technical School of approximately 60 boys, Torgil girls' School which take girls up to the Vureas entrance standard as well as a slower stream of girls, and is also now taking smaller boys so that there are lower classes for teaching training. St. Barnabas Leprosarium which is run from the hospital, and hospital itself.... The European staff for all these stations has had to become more and more specialized over the years as the standard required by the Melanesians has risen. A "Jack of all trades" was one of the handiest men in the past, but, although *very* useful still, the work now requires real specialists. The result has been a great increase in staff. At the beginning of 1956 there were 7 Europeans for all stations, but there are now 21 adults and 13 children.

The St. Barnabas Leprosarium is about 5 minutes walk up a hill behind us on a sort of plateau. Aoba is very hilly and wherever we go we have to climb. The plateau is about the biggest piece of really flat land round these parts and on it is a football field and the Leprosarium. There are usually between 60 and 70 Lepers and they manage their own affairs with help from us. We usually have one sister completely responsible for them, but it is not her only job. Dressers and nurses from the hospital each work there for 2 months of their training which gives them good experience. The lepers themselves, do their own buildings, have a very good pupil school with leper teachers, work their own gardens, have their own twice-

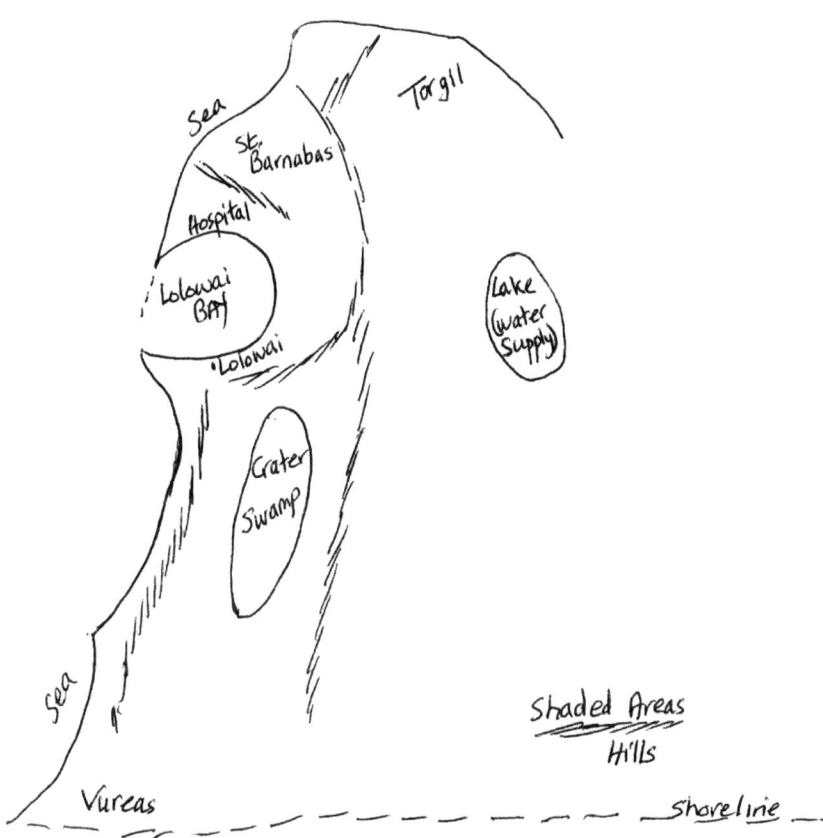

Map of Lolowai Hospital with leprosarium, drawn by Betty Pyatt.

daily services in their own chapel, keep their place very clean and supply 2 men and 2 women for dispensary duties. There is an elected chief and a Head Leper who are the main leaders. Leprosy, diagnosed early, is now curable, and not the frightening disease it used to be.

The leprosarium consists of 14 sleeping houses of various sizes, a dining room/recreation room, kitchen, work shop, store house, Church, classroom and 2 ablutions blocks. The people have their own Melanesian built houses in the bush around, in which they can cook their own way at weekends, etc. They have a delightful beach and a fleet of canoes which gives them a great sense of freedom. 90% of the patients are capable of living fairly normal lives although they have their off and on days. The other 10% are mostly people who had their diseases long before they came here or long before modern drugs were found, so that deformities and ulceration keep them pretty helpless.

[Betty Pyatt]

Chapter Notes

Introduction

1. Information about the worldwide project and leprosy archives can be viewed at www.leprosyhistory.org.
2. R. Edmond, *Leprosy and Empire: A Medical and Cultural History* (Cambridge University Press, 2006).
3. C. J. Austin, *Makogai, Fiji Leprosy Hospital*, Government of the Colony of Fiji, Public Relations Office for the Medical Department (Suva, 1954). Dr. Austin believed that leprosy was dreaded because its manifestations were external and obvious. I. J. Volinn, "Issues of Definitions and Their implications: Aids and Leprosy," *Social Science and Medicine* 29, no. 10 (1989): 1160–1161. Volinn suggests that leprosy stigma relates to its epidemiological and etiological characteristics, being a mutilating, disfiguring and progressive disease.
4. Z. Gussow, *Leprosy, Racism, and Public Health: Social Policy in Chronic Disease Control* (London, 1989), p. 196; A. P. Hattori, *Colonial Disease: U.S. Navy Health Policies and the Chamorros of Guam, 1898–1941* (Honolulu, 2004); K. S. Loh, "Heritage for Whom? Leprosy, Memory and Modernity in Singapore," International Conference on *Heritage in Asia: Converging Forces and Conflicting Values* (8–10 January, 2009).
5. D. Scott Smith, "Leprosy: eMedicine Infectious Diseases" (August, 2008), Stanford University School of Medicine, http://emedicine.medscape.com./article/220455-overview , pp. 1–2.
6. *Ibid.*, pp. 2 and 5.
7. R. Farrugia, Oral history (2006), p. 23. Dr. Farrugia is a retired WHO leprologist and currently the PLF consultant.
8. Smith, p. 3.
9. Farrugia, p. 34; this explains the high incidence of amputees among the leprosy sufferers interviewed.
10. Smith, p. 4.
11. *Ibid.*, pp. 2 and 4–5.
12. W. R. Lang, "Leprosy in Auckland," *The New Zealand Medical Journal* 669 (October 1980): 271.
13. Smith, p. 2.
14. Lang, pp. 271 and 274.
15. M. Eales, Oral history (2007), p. 2; and Smith, p. 2.
16. Z. Gussow and G. Tracy, "Stigma and the Leprosy Phenomenon: The Social History of a Disease in the Nineteenth and Twentieth Centuries," *Bulletin of the History of Medicine* 44, no. 5 (1970): 435–436.
17. J. Buckingham, *Leprosy in Colonial South India: Medicine and Confinement* (Basingstoke and New York, 2002), pp. 91–92.
18. C. M. Gould, "Sister Hilary Ross and Carville: Her Thirty-Seven Year Struggle Against Hansen's Disease," *The Star*, Carville, Louisiana, USA, 50:5, no. 9 (May-June, 1991), pp. 8–9, N. Harris papers, Macmillan Brown Library.
19. *The Star*, Carville, Louisiana, USA, 59:2 (April-June, 2000), N. Harris Papers, Macmillan Brown Library. Featured on back page of the quarterly magazine.
20. Farrugia, p. 23; and Smith, p. 1.
21. WHO, "The Final Push Towards Elimination of Leprosy: Strategic Plan 2000–2005," *The Star* (April-June, 2000), p. 6; and Smith, pp. 1 and 5.
22. Farrugia, p. 23.

23. G. Grice, "Where Leprosy Lurks," *Discover* 21, no. 11 (November 2000): 76–84.
24. Lang, p. 271.
25. Farrugia, p. 36; Smith, p. 4.
26. B. Mackereth, oral history (2007), p. 18.
27. Smith, p. 3.
28. B. T. McMahon, oral history (2006), p. 27.
29. I. J. Volinn, "Aids and Leprosy," pp. 1160–1161.
30. Edmond, pp. 220–244.
31. Z. Gussow and G. Tracy, "The Use of Archival Materials in the Analysis and Interpretation of Field Data: A Case Study in the Institutionalization of the Myth of Leprosy as 'Leper,'" *American Anthropologist* 73, no. 3 (1971): 696.
32. I. J. Volinn, "Health Professionals as Stigmatizers and Destigmatizers of Diseases, Alcoholism and Leprosy as Examples," *Social Science and Medicine*, 17 (1983): 385.
33. J. Miles, *Infectious Diseases: Colonising the Pacific?* (Dunedin, 1997), pp. 38–41.
34. D. A. Lonie, "Trends in Leprosy in the Pacific," Technical Information Circular, No. 32, *South Pacific Commission* (Noumea, New Caledonia, 1959), p. 19.
35. Beckett, "The Striking Hand of God: Leprosy in History," *New Zealand Medical Journal* 100 (1987): 494–497, from an unpublished copy in Harris papers, Macmillan Brown Library, pp. 13–15; and Lang, p. 1.
36. C. J. Austin, "Leprosy in Fiji and the South Seas," *International Journal of Leprosy* 17, no. 4 (1949): 403.
37. Gussow, p. 95.
38. B. T. McMahon, "Medical Advisory Committee," Pacific Leprosy Foundation Annual Review (2005), pp. 5–6.
39. www.leprosyhistory.org.
40. B. Madey and L. Thomas, *Compassionate Exile*, Filmmakers: X-Isle Productions (Suva, 1999).
41. D. McMenamin, "Recording the Experiences of Leprosy Sufferers in Suva, Fiji," *The Fiji Social Workers Journal* 1, no. 1 (November 2005): 27–32; and in *Oral History in New Zealand* 17, (2005): 23–25; and Buckingham, "The Pacific Leprosy Foundation Archive," pp. 81–86.
42. J. Valentine, oral history (2006) and *Hell-Bent for Life* (Oakura, NZ, 2009).
43. E. Silla, *People Are Not the Same: Leprosy and Identity in Twentieth-Century Mali* (Oxford, 1998), p. 2.
44. Gussow and Tracy, "Stigma and the Leprosy Phenomenon," pp. 425–449, and "Myth of Leprosy," pp. 695–705.
45. *The Oxford English Reference Dictionary, Second Edition*, Oxford University Press, 1996.
46. S. L. Gilman, *Picturing Health and Illness: Images of Identity and Difference* (Baltimore, 1995), p. 156.
47. S. G. Browne, "Leprosy in the Bible" (London, 1979); and D. Beckett, "The Striking Hand of God," pp. 1–2.
48. Browne, p. 6.
49. *Ibid.*, pp. 14 and 10.
50. *Ibid.*, pp. 9–10.
51. *Ibid.*, pp. 22–23.
52. *Ibid.*, p. 25.
53. *Ibid.*, p. 26.
54. Beckett, "The Striking Hand of God," pp. 1–2, and Oral history, pp. 1–3.
55. Beckett, "The Striking Hand of God," p. 1.
56. S. N. Brody, *The Disease of the Soul: Leprosy in Medieval Literature* (Ithaca, 1974), p. 11.
57. J. McCurry, "Japanese Leprosy Patients Continue to Fight Social Stigma," *The Lancet* 363, no. 9408 (February 2004): 544.
58. C. L. Marshall, M. Maeshiro and S. P. Korper, "Attitudes Toward Leprosy in the Ryukyu Islands," *Public Health Reports 1896–1970*, 82, no. 9 (September 1967): 795–801.
59. McCurry, p. 544.
60. Farrugia, oral history, p. 24. Yohei Sasakawa publishes his activities of goodwill regularly in *WHO Goodwill Ambassador's Newletter for the Elimination of Leprosy*.
61. Buckingham, *Leprosy in Colonial South India*, pp. 145 and 184; and Gussow and Tracy, "Stigma and the Leprosy Phenomenon," pp. 435–436.
62. Edmond, p. 103.
63. *Ibid.*, p. 101.
64. *Ibid.*, pp. 131–141.
65. *Ibid.*, pp. 125–141 and 220–244.
66. Gussow and Tracy, "Stigma and the Leprosy Phenomenon," pp. 444–446.
67. Edmond, pp. 176–177.
68. Browne, p. 30.
69. Gussow and Tracy, "Myth of Leprosy," p. 446.

70. *Ibid.*, pp. 446–7.
71. Gussow and Tracy, "Stigma and the Leprosy Phenomenon," pp. 428–431.
72. Gussow and Tracy, "Myth of Leprosy," pp. 695 and 702–704.
73. Gussow and Tracy, "Stigma and the Leprosy Phenomenon," pp. 444–445.
74. Gussow and Tracy, "Myth of Leprosy," pp. 702–703.
75. *WHO Goodwill Ambassador's Newsletter for the Elimination of Leprosy* 36 (February 2009), The Nippon Foundation, p. 8.
76. http://www.aifoindia.org/Raoul-Follereau.htm (24 May, 2009).
77. D. J. Rothman, *The Discovery of the Asylum: Social Order and Disorder in the New Republic* (Boston and Toronto, 1971), p. 141.
78. Rothman, pp. xix, 141 and 152–4.
79. Gussow and Tracy, "Myth of Leprosy," p. 446.
80. *Ibid.*, p. 697.
81. *Ibid.*, pp. 699 and 703.
82. Gussow, pp. 209–212.
83. www.culion.net/history/html.
84. M. A. Grosperrin, *The Vocation of the Pioneers* (Rome, 2005), pp. 63–64.
85. J. Morris, "They Came to Makogai: A Community Study," University of Wellington (1956), p. i.
86. Edmond, pp. 210–217.
87. *Ibid.*, pp. 210–211.
88. *Ibid.*, p. 211.
89. *Ibid.*, p. 212.
90. *Ibid.*, pp. 214–215.
91. P. Moblo, "Blessed Damien of Moloka'i: The Critical Analysis of Contemporary Myth," *Ethnohistory* 44, no. 4 (1997): 697.
92. Moblo, pp. 691–5.
93. Gussow, p. 99.
94. C. M. Gould, "Sister Hilary Ross and Carville: Her Thirty-Seven Year Struggle Against Hansen's Disease," in *The Star: Radiating the Light and Truth of Hansen's Disease* 50, no. 5 (May/June, 1991): 9, and 50, no. 6 (July/August 1991): 4–5, N. Harris papers, Macmillan Brown Library.
95. B. Lou, "The Carville Praesidium" (March, 1952), N. Harris papers, Macmillan Brown Library, p. 1.
96. *Ibid.*
97. Fakatava testimony in Madey and Thomas, documentary, *Compassionate Exile*.
98. *Carville*, U.S. Department of Health and Human Services, Public Health Services, Carville, Louisiana, USA, n.d. and *Carville, USA*, The United States Public Health Service Hospital, Federal Security Agency, Carville, Louisiana, n.d., N. Harris papers, Macmillan Brown Library.
99. Gussow and Tracy, "Stigma and the Leprosy Phenomenon," p. 426.
100. Beckett, "The Striking Hand of God," pp. 15–16.
101. Gussow, p. 131.
102. Hattori, pp. 79–82.
103. *Ibid.*, p. 73.
104. *Ibid.*, pp. 72–3.
105. *Ibid.*, pp. 80–82.
106. *Ibid.*, p. 84.
107. *Ibid.*, pp. 86–87.
108. *Ibid.*, pp. 87–88.
109. Buckingham, *Leprosy in Colonial South India*, p. 46.
110. *Ibid.*, pp. 48–9 and 54.
111. *Ibid.*, p. 100.
112. Rudy, oral history (2006), p. 2; and Fusi, Oral history (2006), pp. 2–3.
113. Buckingham, *Leprosy in Colonial South India*, p. 167.
114. *Ibid.*, pp. 59–60.
115. K. S. Loh, "Heritage for Whom? Leprosy, Memory and Modernity in Singapore," p. 6.
116. Loh, "'Our Lives Are Bad but Our Luck Is Good': A Social History of Leprosy in Singapore," 21, no. 2 (3 June, 2008): 289.
117. Loh, "Heritage for Whom?" p. 4, and Stella, p. 19.
118. Loh, "Heritage for Whom? p. 8.
119. Loh, "'Our Lives Are Bad but Our Luck Is Good,'" p. 291.
120. D. McMenamin, Report on visit to Fiji (August, 2004), Macmillan Brown Library.
121. Silla, p. 180.
122. *Ibid.*
123. *Ibid.*, p. 181.
124. *Ibid.*, p. 189.
125. *Ibid.*, p. 190.
126. *Ibid.*, p. 189.
127. *Ibid.*, p. 177.
128. The research was funded in the main by the International Leprosy Association Project, Global Project on the History of Leprosy (funded by the Nippon Foundation) Welcome Unit for the History of Medicine, University of Oxford; and partially by the

Marsden Fund Council, administered by the Royal Society of New Zealand, and partially by my family. The archival material has been deposited at the Macmillan Brown Library at the University of Canterbury, Christchurch, New Zealand. See also J. Buckingham, "The Pacific Leprosy Foundation Archive and Oral Histories of Leprosy in the South Pacific," *The Journal of Pacific History* 41, no. 1 (June 2006): 81–86.

129. P. Fakatava and S. L. Fatiaki testimonies in Madey and Thomas, documentary *Compassionate Exile*.

Chapter 1

1. *Leprosy Trust Board: A Brief Outline of the Development and Operations of the Leprosy Trust Board (The Leper Man Appeal)*, based on a series of talks by Derek Douglas, Secretary of the Board (Christchurch, 1985), pp. 2–3.
2. H. Laracy, *Dictionary of New Zealand Biography*, www.dnzb.govt.nz (accessed 10 Sept., 2007), N. Harris Papers, Macmillan Brown Library, p. 1.
3. *Ibid.*, p. 1.
4. M.P.W. "A Life of Dedication" (n.d.), N. Harris Papers, Macmillan Brown Library.
5. P. Jackson, *Tamahua, Quail Island — a Link with the Past* (Christchurch, 2006), pp. 31 and 35.
6. *Ibid.*, pp. 37–38.
7. *Ibid.*, p. 37.
8. *Ibid.*, pp. 40–42 and 93.
9. *Ibid.*, pp. 37–39.
10. *Ibid.*, pp. 38–41.
11. *Ibid.*, pp. 40–41.
12. *Ibid.*, p. 40.
13. *Ibid.*
14. *Ibid.*, p. 41, and Edmond, p. 173.
15. Jackson, p. 43.
16. Edmond, p. 174.
17. Jackson, p. 43.
18. *Ibid.*, pp. 42–43.
19. P. J. Twomey, MBE, "Ernest — A Leper Hero!" Macmillan Brown Library, IPD No. 14612 PLF Overview (1948), LMB469/228, Macmillan Brown Library.
20. D. McMenamin, "Recording the Experiences of Leprosy Sufferers in Suva, Fiji," *The Fiji Social Workers Journal* 1, no. 1 (November 2005): 29–30; Stella, pp. 104–108; and P.J. Twomey, "Ernest — A Leper Hero!" Harris Papers, Macmillan Brown Library.
21. Sister Mary Stella, SMSM, *Makogai — Image of Hope: A Brief History of the Care of Leprosy Patients in Fiji* (Christchurch, 1978, and 2nd edition, 2006), p. 105.
22. Jackson, p. 43.
23. "Leper Work in New Zealand," Lepers' Trust Board Incorporated (c.1944), Macmillan Brown Library, IPD No. 14612 PLF Overview 1948, LMB469/228, Macmillan Brown Library, University of Canterbury.
24. N. Harris, oral history (2005), pp. 7–8.
25. P. J. Twomey, LTB newsletter (1948), p. 2, N. Harris Papers, Macmillan Brown Library.
26. Harris, p. 7.
27. *Ibid.*
28. *A Brief Outline of the Development and Operations of the Leprosy Trust Board*, pp. 2–3.
29. C. J. Austin, "Leprosy in the British Solomon Islands Protectorate," South Pacific Commission (July, 1952), refers to the figures provided in a survey of the region by Ross Innes in 1937/38, pp. 1–2.
30. "Leper Work in New Zealand," p. 2.
31. M.P.W. "A Life of Dedication," p. 2.
32. P. J. Twomey newsletter, 1948, p. 2.
33. LTB pamphlets (1950 and c.1945), LMB469/228, IPD No. 14612, Macmillan Brown Library.
34. Harris, p. 8, and "Leper Work in New Zealand," p. 2.
35. "Leper Work in New Zealand," p. 2.
36. *Ibid.*, p. 1.
37. *A Brief Outline of the Development and Operations of the Leprosy Trust Board*, p. 3.
38. "Leper Work in New Zealand," p. 1, and *A Brief Outline of the Development and Operations of the Leprosy Trust Board* — "Appendix A," p. 17.
39. Harris, pp. 26–27; and B. Pyatt, Oral history, Tape 2, pp. 2–3.
40. *A Brief Outline of the Development and Operations of the Leprosy Trust Board*, pp. 10 and 18.
41. *A Brief Outline of the Development and Operations of the Leprosy Trust Board*, pp. 6–7.
42. "A Life of Dedication," pp. 3–4.
43. *Ibid.*, pp. 3–4.

44. *Ibid.*, p. 4.
45. Harris, p. 23.
46. Pacific Leprosy Foundation, Financial Statements, Annual Review (2005), pp. 7–8.
47. Gussow, p. 217.
48. *Ibid.*, p. 218.
49. Personal communication with Lala Gittoes, PLF Relations Manager.
50. C. J. Austin, *Fiji Leprosy Hospital Makogai*, brochure, Suva, Public Relations Office for Medical Department (1954), p. 18, Harris Papers, Macmillan Brown Library.
51. Beckett, "The Striking Hand of God," p. 11.
52. *Ibid.*
53. *Ibid.*, p.12; Stella, p. 181.
54. Stella, p. 18–19.
55. Austin, "Leprosy in Fiji and the South Seas," p. 400; D. W. Beckett, "The Striking Hand of God," p.12.
56. Beckett, "The Striking Hand of God," p. 12.
57. *Ibid.*, p. 11.
58. Stella, p. 19.
59. *Ibid.*
60. *Ibid.*
61. *Ibid.*, pp. 21–22.
62. *Ibid.*
63. *Ibid.*, pp. 23–24.
64. *Ibid.*, p. 25.
65. *Ibid.*
66. *Ibid.*, pp. 25–26.
67. *Ibid.*, p. 26.
68. *Ibid.*
69. *Ibid.*, pp. 26–28.
70. *Ibid.*, pp. 28–32 and 31.
71. *Ibid.*, p. 30.
72. *Ibid.*, pp. 32–37.
73. *Ibid.*, p. 36.
74. Browne, pp. 6–14; Gussow and Tracy, "Stigma and the Leprosy Phenomenon," pp. 443–444; and Alison Bashford, *Imperial Hygiene: A Critical History of Colonialism, Nationalism and Public Health* (New York, 2004), p. 87.
75. Browne, p. 8.
76. Parsons, Sister Marietta, personal communication.
77. Stella, p. 46.
78. *Ibid.*, p. 39.
79. *Ibid.*, pp. 45–46.
80. *Ibid.*, pp. 47–49.
81. Austin, 'Leprosy in Fiji and the South Seas,' p. 401.
82. Stella, p. 171; and Austin, *Fiji Leprosy Hospital Makogai*, pp. 4–5.
83. Stella, p. 74, provides a diagram of the island of Makogai, which is reproduced here.
84. Austin, *Fiji Leprosy Hospital Makogai*, p. 3.
85. *Ibid.*, pp. 2–3.
86. Personal communication with SMSM sisters in Samoa.
87. Stella, footnote on p. 94.
88. Stella, p. 50.
89. *Ibid.*
90. *Ibid.*, p. 68–69.
91. *Ibid.*, p. 51.
92. Harris, oral history, p. 14, and personal communication.
93. Stella, p. 51.
94. *Ibid.*, p. 56.
95. *Ibid.*, pp. 55–56.
96. *Ibid.*, p. 93; Morris, p. 80, also mentions "a few suicides" were recorded.
97. Stella, pp. 56
98. Edmond, p. 177.
99. Stella, p. 82.
100. Austin, *Fiji Leprosy Hospital Makogai*, pp. 8–9; Stella, pp. 78–83.
101. Austin, pp. 9–11.
102. Morris, p. 13; and Stella, p. 85.
103. Stella, p. 65.
104. *Ibid.*, p. 64.
105. *Ibid.*, pp. 108–110.
106. Edmond, p. 176.
107. Stella, p. 71.
108. *Ibid.*, p. 100, quote from *Fiji Times*, 2 July, 1962.
109. Stella, p. 71.
110. *Ibid.*, pp. 70–71.
111. *Ibid.*, p. 171.
112. Austin, "Leprosy in Fiji and the South Seas," pp. 399–409; also reported in Morris, p. 19.
113. Stella, p. 96.
114. *Ibid.*, p. 97.
115. *Ibid.*
116. *Ibid.*, p. 98.
117. *Ibid.*, p. 97.
118. Austin, *Fiji Leprosy Hospital Makogai*, pp. 20–21.
119. Morris, p. 22.
120. Beckett, oral history (2007), p. 8.
121. *Ibid.*, p. 9.
122. *Ibid.*, pp. 7–8.
123. "Semisi Maya—the Story of a Leper

Artist," LTB advertisement in Harris Papers, Macmillan Brown Library.

124. *Ibid.*; and M. Holmes, "The Semisi Maya Story," *Spam* 2, no. 1 (1982): 35–37, in Harris papers, Macmillan Brown Library.

125. Madey and Thomas, *Compassionate Exile*, Filmmakers: X-Isle Productions (Suva, 1999).

126. *Ibid.*

127. S. F. Layasewa, oral history (2004), pp. 3–4.

128. Layasewa, p. 5.

129. *Ibid.*, p. 12.

130. *Ibid.*, p. 8.

131. *Ibid.*, p. 10.

132. *Ibid.*, p. 9.

133. *Ibid.*, pp. 13–14.

134. Paras Ram, oral history (2004), p. 1.

135. *Ibid.*, p. 1.

136. *Ibid.*, p. 2.

137. *Ibid.*, pp. 4–5.

138. *Ibid.*, p. 6.

139. *Ibid.*

140. M. ItaTetoariki, oral history (2004), p. 2.

141. *Ibid.*, p. 3.

142. *Ibid.*, pp. 3–4.

143. T. W. Soko, oral history (2004).

144. *Ibid.*, p. 4.

145. *Ibid.*

146. *Ibid.*, p. 6.

147. *Ibid.*, p. 10.

148. S. Tiko, oral history (2004), pp. 1–2.

149. *Ibid.*, p. 3.

150. *Ibid.*

151. *Ibid.*

152. *Ibid.*, p. 5.

153. L. Musuka, oral history (2004), p. 7.

154. *Ibid.*, p. 9.

155. A recording of the residents singing is filed with the McMenamin Pacific Papers, Macmillan Brown Library.

156. V. Metuisela, Oral history (2004), pp. 1–2.

157. *Ibid.*, p. 3.

158. *Ibid.*, pp. 5–6.

159. *Ibid.*, p. 4.

160. Pacific Leprosy Foundation, Annual Review (2007–8), pp. 2 and 5.

161. J. Mai and V. Meto, Interview notes (2004), McMenamin Pacific Papers, Macmillan Brown Library.

162. J. Singh, oral history (2004), pp. 4–5.

163. W. Moira, oral history (2004), pp. 3–4.

164. *Ibid.*, p. 5.

165. *Ibid.*

166. *Ibid.*, p. 10.

167. *Ibid.*

168. *Ibid.*, p. 8.

169. *Ibid.*, pp. 6 and 10.

170. *Ibid.*, p. 11

171. *Ibid.*, p. 13.

172. *Ibid.*, pp. 13–14.

173. *Ibid.*, p. 14.

174. *Ibid.*, p. 15. Sadly, Josephine died in 2008.

175. *Ibid.*

176. *Ibid.*

Chapter 2

1. P. Bobin, "La Lepre en Nouvelle-Caledonie: Rappel Historique" (Noumea, 1999), McMenamin Pacific Papers, Macmillan Brown Library, p. 1. Bobin created the small museum now in existence at Ducos. Also see M. Crouzat, "Situation de la Lepre en Nouvelle-Caledonie" (Noumea, 2001), McMenamin Pacific Papers, Macmillan Brown Library, pp. 1–2.

2. Bobin, pp. 1–2.

3. McMenamin Pacific Papers deposited in the Macmillan Brown Archives.

4. Lonie, pp. 14 and 23.

5. *Ibid.*, p. 19.

6. Bobin, pp. 1–2.

7. *Ibid.*, p. 1.

8. Grosperrin, *The Vocation of the Pioneers*, pp. 34–35.

9. Bobin, p. 1. The term "lazaret" derived from Jesus healing Lazarus of leprosy in the New Testament.

10. Bobin, p. 1.

11. *Ibid.*

12. *Ibid.*

13. *Ibid.*

14. Silla, p. 179.

15. H. Tourte, oral history, p. 2.

16. Bobin, pp. 1–2.

17. Grosperrin, pp. 63–64. Sister Marie de la Croix was awarded medals of honor for her work in New Caledonia. Six hundred of her letters are filed at the SMSM archives in Rome.

18. *Ibid.*, p. 64.

19. *Ibid.*, p. 70.
20. McMenamin Report, SMSM archive notes and communication with Sister Aquin, SMSM archivist; and Stella, p. 36.
21. Stella, pp. 14–15.
22. McMenamin Report, SMSM archive notes.
23. C. M. Gould, "Sister Hilary Ross and Carville: Her Thirty-Seven Year Struggle Against Hansen's Disease, Part II," *The Star* (Carville, July/August 1991), Harris papers, Macmillan Brown Library, p. 5.
24. C. M. Gould, "Sister Hilary Ross and Carville: Her Thirty-Seven Year Struggle Against Hansen's Disease, Part I," *The Star* (Carville, May/June 1991), p. 8; and "Part II," Harris papers, Macillan Brown Library, p. 4.
25. Edmond, p. 176–177.
26. Sister N. Thiossey, oral history (2006), p. 3.
27. Tourte, pp. 1 and 5.
28. M. Crouzat and N. Forrest, *L'hymne à la vie: des pensionnaires du Centre Raoul Follereau, Une page d'histoire calédonienne*, no date or publisher (Book Launch 2006).
29. Tourte, pp. 3–5.
30. *Ibid.*, p. 5.
31. Crouzat and Forrest, p. 20.
32. Tourte, p. 1.
33. *Ibid.*, p. 2.
34. *Ibid.*, p. 3.
35. *Ibid.*
36. *Ibid.*
37. Stella, p. 97.
38. The later testimony of Dr. Farrugia will indicate these ideas in Ducos and Noumea.
39. Bobin, p. 1; and D. McMenamin, SMSM archives report (October 2006).
40. Tourte, p. 5; and A. H. T. Rose, "Early Days of Mr. Twomey in New Caledonia" (Christchurch, 1987), Harris papers, Macmillan Brown Library, p. 3.
41. A. Grennell, "Portrait from Life P. J. Twomey, MBE," radio interview (1958), Harris papers, Macmillan Brown Library, p. 6. Another SMSM sister, Sister Mary Joseph, daughter of an Australian farmer at Tetere leprosarium on Guadalcanal, is reported to be a competent driver of trucks or tractors, carrying out all repairs herself, and that her relaxation was shooting, often going out after crocodiles or bringing home a brace of pigeons for the pot! Yet, he maintained, Sister Joseph retained the charm of a refined woman, of whom the locals sang praises, and she was awarded an MBE in 1955 (p. 5).
42. Tourte, p. 5.
43. *Ibid.*
44. Crouzat and Forrest, p. 20; and Farrugia, oral history, pp. 10–11.
45. Médecin-Capitaine des Troupes Coloniales Lacour, Directeur de l'Institut Pasteur de Nouméa, "An Attempt to Control Leprosy by B.C.G. Vaccine in the Loyalty Islands," McMenamin Papers, Macmillan Brown Papers, p. 6.
46. M. Crouzat, "The Disease of Hansen in New Caledonia," report of Director of Dermatology on the website of the Territorial Hospital complex of Noumea, July 1999, McMenamin Pacific Papers, Macmillan Brown Library.
47. R. G. Farrugia, oral history (2006), p. 7; and R. G. Farrugia *"Curriculum vitae,"* McMenamin Pacific Papers, Macmillan Brown Archives, p. 1.
48. Crouzat and Forrest, p. 21.
49. *Ibid.*, pp. 26–28.
50. *Ibid.*, pp. 21 and 29.
51. *Ibid.*, p. 26.
52. Rose, p. 1.
53. *Ibid.*
54. Crouzat and Forrest, p. 29.
55. "A Few Facts About the Leprosy Trust Board in New Caledonia," n.d., Harris Papers, Macmillan Brown Library, pp. 1–2.
56. *Ibid.*
57. Photographed in 2006 and included with McMenamin Pacific Papers, Macmillan Brown archives.
58. Crouzat and Forrest, p. 29.
59. Photographs taken at RFC cemetery, included with McMenamin Pacific Papers.
60. Rose, p. 4.
61. Crouzat and Forrest, p. 39.
62. *Ibid.*, p. 39.
63. Personal communications, McMenamin report on visit to New Caledonia (September 2006), p. 1
64. *Ibid.*
65. Thiossey, pp. 2–3.
66. McMenamin report on visit to New Caledonia.
67. Thiossey, pp. 3 and 7.
68. *Ibid.*, p. 3.
69. R. Farrugia, oral history, pp. 6–7.
70. *Ibid.*, p. 9.

71. *Ibid.*, pp. 6 and 13.
72. *Ibid.*, p. 7.
73. *Ibid.*, pp. 8–9.
74. *Ibid.*, pp. 10–11.
75. *Ibid.*, p. 10.
76. *Ibid.*, pp. 10–11.
77. *Ibid.*, p. 14. Dr. Farrugia had also worked with leprosy in the Philippines, China, Japan, Laos and Vietnam.
78. *Ibid.*, p. 11.
79. *Ibid.*, p. 12.
80. *Ibid.*, p. 11.
81. Crouzat and Forrest, p. 20.
82. Thiossey, p. 5.
83. *Ibid.*, p. 4.
84. *Ibid.*, p. 8.
85. *Ibid.*
86. *Ibid.*, p. 4.
87. *Ibid.*, p. 5.
88. *Ibid.*, p. 9.
89. M. Crouzat, "Situation de la Lepre en Nouvelle-Caledonie" (Dec. 2001), p. 5.
90. Farrugia, oral history, p. 30.
91. *Ibid.*, p. 16.
92. M. Crouzat, "The Disease of Hansen in New Caledonia," p. 1.
93. M. Crouzat, "Situation de la Lepre en Nouvelle-Caledonie" (Dec. 2001), McMenamin Pacific Papers, Macmillan Brown Archives.
94. M. Crouzat, "The Disease of Hansen in New Caledonia," p. 1.
95. Crouzat and Forrest, p. 43.
96. *Ibid.*, p. 43.
97. Farrugia, oral history, p. 35.
98. *Ibid.*
99. New Caledonia is the world's second largest nickel producer.
100. Crouzat and Forrest. Additionally, photographs were taken of the Raoul Follereau Center at Ducos, and the interior of the museum.

Chapter 3

1. S. Akeli, "Leprosy in Samoa 1890 to 1922: Race, Colonial Politics and Disempowerment" (Masters thesis, University of Canterbury, 2007), pp. 4–5 and 7–9.
2. N. Sloan, "Leprosy in Western Samoa and the Cook Islands: A Survey" (Noumea, 1954), p. 4; and Akeli, pp. 64–71.
3. Akeli, pp. 71 and 73.
4. *Ibid.*, pp. 73–74.
5. *Ibid.*, pp. 46–47.
6. *Ibid.*
7. *Ibid.*, pp. 78–84.
8. *Ibid.*, pp. 97–99.
9. *Ibid.*, p. 169.
10. *Ibid.*, p. 42.
11. *Ibid.*, p. 51.
12. Dr. Daulako, "Workshop Notes" (1984 file in Box 6/3 Western Samoa 1980–1986, PLF archives, Macmillan Brown Library).
13. Akeli, p. 99.
14. *Ibid.*, pp. 101–102.
15. *Ibid.*, p. 107.
16. *Ibid.*, p. 109.
17. M. A. Grosperrin, *The Vocation of the Pioneers*, pp. 4 and 64.
18. Akeli, pp. 110–112.
19. *Ibid.*, p. 110.
20. Edmond, pp. 176–177.
21. *Ibid.*, p. 113.
22. *Ibid.*, p. 136.
23. *Ibid.*, pp. 114–116 and 136.
24. *Ibid.*, pp. 161–162.
25. *Ibid.*, p. 135.
26. *Ibid.*, pp. 119–120.
27. *Ibid.*, pp. 117–118.
28. *Ibid.*, p. 135.
29. *Ibid.*, pp. 135–36.
30. *Ibid.*, p. 139.
31. *Ibid.*, p. 137 and 142.
32. P. Moblo, "Leprosy, Politics, and the Rise of Hawaii's Reform Party 1887–1892," *The Journal of Pacific History* 34, no. 1 (June 1999): 75–89.
33. Akeli, pp. 145–46.
34. Stella, p. 72. Rates were estimated at 70 per annum for part-Europeans, 60 for Chinese and 40 for Samoans, with transport costs paid by the Samoan government.
35. Akeli, p. 155. See also Stella, p. 73. Akeli maintains that twelve patients were transferred, while Stella records thirteen patients being received in two separate sailings from Samoa to Makogai.
36. Akeli, pp. 159–160; and Stella, p. 73.
37. Akeli, p. 160.
38. McFarland, oral history (2006), p. 3.
39. *Ibid.*, p. 2.
40. *Ibid.*, p. 3.
41. *Ibid.*
42. Anonymous (1), p. 2; and Anonymous (2), pp. 1–2.

43. Anonymous (1), p. 1; and Anonymous (2), pp. 5–6.
44. Anonymous (2), pp. 2–3.
45. *Ibid.*, pp. 2–4.
46. *Ibid.*, p. 5.
47. McFarland, p. 4.
48. *Ibid.*
49. *Ibid.*, p. 5.
50. *Ibid.*, p. 7.
51. *Ibid.*, p. 8.
52. *Ibid.*
53. *Ibid.*, p. 9.
54. Stella, pp. 110–112.
55. Manu Ah Chong, oral history (2006), pp. 2 and 6.
56. Marietta, oral history (2005), p. 11.
57. Anonymous (2), p. 6.
58. Marietta, p. 6.
59. Dick Nansen, oral History (2006), p. 2.
60. *Ibid.*, pp. 2–3.
61. *Ibid.*, p. 6. Photos of the family in *PLF Newsletter* (May 2005), p. 2. His five-year-old daughter is named Marietta, after Sister Marietta, who discovered the family and offered PLF assistance to them in 1999.
62. Marietta, p. 13.
63. Personal communications with Sister Marietta, and conversations with the children and Fiapotu.
64. Nansen, p. 5.
65. L. Laulu, oral history (2006), pp. 2–3.
66. *Ibid.*, p. 2.
67. *Ibid.*, pp. 3–4.
68. *Ibid.*, p. 5.
69. *Ibid.*, p. 6.
70. *Ibid.*
71. *Ibid.*, p. 7.
72. Marietta, pp. 2–3.
73. *Ibid.*, p. 13.
74. *Ibid.*
75. *Ibid.*, p. 14.
76. *Ibid.*, p. 16.
77. Personal communication with Sister Marietta, December 6, 2008.
78. Marietta, p. 13; and Dick, p. 5.
79. Marietta, p. 13.
80. *Ibid.*
81. W. R. Lang, "Seminar on the Medical and Surgical Treatment of Hansen's Disease" (June 1977), in Harris Papers, Macmillan Brown Library, p. 10; B. T. McMahon, "Medical Advisory Committee Report," *PLF Annual Review 2007–2008*, p. 7.
82. McFarland, p. 14.
83. McMahon, *PLF Annual Review, 2007–2008*, p. 7.
84. McFarland, p. 15.
85. Laulu, p. 21.
86. B. T. McMahon, "Medical Advisory Committee Report," *PLF Annual Review* (2005), p. 11.
87. McMahon, *PLF Annual Review 2007–2008*, p. 7; WHO, "The Final Push Towards Elimination of Leprosy: Strategic Plan 2000–2005," *The Star* (April-June, 2000), p. 5.

Chapter 4

1. I. C. Campbell, *Island Kingdom: Ancient & Modern* (Christchurch, 1992), p. 33; and J. Siers, *Tonga* (Wellington, 1978), p. 6.
2. Siers, p. 6.
3. Campbell, p. 35.
4. *Ibid.*, pp. 52–54.
5. *Ibid.*, p. 55.
6. *Ibid.*, pp. 56–58.
7. Latukefu, *Church and State in Tonga*, p. 136.
8. *Ibid.*, pp. 146–47.
9. Noel Rutherford, *Shirley Baker and the King of Tonga* (Melbourne, 1971), p. 16.
10. *Ibid.*, p. 3.
11. Latukefu, pp. 45, 58 and 73.
12. Rutherford, p. 13.
13. *Ibid.*, p. 22. On p. 135 it is noted that the dollar is a Spanish dollar, equivalent to four shillings.
14. *Ibid.*, p. 2.
15. *Ibid.*, p. 78.
16. *Ibid.*, p. 50.
17. *Ibid.*
18. Present-day Hawaii and Efate in Vanuatu were formerly known as the Sandwich Islands. Quote from Latukefu, *The Tongan Constitution: A Brief History to Celebrate Its Centenary* (Nuku'alofa, 1975), p. 90; see also Latukefu, *Church and State in Tonga*, pp. 207, 252–3.
19. T. Lutui, email from 8 December, 2006, McMenamin Pacific Papers, Macmillan Brown Library.
20. Akeli, pp. 78–79.
21. *Ibid.*, p. 80. Cites letters exchanged by Whitcombe and Schmidt, August 1986 Samoa SG/2/3e, concerning leprosy 1891–1896, Archives New Zealand.

22. *Ibid.* Cites letter from C.D. Whitcombe to Eric Schmidt, 21 August, 1896, Samoa SG/2/3e, Archives New Zealand.

23. T. Lutui, email from 6 December, 2006, McMenamin Pacific Papers, Macmillan Brown Library.

24. Stella p. 171; and D. McMenamin report on visit to Tonga (October, 2006), McMenamin Pacific Papers, Macmillan Brown Library.

25. T. Poluka, "Leprosy Reports 1957–1965," McMenamin Pacific Papers, Macmillan Brown Library.

26. TB & Leprosy Control Officer Memorandum, Niu'ui Hospital (25 June, 1965), McMenamin Pacific Papers, Macmillan Brown Library.

27. Farrugia reports, "Tonga," McMenamin Pacific Papers, Macmillan Brown Library.

28. B. T. McMahon, "Medical Advisory Committee Report," Pacific Leprosy Foundation Annual Review 2007–2008, p. 7

29. McMenamin report on visit to Tonga, November 2006, sighting Minute Books and SMSM records re Leprosy Trust held by Sister Joan Marie SMSM at Mau'Faanga, Nuku'alofa.

30. K. Tu'a Leketi, oral history (2006), p. 2.

31. F. Takeifanga, oral history (2006), p. 2.

32. D. McMenamin, "Report on Visit to Tonga" (2006), p. 4.

33. *Ibid.*, p. 1.

34. Lutui, email 6 December, 2006.

35. Lutui, email 8 December, 2006.

36. Lutui, McMenamin report on visit to Tonga, p. 4.

37. Tu'aLeketi, p. 2.

38. Lutui, email 6 December, 2006.

39. Two interviews in Nuka'alofa, four in the island of Vava'u, and one at Twomey hospital, Fiji.

40. Madey and Thomas, *Compassionate Exile*.

41. P. Fakatava, oral history (2004), p. 3.

42. *Ibid.*, p. 2.

43. *Ibid.*, pp. 2–3.

44. *Ibid.*, p. 6.

45. *Ibid.*, pp. 4–5.

46. *Ibid.*, p. 4.

47. *Ibid.*, p. 5.

48. *Ibid.*, p. 6.

49. *Ibid.*, p. 5.

50. *Ibid.*, p. 7.

51. T. Sanft, oral history (2006), pp. 2–3.

52. *Ibid.*, p. 3.

53. *Ibid.*, p. 2.

54. *Ibid.*, pp. 2–3.

55. *Ibid.*, p. 1.

56. *Ibid.*

57. *Ibid.*

58. M. Nunu, oral history (2006), pp. 1–2.

59. *Ibid.*, p. 2.

60. *Ibid.*

61. *Ibid.*, p. 4.

62. *Ibid.*, p. 5.

63. *Ibid.*, p. 2.

64. *Ibid.*, p. 4.

65. *Ibid.*

66. *Ibid.*

67. *Ibid.*, p. 5.

68. *Ibid.*

69. Takeifanga, pp. 3–4.

70. M. Moli Moli, oral history (2006) p. 2.

71. *Ibid.*, p. 3.

72. *Ibid.*, p. 4.

73. *Ibid.*, p. 3.

74. *Ibid.*, p. 6.

75. *Ibid.*

76. Tu'a Leketi, p. 1.

77. *Ibid.*

78. *Ibid.*, p. 2.

79. *Ibid.*, p. 3.

80. *Ibid.*, p. 4. Kulaea does not say she divorced and then married Tofa; it is more likely to have been a defacto relationship.

81. *Ibid.*

82. *Ibid.*

83. *Ibid.*, pp. 4–5.

84. *Ibid.*, p. 5.

85. *Ibid.*, p. 6.

86. P. Tu'amelie, oral history (2006), p. 2.

87. *Ibid.*

88. *Ibid.*, p. 3.

89. *Ibid.*

90. *Ibid.*

91. *Ibid.*, p. 4.

92. *Ibid.*

93. *Ibid.*

94. M. Fonoga, oral history (2006), p. 1.

95. *Ibid.*, p. 2.

96. Gussow and Tracey, "Myth of Leprosy," pp. 702–703.

97. Fonoga, p. 1.

98. *Ibid.*, p. 3.
99. *Ibid.*
100. *Ibid.*, p. 4.
101. *Ibid.*
102. *Ibid.*, pp. 4–5.
103. *Ibid.*, p. 6.
104. *Ibid.*
105. Moli Moli, p. 6.

Chapter 5

1. J. K. Laing, "The Development of Medical and Health Services in New Hebrides and Vanuatu," McMenamin Pacific Papers, Macmillan Brown Library, p. 129.
2. J. Miles, *Infectious Diseases: Colonising the Pacific?* (Dunedin, 1997), p. 38; and J. Z. Montgomerie, "Leprosy in New Zealand," *Journal of the Polynesian Society* 97, no. 2 (1988): 139. According to Miles, because of the appearance of islanders on Aoba and Maewo, the islands were named Isles des Lepreux.
3. J. G. Miller, *Live: A History of Church Planting in the Republic of Vanuatu, Book 4* (Vanuatu, 1989), pp. 2–3.
4. Laing, pp. 135–137.
5. Miller, p. 1.
6. Laing, pp. 130–131.
7. Miller, p. 2.
8. Laing, pp. 134–135.
9. *Ibid.*, pp. 130–133.
10. *Ibid.*, p. 131.
11. *Ibid.*, pp. 130–3.
12. *Ibid.*, p. 139.
13. R. Godden, *Lolowai: The Story of Charles Godden and the Western Pacific* (Sydney, 1967), pp. 2 and 169–170.
14. A. Tevi, oral history (2006), p. 2.
15. D. W. Beckett, "The Striking Hand of God: Leprosy in History," p. 9.
16. Lone, p. 13.
17. Miller, pp. 102–4; Nicholson's work is also referred to in John Garrett, *Footsteps in the Sea: Christianity in Oceania to World War II*, University of the South Pacific, Institute of Pacific Studies, 1992, pp. 96–97.
18. Miller, p. 103.
19. More recent Presbyterian Mission archives are held at Knox College, Dunedin, New Zealand.
20. Miller, pp. 166–167.
21. *Ibid.*
22. *Ibid.*, p. 167.
23. Laing, "Leprosy in the South Pacific and the Origins the Leprosy Trust Board," McMenamin Pacific Papers, Macmillan Brown Library, pp. 21–22.
24. *Ibid.*, pp. 23 and 30.
25. Lonie, p. 13; and A. J. Davies, "Looking for Lepers in the New Hebrides," undated copy in Harris Papers, Macmillan Brown Library.
26. Laing, p. 29.
27. *Ibid.*
28. Lonie, p. 21.
29. In 1939 this was reported by the leprologist Dr. Innes, reported in Lonie, p. 23–4.
30. Miller, pp. 166–167.
31. Laing, p. 26, cites the "Report of the First LTB Conference in Christchurch," 10 February, 1947, pp. 18.
32. B. Pyatt, oral history (1999), tape 1, p. 7.
33. Her eldest brother subsequently became Bishop Pyatt in New Zealand.
34. Edmond, p. 176–177.
35. Pyatt, tape 2, oral history (2007), p. 2; and N. Harris, undated report, memoir, p. 3.
36. Pyatt, tape 2, p. 3.
37. *Ibid.*, p. 21.
38. *Ibid.*, p. 4.
39. Pyatt, tape 1, p. 10.
40. *Ibid.*, pp. 10–11.
41. *Ibid.*, p. 10.
42. *Ibid.*, p. 11.
43. Pyatt, tape 2, p. 5.
44. An undated letter from Betty Pyatt describing in more detail the hospital and small leprosarium is filed with McMenamin Pacific Papers, Macmillan Brown Library. Typed copy is Appendix I herein.
45. Pyatt, tape 2, p. 3.
46. *Ibid.*, p. 8.
47. *Ibid.*, p. 3.
48. *Ibid.*, p. 8.
49. *Ibid.*, p. 5.
50. *Ibid.*, p. 6.
51. *Ibid.*, p. 9.
52. *Ibid.*, pp. 6–7.
53. *Ibid.*, p. 7.
54. *Ibid.*, p. 9.
55. *Ibid.*, pp. 12–13.
56. *Ibid.*, p. 12.
57. *Ibid.*, pp. 7–8.

58. *Ibid.*, p. 17.
59. *Ibid.*, pp. 13–14.
60. B. and C. Mackereth, oral history (2007), p. 11.
61. *Ibid.*
62. *Ibid.*, p. 14.
63. *Ibid.*, pp. 14–15.
64. *Ibid.*, pp. 16–17.
65. *Ibid.*, p. 17.
66. *Ibid.*, pp. 18–19.
67. Pyatt, Tape 2, pp. 27–28.
68. *Ibid.*, p. 13.
69. Pyatt, Tape 1, p. 11.
70. Tevi, p. 5.
71. J. Woi Tarisesei, oral history (2006), p. 1.
72. *Ibid.*
73. McMenamin, report on visit to Vanuatu (2006), p. 10.
74. Pyatt, Tape 2, p. 10.
75. McMenamin, report on visit to Vanuatu, p. 3.
76. *Ibid.*, p. 11.
77. *Ibid.*
78. Laing, p. 31.
79. *Ibid.*
80. *Ibid.*, pp. 31–32.
81. *Ibid.*, p. 32.
82. Personal communication with Dr. R. Farrugia.
83. Farrugia, oral history, pp. 32–33.
84. *Ibid.*, p. 34.
85. *Ibid.*
86. *Ibid.*, p. 35.
87. *Ibid.*
88. Oral histories recorded with six of the leprosy suffers, but only notes recorded relating to Charlie Vuti.
89. B. Varu, oral history (2008), p. 2.
90. *Ibid.*, p. 1.
91. *Ibid.*, p. 2.
92. E. Vira, oral history (2008), p. 1.
93. M. A. Namtaktak, oral history (2008), p. 2.
94. *Ibid.*, p. 2.
95. R. Abana, oral history (2008), p. 4.
96. *Ibid.*
97. R. Andrew, p. 1.
98. *Ibid.*, p. 2–3.
99. *Ibid.*, p. 2.
100. C. Vuti, notes of interview (2008), p. 1.
101. V. Stephens, oral history (2008), pp. 1–2.
102. *Ibid.*, p. 3.
103. B. Varu, p. 3.
104. Personal communication, detailed in McMenamin report on visit to Vanuatu, p. 7.
105. Andrew, oral history (2008), p. 2.

Conclusion

1. Stella, pp. 65, 80–81, 96–97, 128, and 144–145; and in photograph albums in the SMSM archives in Auckland, as well as negatives of photographs archived in the Macmillan Brown Library.

Bibliography

Primary Sources

ORAL HISTORIES (Recorded by D. McMenamin, unless otherwise stated, and filed at the Macmillan Brown Library, Christchurch, New Zealand)

Abana, Rere. Kole, Santo, Vanuatu, July 2008.
Ah Chong, Manu. Taufusi, Samoa, January 2006.
Andrew, Rocky. Santo, Vanuatu, July 2008.
Anonymous (1), (2), (3) and (4). Samoa, January 2006.
Beckett, Dr. Desmond W. Auckland, New Zealand, May 2007.
Eales, Marilyn M. Auckland, New Zealand, April 2007.
Fakatava, Polutele. Suva, Fiji, August 2004.
Farrugia, Dr. Roland G. Port Vila, Vanuatu, October 2006.
Fonoga, Mele. Vava'u, Tonga, November 2006.
Harris, Noeline Theresa. Christchurch, New Zealand, May 2005.
Gwero, James (dvd and notes only). Port Vila, Vanuatu, October 2006.
Laulu, Ierone Lome. Falefa, Samoa, January 2006.
Layasewa, Susau Fatiaki. Suva, Fiji, August 2004.
Mackereth, Dr. M. Bruce and Catherine M. Whitianga, New Zealand, April 2007.
Madigi, Tomasi (notes only). Suva, Fiji, August 2004.
McFarland, Rudy. Aleisa, Samoa, January 2006.
McMahon, Dr. Brian. Christchurch, New Zealand, July 2006.
Mei, Josefa (notes only). Suvavou, Fiji, August 2004.
Metuisela, Volau. Suva, Fiji, August 2004.
Moli Moli, Manitepi. Longomapu, Vava'u, Tonga, November 2006.
Moria, Wati. Valelavu, Suva, Fiji, August 2004.
Musuka, Lenaitasi. Suva, Fiji, August, 2004.
Namtaktak, Mary Alma. Santo, Vanuatu, July 2008.
Nansen, Dick. Apia, Samoa, January 2006.
Nunu, Maliakalemeli. Nuku'Alofa, Tonga, November 2006.
Parsons, Sr. Marietta J. Christchurch, New Zeland, November 2005.
Pyatt, Sister Betty. (Interview 1) Auckland, New Zealand, interviewed by Noelene Shore, July 1999; tape copied, uploaded onto CD and filed with Interview 2.
Pyatt, Sr. Betty. (Interview 2) Auckland, New Zealand, April 2007.
Ram, Paras. Suva, Fiji, August 2004.
Rarawa, Siteri. Suva, Fiji, August 2004.
Sanft, Taliai. Halalaufuli, Vava'u, Tonga, November 2006.
Singh, Sher Bahadur (John). Narere, Suva, Fiji, August 2004.
Soko, Tevita Vuniwaqa. Suva, Fiji, August 2004.
Spooner, Dr. Frank Bakeo (notes only). Port Vila, Vanuatu, October 2006.
Stephen, Vearu. Sarere, Santo, Vanuatu, July 2008.
Takeifanga, Fusi. Vava'u, Tonga, November 2006.

Tarisesei, Jean Woi. Port Vila, Vanuatu, October 2006.
Tetoariki, Maria. Ita, Suva, Fiji, August 2004.
Tevi, Anna Mugita. Port Vila, Vanuatu, October 2006.
Thiossey, Sister Noëllie. Noumea, New Caledonia, September 2006.
Tiko, Salote. Suva, Fiji, August 2004.
Tourte, Honoré. Ducos, New Caledonia, September 2006.
Tua Leketi, Kulaea. Longomapu, Tonga, November 2006.
Tu'amelie, Pepetua. Popua, Tongatapu, Tonga, November 2006.
Valentine, Dr. John. Christchurch, New Zealand, March 2006.
Varu, Bialoloso. Vibue, Santo, Vanuatu, July 2008.
Vira, Emrere. Sarere, Santo, Vanuatu, July 2008.
Venaisi, Bosenandrau Meto (notes only). Suvavu, Fiji, August 2004.
Vuti, Charlie (notes only). Santo, Vanuatu, July 2008.
Wainigolo, Viliame (notes only). Suva, Fiji, August 2004.

Unpublished Papers and Manuscripts

"Activities of L.T.B. in New Caledonia." No date, archived with Noeline Harris papers at Macmillan Brown Library, Christchurch, New Zealand.
Austin, C. J. *Fiji Leprosy Hospital Makogai* brochure. Suva, Public Relations Office for Medical Department (1954), archived with Noeline Harris papers at Macmillan Brown Library, Christchurch, New Zealand.
Bobin, P. "La Lepre en Nouvelle-Caledonie: Rappel Historique." Service de Dermatologie CHT Noumea, 11 March, 1999, archived with D. McMenamin papers at Macmillan Brown Library, Christchurch, New Zealand.
———. "La Lepre en Nouvelle-Caledonie: Rappel Historique." Service de Dermatologie CHT Noumea, undated, archived with D. McMenamin papers at Macmillan Brown Library, Christchurch, New Zealand.
Boyer, Sylvette. "La Lepre en Nouvelle-Caledonie." Dossier C (in French), undated, archived with D. McMenamin papers at Macmillan Brown Library, Christchurch, New Zealand.
Corre, Bruno. "La Lèpre en Nouvelle-Calédonie." Dossier B (in French), undated, archived with D. McMenamin papers at Macmillan Brown Library, Christchurch, New Zealand.
Crouzat, Dr. Maryse. "The Disease of Hansen in New Caledonia." Service of Dermatology, Website of the Territorial Hospital complex of Noumea, printout from July 1999. http://64.233.179.104/translate_c?hl=en&sl=Fr&u=htp://www.cht.nc/Actu/Leprel99907.
———. "Situation de la Lepre en Nouvelle-Caledonie." Pasteur Hospital report, December 2001, archived with D. McMenamin papers at Macmillan Brown Library, Christchurch, New Zealand.
Davies, E. J. "Looking for Lepers in the New Hebrides." Leprosy Survey 1948–1951 (n.d., part copy), archived with Noeline Harris papers at Macmillan Brown Library, Christchurch, New Zealand.
Eales, M. M. "What Goes Around Comes Around." Long abstract of address given at the Pacific Leprosy Foundation AGM, May 2006, archived with D. McMenamin papers at Macmillan Brown Library, Christchurch, New Zealand.
Farrugia, Dr. Roland. Copies of reports relating to Pacific region [Confidential], archived with D. McMenamin papers at Macmillan Brown Library, Christchurch, New Zealand.
"A Few Facts About the Leprosy Trust Board in New Caledonia." No date, archived with Noeline Harris papers at Macmillan Brown Library, Christchurch, New Zealand.
Foester, Fraser. Notes on Radio NZ interview re New Caledonia, March 1987, archived with Noeline Harris papers at Macmillan Brown Library, Christchurch, New Zealand.
Grennell, Airini. Radio feature "Portrait from Life: P. J. Twomey, M.B.E." Un-

dated interview (probably conducted in 1958, as P. J. Towmey's age is given as 66 years), archived with Noeline Harris papers at Macmillan Brown Library, Christchurch, New Zealand.

Lang, W. R. "Seminar on the Medical and Surgical Treatment of Hansen's Disease." June 1977, archived with Noeline Harris papers at Macmillan Brown Library, Christchurch, New Zealand.

"Leper Work in New Zealand." Lepers' Trust Board Incorporated (c.1944), IPD No. 14612, PLF Overview 1948, LMB 469/228, Macmillan Brown Library.

LTB pamphlets. 1950 and c.1945, LMB469/228, IPD No. 14612.

Lutui, Dr. Taniela. Emails to and from D. McMenamin dated 6 and 8 December, 2006, archived with D. McMenamin papers at Macmillan Brown Library, Christchurch, New Zealand.

Mackereth, Dr. Bruce. Collection of letters to home from Lolowai, Vanuatu, archived with D. McMenamin papers at Macmillan Brown Library, Christchurch, New Zealand.

McMenamin, Dorothy. Reports on visits to Suva, Fiji, August, 2004; Nouméa, New Caledonia, (inc. notes re Jacques Michaudel), September 2006; Port Vila, Vanuatu, October 2006; Apia, Samoa, January 2006; Nuku'alofa and Vava'u, Tonga, November 2006; SMSM Archives, Auckland, April 2007. All archived with D. McMenamin papers at Macmillan Brown Library, Christchurch, New Zealand.

Médecin-Capitaine des Troupes Coloniales Lacour, Directeur de l'Institut Pasteur de Nouméa. *An Attempt to Control Leprosy by B.C.G. Vaccine in the Loyalty Islands,* 1955. Archived with D. McMenamin papers at Macmillan Brown Library, Christchurch, New Zealand.

M.P.W. "A Life of Dedication." No date, archived with Noeline Harris papers at Macmillan Brown Library, Christchurch, New Zealand.

Pacific Leprosy Foundation Archives, Macmillan Brown Library. 1984 file in Box 6/3 Western Samoa 1980–1986.

Pyatt, Betty M. Copy of letter describing Lolowai Hospital. Undated (c. 1964), archived with D. McMenamin papers at Macmillan Brown Library, Christchurch, New Zealand.

Poluka, Dr. Tili. "Leprosy Records 1957–1964." Provided by his son, Dr. Mappa Poluka, in Nuku'alofa, posted to D. McMenamin.

Twomey, P. J. LTB Newsletter (1948); and "Ernest – A Leper Hero!"

Published Primary Sources

Allan, Colin H. *Solomons Safari 1953–58, Part I.* Christchurch: Nag's Head Press, 1989.

Austin, C. J. "Leprosy in Fiji and the South Seas." *International Journal of Leprosy* 17, no. 4 (1949): 399–409.

———. "Leprosy in the British Solomon Islands Protectorate." *South Pacific Commission* (July, 1952).

Browne, Stanley G. "Leprosy in the Bible." London, Christian Medical Fellowship Publications, 157 Waterloo Road, Third Edition, 1979.

"Countries Mark World Leprosy Day." *WHO Goodwill Ambassador's Newsletter for the Elimination of Leprosy* 36 (February 2009), The Nippon Foundation.

Crouzat, Dr. Maryse, and Forrest, Nicole. *L'hymne à la vie: des pensionnaires du Centre Raoul Follereau.* Une page d'histoire calédonienne, no date or publisher (Book Launch 2006).

De Mijolla, Marie Cécile. *Marie Françoise Perroton: A Woman from Lyons* (Trans. Sisters Yvette Marie and Lamerand). Rome: Missionary Sisters of the Society of Mary, 1997.

Grosperrin, Sister Marie Ancilla. *The Vocation of the Pioneers* (Trans. Sister Marie Lamerand). Rome: Missionary Sisters of the Society of Mary, 2005.

Lang, W. R. "Leprosy in Auckland." *The New Zealand Medical Journal* 669 (October 8, 1980): 271.

Leprosy Trust Board: A Brief Outline of the Development and Operations of the Leprosy Trust Board (The Leper Man Appeal). Based on a series of talks by Derek Doug-

las, Secretary of the Board, Christchurch, New Zealand, 1985.
Pacific Leprosy Foundation. *Annual Review*, 2005, and 2007–2008.

Unpublished Secondary Sources

Akeli, Safu. "Leprosy in Samoa, 1890 to 1922: Race, Colonial Politics and Disempowerment." MA History, University of Canterbury, 2007.
Beckett, D. W. "The Striking Hand of God: Leprosy in History." Pre-publication copy, archived with Noeline Harris papers at Macmillan Brown Library, Christchurch, New Zealand.
Laing, J. "The Development of Medical and Health Services in New Hebrides and Vanuatu." Sponsor Malama Meleisea, Ph.D, archived with Noeline Harris papers at Macmillan Brown Library, Christchurch, New Zealand.
_____. "Leprosy in the South Pacific and the Origins and Development of the Leprosy Trust Board." Research essay, History, University of Canterbury, 1989, archived with Noeline Harris papers at Macmillan Brown Library, Christchurch, New Zealand.
Leprosy Trust Board. "Semisi Maya — the Story of a Leper Artist" advertisement. Archived with Noeline Harris papers at Macmillan Brown Library, Christchurch, New Zealand.
Loh, Kah Seng. "Heritage for Whom? Leprosy, Memory and Modernity in Singapore." Paper presented at the International Conference on *Heritage in Asia: Converging Forces and Conflicting Values*, 8–10 January, 2007, Asia Research Institute, National University of Singapore.
Lou, Betty. "The Carville Praesidium." March 1952, archived with Noeline Harris papers at Macmillan Brown Library, Christchurch, New Zealand.
Morris, Joan M. *They Came to Makogai: A Community Study*. Dept. Soc. Sci., University of Victoria, 1956.
Rose, A. H. T. "Early Days of Mr. Twomey in New Caledonia." January 1987, archived with Noeline Harris papers at Macmillan Brown Library, Christchurch, New Zealand.

Published Secondary Sources

Bashford, Alison. *Imperial Hygiene: A Critical History of Colonialism, Nationalism and Public Health*. New York: Palgrave, 2004.
Beckett, Desmond. "The Striking Hand of God: Leprosy in History." *New Zealand Medical Journal* 100 (1987): 494–497.
Brody, S. N. *The Disease of the Soul: Leprosy in Medieval Literature*. Ithaca: Cornell University Press, 1974.
Buckingham, Jane. *Leprosy in Colonial India: Medicine and Confinement*. Basingstoke and New York: Palgrave Publishers Ltd., 2002.
_____. "The Pacific Leprosy Foundation Archive and Oral Histories of Leprosy in the South Pacific." *The Journal of Pacific History* 41, no. 1 (June 2006): 81–86.
Campbell, I. C. *Island Kingdom: Tonga Ancient & Modern*. Christchurch: Canterbury University Press, 1992.
Carville. U.S. Department of Health and Human Services, Public Health Services, Carville, Louisiana, USA, n.d, archived with Noeline Harris papers at Macmillan Brown Library, Christchurch, New Zealand.
Carville, USA. The United States Public Health Service Hospital, Federal Security Agency, Carville, Louisiana, n.d., archived with Noeline Harris papers at Macmillan Brown Library, Christchurch, New Zealand.
Cochrane, R. G. "Biblical Leprosy: A Suggested Interpretation." *Christian Medical Fellowship*, Tyndale Press, 1963.
_____. *A Practical Textbook of Leprosy*. London: Oxford University Press, 1947.
Compassionate Exile. Documentary/Video produced by Bob Madey and Larry Thomas, Publisher: Regional Media Centre (Suva, 1999).
Edmond, Rod. *Leprosy and Empire: A Medical and Cultural History*. Cambridge: Cambridge University Press, 2006.
Fiji history and discovery at http://www.

polynesia.com/fiji/history-and-discovery.html.
Gilman, Sander L. *Picturing Health and Illness: Images of Identity and Difference*. Baltimore: The John Hopkins University Press, 1995.
Global Project on the History of Leprosy. International Leprosy Association website, http://www.leprosyhistory.org.
Godden, Ruth. *Lolowai: The Story of Charles Godden and the Western Pacific*. Sydney: The Wentworth Press, 1967.
Gould, Cynthia M. "Sister Hilary Ross and Carville: Her Thirty-Seven Year Struggle Against Hansen's Disease." *The Star: Radiating the Light and Truth of Hansen's Disease, Part I* 50, no. 5 (May/June, 1991), and no. 6 (July/August, 1991), archived with Noeline Harris papers at Macmillan Brown Library, Christchurch, New Zealand.
Grice, Gordon. "Where Leprosy Lurks." *Discover* 21, no. 11 (November 2000): 76–84.
Gussow, Zachary. *Leprosy, Racism, and Public Health: Social Policy in Chronic Disease Control*. Boulder, CO: Westview Press, Inc., 1989.
Gussow, Z., and Tracy, G. "Stigma and the Leprosy Phenomenon: The Social History of a Disease in the Nineteenth and Twentieth Centuries." *Bulletin of the History of Medicine* 44, no. 5 (1970): 425–449.
_____. "The Use of Archival Materials in the Analysis and Interpretation of Field Data: A Case Study in the Institutionalization of the Myth of Leprosy as 'Leper.'" *American Anthropologist* 73, no. 3 (1971): 695–705.
Hamilton, Bernard. *The Leper King and His Heirs: Baldwin IV and the Crusader Kingdom of Jerusalem*. Cambridge: Cambridge University Press, 2000.
Hattori, Anne Perez. *Colonial Dis-ease: U.S. Navy Health Policies and the Chamorros of Guam, 1898–1941*. Honolulu: University of Hawaii Press, 2004.
Holmes, Malcolm. "The Semisi Maya Story." *Spam* 2, no. 1 (1982): 35–37.
Jackson, Peter, *Tamahua, Quail Island—a Link with the Past, 2nd Edition*. Christchurch, New Zealand: Tamahua/Quail Island Trust, 2006.
Laracy, H. *Dictionary of New Zealand Biography*. www.dnzb.govt.nz (accessed 10 September, 2007).
Latukefu, Sione. *Church and State in Tonga: The Wesleyan Methodist Missionaries and Political Development, 1822–1875*. Canberra: Australian National University Press, 1974.
_____. *The Tongan Constitution: A Brief History to Celebrate Its Centenary*. Nuku'alofa: Tonga Traditions Committee Publication, 1975.
Loh, Kah Seng. "'Our Lives Are Bad but Our Luck Is Good': A Social History of Leprosy in Singapore." *Social History of Medicine*, no. 2 (3 June, 2008): 291–309.
Lonie, D. A. "Trends in Leprosy in the Pacific." *Technical Information Circular* 32. Noumea, New Caledonia: South Pacific Commission, 1959.
McCurry, Justin, "Japanese Leprosy Patients Continue to Fight Social Stigma." *The Lancet* 363, no. 9408 (February 14, 2004): 544.
McMenamin, Dorothy. "Recording the Experiences of Leprosy Sufferers in Suva, Fiji." *The Fiji Social Workers Journal* 1, no. 1 (November 2005): 27–32; and in *Oral History in New Zealand* 17 (2005): 23–25.
Miles, John. *Infectious Diseases: Colonising the Pacific?* Dunedin, University of Otago Press, 1997.
Miller, J. Graham. *Live: A History of Church Planting in the Republic of Vanuatu, Book 6, The Northern Islands 1881–1948*. Vanuatu: The Presbyterian Church of Vanuatu, 1989.
Moblo, Pennie. "Leprosy, Politics, and the Rise of Hawaii's Reform Party." *The Journal of Pacific History* 34, no. 1 (1999): 75–89.
Moran, Michelle T. *Imperialism and the Politics of Public Health in the United States*. Chapel Hill: University of North Caroline Press, 2007.
Perks, Robert, and Thomson, Alistair (eds.). *The Oral History Reader*. New York: Routledge, 1998.
Portelli, Alessandro. "What Makes Oral

History Unique." In *The Oral History Reader, 2nd Edition*, edited by Robert Perks and Alistair Thomson, 32–42k. London: Routledge, 2006.
Raoul Follereaum. AIFI website, http://www.aifoindia.org/RaoulFollereau.htm.
Rees, R.J.W. "New Prospects for the Study of Leprosy in the Laboratory." *Bulletin World Health Organization* 40 (1969): 785–800.
Rothman, David J. *The Discovery of the Asylum: Social Order and Disorder in the New Republic*. Boston and Toronto: Little, Brown & Company, Ltd., 1971.
Rutherford, Noel. *Shirley Baker and the King of Tonga*. Melbourne: Oxford University Press, 1971.
Scott Smith, D. "Leprosy: eMedicine Infectious Diseases." Stanford: Stanford University, August 2008. http://emedicine.medscape.com/article/220455-overview (accessed 28 June, 2009).
Siers, James. *Tonga*. Wellington: Millwood Press, 1978.
Silla, Eric. *People Are Not the Same: Leprosy and Identity in Twentieth-Century Mali*. Social History of Africa Series, Heinemann, Portsmouth, NH, and James Curry, Oxford, 1998.
Stella, Sister Mary S.M.S.M. *Makogai — Image of Hope: A Brief History of the Care of Leprosy Patients in Fiji*. Christchurch: Lepers' Trust Board, 1978.
Thelen, David. "Memory and American History." *The Journal of American History* 75, no. 4 (March, 1989): 1117–29.
Thompson, Paul. *The Voice of the Past: Oral History*. Oxford: Oxford University Press, 1978; and 3rd edition, Oxford University Press, 2000.
Valentine, John. *Hell-Bent for Life*. Oakura, New Zealand: John Valentine Publishing, 2009.
Volinn, Ilse J. "Health Professionals as Stigmatizers and Destigmatizers of Diseases: Alcoholism and Leprosy as Examples." *Social Science and Medicine* 17, no. 7 (1983): 385–393.
_____. "Issues of Definitions and Their Implications: Aids and Leprosy." *Social Science and Medicine* 29, no. 10 (1989): 1157–1162.

Index

Numbers in ***bold italics*** indicate pages with photographs.

Ah Chong, Manu ***111***
AIDS 7, 12
Ake, Dr. Malaki 130
Akeli, Safua 10, 99–101, 210*n*35
Alia, Samoa 101–103, 122, 195–196
American Samoa 98, 119
amputations 5, 39, 58–62, 65–66, 116, 117, 187, 196–197
Andrew, Rocky 179, 185, ***186***, 188–189, 197
Anglican Melanesian Mission 18–19, 36, 156, 159; *see also* Melanesian Mission
asylums 10, 17, 43
Austin, Dr. C.J. 9, 40–41, 45, 50, 83, 203*n*3
Ayurvedic 6

Baha'i 28
BCG vaccine 81, 90–91
Beckett, Dr. Desmond vi, 13, 21, 51–52, 56, 88
Belep, New Caledonia 73, 75–76, 84–85, 195
Ben-Hur 3
Benemerenti 38
Beqa, Fiji 42–45
Bible 12, 13–15, 44, 100, 126, 131, 138, 151, 162
Biblical stigma 2, 4, 12–13, 15–16, 92, 100, 104, 131, 138, 142, 148, 150, 192–193
blackbirding 73, 155, 174
Bobin, P. 24–25, 75–76, 82
Boeck 13
bokola 41
Bonneaud, Henri 82
Bough, Carren vi, 28
Bowie, Dr. 158–159
British Medical Journal 19
Brody, S.N. 13
Buckingham, Jane v, 9–10, 23, ***57***

camaraderie 1, 25, 61, 71–72, 109, 135–137, 141, 153, 191, 195–196
Carville, USA 6, 11, 16, 18–19, 21, 58, 77
Catholicism 18, 32, 34, 36–37, 43–44, 47, 93, 98, 101–102, 118, 120, 124, 139, 156, 158, 193, 198
charity 1, 4, 15, 18–20, 23, 25, 31, 33–36, 38–39, 77, 81, 120
chaulmoogra oil 6, 77–78, 87, 162
Chevalier of the Legion of Honor 38
China 8, 75, 91–92, 99, 111, 126
Christianity 4, 12–13, 18, 24, 44, 98–100, 124–126, 134, 156, 158–159, 162, 192–193
claw hand 39, 66, 185
clofazimine viii, 7
Cluny Sisters 76, 84, 86, 95, 193
colonialism 8, 10–11, 16, 21, 24–25, 40–43, 52, 73, 99–100, 155–156, 192–193
Compassionate Exile 55, 132, 204–206
Cook Islands 37
Corney, Dr. Bolton 41, 43
Crouzat, Dr. Maryse vi, 10, 95, 97
Culion, Philippines 18–19, 21–22

Daly, Numa 82
Danielssen 13
Dapsone 6–7, 58–59, 86–87, 110, 132, 169
Daughters of Charity of St. Vincent de Paul 18, 20, 77
Daulako, Dr. 100
Davies, Dr. Jean 158
DDS 6, 51, 53, 55, 58, 128, 132
diagnosis v, 3, 6, 12, 14–16, 22, 39–40, 54–55, 58, 87–88, 95, 105, 108, 112, 116, 123, 125, 127, 131, 132, 143, 151, 168–169, 176, 180, 185, 191, 194–195
disabilities 3, 5–6, 8, 23–24, 26, 36, 40, 53, 58, 61, 77, 81, 96, 110, 118, 123, 136, 138, 142, 185, 189, 196, 198
Ducos 10, 23, 27, 73–79, 81, ***82***, 83–88, 90–91, 94–97, 171, 175–176, 193, 195–196; *see also* RFC Centre

Eales, Marilyn vi
Edmond, R. 8, 11, 15, 19, 33, 47, 49, 77, 93

Index

Espiritu Santo 28, 157, 176–177, 179, 182, 185, 189, 190, 192, 197, 199–200
eye problems 39, 55, 59, 60, 67, 80, 113, 116, 122, 146

Fale'ofa leprosy station, Tonga 27, 126, 128–131, 141, 146, 150–151, 175, 196–197
Farrow, Christine M. 34
Farrugia, Dr. Roland vi, 7, 28, 74, 81, 85–97, 122, 157, 176–178, 180, 185–188, 203*n*7&9
Fatakava, Polutele 54–55, 127, 131–138, 151, 153
Father Damien 10, 16, 20, 49, 99
Father Le Jeune 49
Father Nicouleau 49
Fiji vi, 1–2, 4–5, 9, 11, 15, 17–21, 24–26, *31–72*, 76, 82, 90, 94, 98, 101, 103–104, 109, 125, 129, 131–134, 138, 142–145, 151, 155, 160, 164, 166, 171, 187, 191–198
Fini 147
Fonoga, Mele 146, 151–153, 197
French Polynesia 37, 39
fumigate 55

Geddes, A.S. 38
Gilbertese 45, 60, 134
Global Project on the History of Leprosy vii, 4
Godden Memorial Hospital 36, 156–157, 159, 199
Gousmett, Michael v, 118
Gussow, Z. 11, 15–16, 25, 151

Hall, Dr. 44
Hansen, G.H.A. 5, 6, 13, 14, 16, 99, 193
Hansen's Disease 5, 16, 51
Harris, Noeline (née Kieley) v, *33*, 34–38, 46, 160
Hattori, Anne Perez 10, 22
Hydebrand, Fritz 112
hydrotherapy pool 37
hygiene 11, 14, 50, 73–74, 79, 87, 112, 169, 182, 189, 194

Ile aux Chèvres (Isle of Goats), New Caledonia 75
Innes, Dr. R. 158
International Association for Integration, Dignity and Economic Advancement (IDEA) 39
International Federation Assisting Leprosy (ILEP) 27
International Leprosy Association Project vii, 4
International Leprosy Conference, Berlin 1897 6, 19, 73, 101, 193
Isle of Lepers 155, 157

Japan 13–14, 58, 84, 131, 151, 197

Kalaupapa 20; *see also* Molokai
Kokere, Jimmy 32

Laulu, Lome Ierone 116, *117*, 118, 120–121, 197
Layasewa, Fatiaki Susau 55–56, *57*, 58, 194
lazar homes 17
lazarette 17, 82, 159
Lazarus 17, 38, 104
lepela 116, 119–120, *121*, 122
Leper Island 102, *103*
The Leper Man *see* Twomey, P.J.
Leper Ordinance, 1899, Fiji 41
Lepers' Ordinance, 1897, Singapore 24
leprologist 7, 18, 24, 28, 39, 74–76, 85, 90, 100, 157, 162–163, 165, 176, 193, 198
lepromatous leprosy 6, 74, 168
leprosaria 1–2, 4–5, 10, 15, *17–25*, 28, 35, 37, 43–44, 53, 58, 61–62, 71, 73–74, 79–81, 99–101, 103–104, 128, 136, 155, 163, 166, 168, 171, 173–174, 176, 191–196
leprosarium 1, 5, 7, 9–11, 13, *15–28*, 194–195; New Caledonia *74–86*, 90–92, 95; New Zealand and Fiji 31, *33–53*, 68, 71; Samoa 97, 100, *101–103*, 109; Tonga *126–130*, 131, 132–135, 140; Vanuatu 149, 156–157, *159–174*, 175–176, 180–183, 185, 187, 189, 200–201
leprosy clinic 37, 111, 121, 123, 128–129, 146, 175, 197
leprosy colony 3, 18, 34, 42, 75, 76
Leprosy Day 17, 83, 122, 142, 145, 148, 153
leprosy station 18, 20, 27, 42–43, 84, 101–103, 195–196
Leprosy Training Center for South Pacific 53, 67
Leprosy Trust Board (LTB) 31, 33, 35–39, 45, 47, 53, 74, 81–83, 140, 158, 160, 162–163; *see also* PLF
Leviticus (Old Testament) 44, 100, 126, 131, 142, 193
Lions Club 38, 82
Loh, Kah Seng 23
Lolowai 7, 19, 28, 36, 156–157, 159–160–176, 180–188, 193–194, 199–201; *see also* St. Barnabas leprosarium
London Missionary Society (LMS) 98–99, 100, 155–156
Longomapu Village, Tonga 141–148, 153, 197
Lonie, D.A. 74–75, 159
Lopez-Bravo, Dr. 168, 176
Louisiana Home 11, 20–21
Loyalty Islands 73, 81, 87, 90
Lutui, Dr. Taniela 126–127, 130–131, 134, 138, 142, 148, 193

Mackereth, Dr. Bruce vi, 7, 28, 157, 159, 168–169, *170–172*, 173–177, 180–181, 188, 194
Mackereth, Catherine vi, 157, 159, 169–*170*, *172*, 173
Macmillan Brown Library 4, 10, 38, 128
Madey, Bob 9
Madras, India 23
Makogai, Fiji 5, 9, 13, 15, 18–20, 22, 24, 26, 31, 33–36, 40–47, *48*, 49–79, 82–83, 88,

94, 101, 103–114, 120–122, 127–145, 151, 166, 175, 180, 182, 191, 193–197
Makondane, Zanzibar 13
Mali, Africa 11, 24–25, 58, 76, 161
Marsden Fund vii
matelevu 67
Maya, Semesi 52–53
McFarland, Rudy 105, *106*, 107–111, 118, 120–122, 197
McMahon, Dr. Brian vi, 7, 38, 122
measles 40
medical officials 1, 37
Melanesia 4, 8, 28, 38, 74–75, 83–84, 87, 91, 93, 155–161, 164, 170, 172–174, 177–178, *180*, 187, 189, 193, 200–201
Melanesian Mission vi, 18–19, 36–37, 44, 156, 158–160, 169, 188, 193; *see also* Anglican Melanesian Mission
Methodism 36, 37, 41, 47, 98, 100
Metuisela, Volau *64*, 65–66
Michaudel, Dr. Jacques vi, 74, 83–84
Micronesia 8, 22
Miles, John 10
Mission to Lepers 18
Missionary Sisters of the Society of Mary (SMSM) vi, 1, 18–19, 26–27, 37, 42–49, 52–53, 55, 57, 71, 74–76, 79, 84, 91, 95–97, 101, 104, 118–119, 129, 133–141, 144–145, 193
Molimoli, Manitepi 131–132, 141–142, *143*, 144–145, 153, 197
Molokai, Hawaii 10, 15–16, 19–20, 43, 49, 99, 102
Moria, Wati *64*, 67–71, 194
Motorcycle Diaries 3
multi-bacillary 6, 108
Multi Drug Therapy (MDT) 2, 7, 9, 14, 21, 24, 87, 96–97, 122, 128, 145, 153–154, 195, 198
Musuka, Lenaitasi *64*, 65
Mycobacterium leprae 5–7, 16, 99
Mycobacterium tuberculosis 5
myth 11, 16, 41

Namtaktak, Mary Alma 28, 179, 180, 181, *182*, 186
Nansen, Dick 113, *114–115*, 116, 118, 120
nerve damage 5–6, 59–61, 169, 190, 196, 198
New Caledonia vi, 1, 4–5, 9–11, 17–19, 21–25, 27, 35–37, 50, *73–97*, 101, 155, 166, 171, 175–176, 178–179, 190–191, 193, 195–196, 198, 208n99
New Hebrides 32, 36–38, 155–156, 192, 199–200, 213; *see also* Vanuatu
New Zealand vi, 1, 4, 9, 15, 28, *31–40*, 59, 71, 82–83, 92, 96, 98–99, 102–104, 112, 114, 119, 135, 149, 156–159, 161, 165, 169, 172–174
New Zealand House, Ducos *82*
Ngu Hospital, Vava'u, Tonga 128–131, 138, 141, 146, 149, 151
Nicholson, Dr. J. Campbell 157–158

Nippon Foundation 4, 14
Niu'ui Hospital, Tonga 128, 212
Nunu, Maliakalemeli 131–132, *139*–141
Nu'utele Leper Island, Samoa 101–102, *103*, 122, 196

oral history v, 1, 4–5, 8–10, 12, 15, 26, 29, 31, 35, 37–38, 46, 49, 54, 93, 98, 104–105, 128, 157, 178–179, 187, 189, 191
Order of St. Lazarus of Jerusalem 38, 104
Oxford Project 4, 9–10, 38; *see also* Global Project on the History of Leprosy (funded by Nippon Foundation); International Leprosy Association Project; Welcome Unit for the History of Medicine

Pacific flying boat service 40
Pacific Leprosy Foundation (PLF) v–vi, 1–2, 4, 7, 15, 24–28, 31, 37–38, 40, 44, 48, 52, 54–55, 58, 64, 66–67, 70–72, 74, 86, 96, 104, 110–123, 128–129, 136–137, 141–142, 145, 148, 150, 152–153, 157, 174, 176–177, 185–186, 188, 190, 196–198; *see also* LTB
paralysis 5, 91, 169, 177
Paton Presbyterian Hospital 157, 170
pauci-bacillary 6, 108
penitentiaries 21, 73; *see also* prisons
physiotherapy 37, 39, 62, 91
Poluka, Dr. Mappa 130
Poluka, Dr. Tilitili 130, 149, 212
Polynesia 4, 8, 28, 33, 37, 98, 124, 128, 156
Potter, Monsieur 82–83
Pratt, Benjamin 32, 34, 38
Presbyterian *Live* publications 158
Presbyterian Melanesian Mission 156, 158
prisons 10, 21, 166; *see also* penitentiaries
prosthetics 67, 110, 121
public health 10–12, 14–15, 40, 58–59, 97, 130, 156, 169

Quail Island, New Zealand 31–34, 45

Ram, Paras 58–59
Raoul Follereau 17, 19, 25, 82–83
Raoul Follereau Centre (RFC) 10, 19, 27, 77, 81, 83, 85–86, 91–97, 171, 195–196; *see also* Ducos
Red Cross 38, 82, 107, 129
religious orders 5, 15, 18–19, 49, 52, 75, 77, 101
Rere Abana 179, *183*, *184*, *188*
rifampicin vii, 7
Robben Island 43
Robertson, Jo v
Rose, A.H.T. 38
Rue P.J. Twomey, Bienfaiteur, Noumea 83
Ryukyu Islands, Japan 13, 58

St. Barnabas Leprosarium 19, 36, 157, 159, 162, 166–169, 171, 174–176, 180–182, 188, 194, 200; *see also* Lolowai

St. Elizabeth leprosy home, Suva 52–53, 55, 70, 144
sakuku 41
Samoa vi, 1–2, 4–5, 9–11, 17, 19, 23, 25–27, 37, 39, 44–45, 61, 66, **98–123**, 126, 133–135, 155–156, 166, 190–193, 195–198
Sanft, Taliai 127, 131–132, 136, *137*, 138
sanitation 14, 169
ṣra'at 13
Sasakawa Yohei 14
segregation 8, 10, 13–15, 18, 20, 22–23, 42–43, 47, 51, 53, 73, 79, 83, 94, 97, 101–102, 104, 107, 112, 134, 140, 144, 158, 163–164, 166, 168, 175, 183, 192–195
self stigma 16–17, 25, 112, 136, 138, 151, 192, 196
Seventh Day Adventists 36
sickness 107, 119–121, 132, 135, 150, 155, 163, 185
Silla, Eric 11, 24–25, 161
sin 4, 100, 104, 192–193
Singapore 19, 23–24, 58
Singh, Sher Bahadur (John) 67
Sister Betty Pyatt vi, 28, 36, 44, 157, 159–161, 163–164, *165*, 166, 168–169, 173–176 181–183, 188, 199–201
Sister Goretti vi, 27, 129, 136, *137*, 142, 144–146, 151–153
Sister Hilary Ross 77
Sister Ives 86–87, 90–91
Sister Joan Marie vi, 27, 141–142, 148
Sister Joan Morris 9, 18, 51
Sister M. Irma 79
Sister M. Othilde 79–80
Sister M. Suzanne 76–77
Sister Marie de la Croix 76, 84, 101, 208n17
Sister Marie Stanislaus 76
Sister Marietta vi, 26–27, 44, 104–105, 111–113, 116, 117, 118–120, *121*, 198
Sister Mary Joseph 209n41
Sister Mary Stella 9, 42, 45, 49, 112, 127, 133, 194, 210n34&35
Sister Nöellie Thiossey vi, 27, 74, 77, 84, *85*, 90–94, 97
Sisters of St. Paul of Chartres 18
Soko, Tevita Vuni Waqa 58, 61–62, 64
Solomon Islands 35–37, 39, 45, 144, 156, 158, 160–161
Spooner, Dr. Frank 176
Stacey, Margaret v
Stephen, Vearu 179, *181*, 186, *187*, 188
sulphones 6, 9, 16, 23, 46, 71, 78, 81, 110, 113, 133, 163, 166, 168, 173, 194–195
sumptuary laws 8

Takeifanga, Fusi 141–142

Tamavua, Fiji 53, 144
Tarisesei, Jean Woi 174, 175, 182
Tetoariki, Maria Ita *57*, 60–61
Tevi, Anna 157, 174, *175*, 181
Thomas, Larry 9
Tiko, Salote *57*, 58, 62–64, 68
Tinian, Mariana Islands 10
Tonga vi, 1–2, 4–5, 9, 11, 17, 19, 22–23, 25, 27, 34, 37, 39, 45, 54–55, 61, 98–100, *124–154*, 166, 175, 191–198
Tourte, Honoré 74, 77–80, *85*, 91, 96
Tracy, G. 11, 15, 16, 25
Tu'a Leketi, Kulaea 141, 146, *147*, 148, 150, 154, 197
Tu'amelie, Pepetua 146, *149*, 150
tuberculoid leprosy 6
Tumon colony 22
Twomey Memorial Hospital vi, 24, 26, 43, *53–56*, 58, 69–72, 79, 94, 100, 110, 121, 131–132, 135–136, 144, 151, 171, 195–196, 198
Twomey, P.J. vi, *31–38*, 82–83, 120, 158, 160, 162, 206; *see also* The Leper Man

ulcers 59, 65–66, 92, 107, 119, 142, 163, 189, 197; plantar ulcers 5, 61, 66, 119, 178, 190, 197
unclean 2, 4, 13, 100, 104, 126, 131, 152, 192–193

Valentine, Dr. John 10
Vallane, Will 32
Vanuatu vi, 1, 4–5, 7, 9, 11, 19, 23, 25, 27–28, 36–39, 44, 94, 96, *155–190*, 191, 192–194 197–198; *see also* New Hebrides
Varu, Bialoloso 179, *180*, 187, 192
Vatu ni sakuku 41
Vava'u 27, 128–132, 138, 141, 143, 146, 149–152, 196
Vira, Emrere 179, 180, *181*, 183, *187*
vukavuk 41
Vuti, Charlie 179, 180, 186

Walu Bay, Fiji 41–43, 52, 70
Watson, G.D. 38
Welcome Unit for the History of Medicine vii, 4
Wesleyan 43, 124–127
Whitley, Tony vi, 28, 176–177
Wolfgram, Ernest 33–34, 46–47, 109, 112
Woodham Ferrers, UK 19
World Health Organisation (WHO) 7, 9, 28, 39, 53, 74, 85, 95, 122, 128, 176, 189, 203–206, 209, 211
World War II 28, 40, 81, 98, 102, 160, 179, 183

www.ingramcontent.com/pod-product-compliance
Ingram Content Group UK Ltd.
Pitfield, Milton Keynes, MK11 3LW, UK
UKHW041948140426
5217IPUK00014B/706